SAUNDERS
STRATEGIES FOR SUCCESS
for the NCLEX-RN®
EXAMINATION

SAUNDERS
STRATEGIES FOR SUCCESS
for the NCLEX-RN®
EXAMINATION

LINDA ANNE SILVESTRI, MSN, RN

Instructor of Nursing
Salve Regina University
Newport, Rhode Island

President
Nursing Reviews, Inc.
and
Professional Nursing Seminars, Inc.
Charlestown, Rhode Island

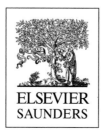

ELSEVIER
SAUNDERS

**ELSEVIER
SAUNDERS**
An imprint of Elsevier

The Curtis Center
Independence Square West
Philadelphia, Pennsylvania 19106

NOTICE

Pharmacology is an ever-changing field. Standard safety precautions must be followed,
but as new research and clinical experience broaden our knowledge, changes in
treatment and drug therapy may be necessary or appropriate. Readers are advised to
check the most current product information provided by the manufacturer of each drug
to be administered to verify the recommended dose, the method and duration of
administration, and contraindications. It is the responsibility of the licensed health care
provider, relying on experience and knowledge of the patient, to determine dosages and
the best treatment for each individual patient. Neither the publisher nor the editor
assume any liability for any injury and/or damage to persons or property arising from
this publication.

Director, Review and Testing: Loren S. Wilson
Managing Editor: Nancy O'Brien
Associate Developmental Editor: Charlene R.M. Ketchum
Publishing Services Manager: Melissa Lastarria
Project Manager: Kelly E.M. Steinmann
Designer: Jyotika Shroff

ISBN-13: 978-1-4160-0095-2

ISBN-10: 1-4160-0095-X

Printed in the United States of America

Last digit is the print number: 9 8 7 6 5 4 3

To all nursing students,

Your commitment to becoming successful and your dedication to the profession of nursing will bring never-ending rewards!

About the Author

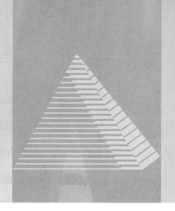

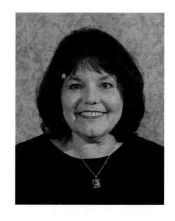

Linda Anne Silvestri received her diploma in nursing at Cooley Dickinson Hospital School of Nursing in Northampton, Massachusetts. Afterwards, she worked at Baystate Medical Center in Springfield, Massachusetts. At Baystate Medical Center, she worked in acute medical-surgical units, the intensive care unit, the emergency department, pediatric units, and other acute care units. She later received an associate degree from Holyoke Community College in Holyoke, Massachusetts, and then received her BSN from American International College in Springfield, Massachusetts.

A native of Springfield, Massachusetts, Linda began her teaching career as an instructor of medical-surgical nursing and leadership-management nursing at Baystate Medical Center School of Nursing in 1981. In 1985, she earned her MSN from Anna Maria College, Paxton, Massachusetts, with a dual major in Nursing Management and Patient Education. Linda is a member of Sigma Theta Tau.

Linda relocated to Rhode Island in 1989 and began teaching advanced medical-surgical nursing and psychiatric nursing to RN and LPN students at the Community College of Rhode Island. While she was teaching at the Community College of Rhode Island, a group of students approached Linda, asking her to help them prepare for the NCLEX examination. Based on her experience as a nursing educator and as an NCLEX item writer, she developed a comprehensive review course to prepare nursing graduates for the NCLEX examination. In 1994, Linda began teaching medical-surgical nursing at Salve Regina University in Newport, Rhode Island. She also prepares nursing students at Salve Regina University for the NCLEX-RN examination.

In 1991, Linda established Professional Nursing Seminars, Inc., and in 2000, she established Nursing Reviews, Inc. Both companies are dedicated to conducting NCLEX-RN and NCLEX-PN review courses and assisting nursing graduates to achieve their goals of becoming Registered Nurses and/or Licensed Practical/Vocational Nurses.

Today, Linda Silvestri's companies conduct NCLEX review courses throughout New England. She is the successful author of numerous NCLEX-RN and NCLEX-PN review products, including *Saunders Comprehensive Review for the NCLEX-RN Examination, Saunders Q&A Review for the NCLEX-RN Examination, Saunders Computerized Review for the NCLEX-RN Examination, Saunders Instructor's Resource Package for the NCLEX-RN, Saunders Comprehensive Review for the NCLEX-PN Examination, Saunders Q&A Review for the NCLEX-PN Examination, Saunders Review Cards for the NCLEX-PN Examination,* and

Saunders Instructor's Resource Package for NCLEX-PN. Linda has also authored several online products including the online specialty tests titled *Adult Health, Mental Health, Maternal-Newborn, Pediatrics, and Pharmacology,* and the *Saunders Online Review Course for the NCLEX-RN Examination.*

Reviewers

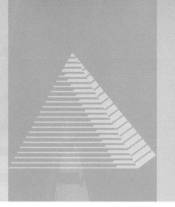

Faculty Reviewers

Bethany Hawes Sykes, EdD, RN, CEN
Adjunct Professor, Department of Nursing
Salve Regina University
Newport, Rhode Island

Jo Ann Barnes Mullaney PhD, APRN, BC
Professor, Department of Nursing
Salve Regina University
Newport, Rhode Island

Student Reviewers

Paul Lovely
Salve Regina University
Newport, Rhode Island

Joanna Bort
Salve Regina University
Newport, Rhode Island

Preface

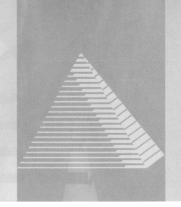

Welcome to Saunders Pyramid to Success!

Saunders Strategies for Success for the NCLEX-RN® Examination is one of a series of products designed to assist you in achieving your goal of becoming a registered nurse. This product provides you with all of the test-taking strategies that will help you pass your nursing examinations and the NCLEX-RN examination.

Organization

Saunders Test-Taking Strategies for Success for the NCLEX-RN Examination contains 4 parts and 15 chapters. The chapters that describe the test-taking strategies include several sample questions that illustrate how to use the test-taking strategy. The sample questions represent all types of question formats including multiple choice, fill in the blank, multiple response, prioritizing (ordered response), and questions that contain a figure or illustration. In addition to the sample questions in the chapters, there are a total of 500 practice questions that accompany this book. There are 265 practice questions in the book. The software contains the 265 practice questions from the book along with an additional 235 practice questions. All of the practice questions are reflective of the framework and the content identified in the 2004 NCLEX-RN test plan. The practice questions in this book relate to each Client Needs category and each Integrated Process of the NCLEX-RN examination. The Client Needs categories include Safe, Effective Care Environment; Health Promotion and Maintenance; Psychosocial Integrity; and Physiological Integrity. The Integrated Processes include Caring, Communication and Documentation, Nursing Process, and Teaching/Learning.

PART I: The NCLEX-RN Examination

Chapter 1 THE TEST PLAN:

The information contained in this chapter focuses on the development and components of the Test Plan. The Levels of Cognitive Ability, Client Needs categories, and the Integrated Processes are identified.

Chapter 2 THE EXAMINATION PROCESS:

This chapter discusses several issues related to the examination process. These include Computerized Adaptive Testing and how it works to determine competency; registration procedures for the NCLEX-RN examination; procedures for scheduling a test date; how to request special accommodations for testing; and procedures that take place at the test center. The procedure for processing examination results, candidate performance reports, and interstate endorsement are also discussed.

Chapter 3 CLIENT NEEDS:

The National Council of State Boards of Nursing identifies four Client Needs categories in the NCLEX-RN examination. This chapter identifies these Client Needs categories and any sub-categories, along with the percentage of test questions and the content addressed in each category.

Chapter 4 INTEGRATED PROCESSES:

The National Council of State Boards of Nursing identifies four Integrated Processes that are fundamental to the practice of nursing and are integrated throughout the categories of Client Needs. This chapter reviews these Integrated Processes and illustrates how these processes are incorporated into examination questions.

Chapter 5 TYPES OF QUESTIONS ON THE EXAMINATION:

This chapter reviews the types of questions that may be administered on the NCLEX-RN examination. These include multiple choice, fill in the blank, multiple response, prioritizing (ordered response), and questions that contain a figure or illustration.

PART II: Strategies for Success

Chapter 6 NONACADEMIC PREPARATION: YOUR PATH TO SUCCESS:

This chapter discusses the issue of test preparation from a nonacademic view and emphasizes a holistic approach for your individual test preparation. This chapter identifies the components of a structured study plan and pattern, anxiety-reduction techniques, and personal focus issues.

Chapter 7 HOW TO AVOID "READING INTO THE QUESTION":

One of the pitfalls that can cause a problem with answering a question correctly is "reading into the question." What "reading into the question" means is that you are considering issues beyond the information that is presented in the question. This chapter describes the strategies to use when answering a question to prevent this from happening.

Chapter 8 TRUE OR FALSE RESPONSE QUESTIONS:

This chapter describes the differences between a true response question and a false response question. Key words or phrases that indicate whether the question is a true response question or a false response question are identified.

Chapter 9 QUESTIONS THAT REQUIRE PRIORITIZING:

Many of the test questions in the examination will require you to use the skill of prioritizing nursing actions. Prioritizing questions can address content in any nursing area. These types of questions can be difficult because when a question requires prioritization, all of the options may be correct and you will need to determine the correct order of action. This chapter describes the test-taking strategies that you can use to assist in answering prioritizing questions correctly. Also included are the strategies for determining the need to contact the physician.

Chapter 10 LEADERSHIP, DELEGATING, AND ASSIGNMENT-MAKING QUESTIONS:

Some of the test questions will relate to the nurse's responsibilities regarding delegating care and assignment-making and the supervisory role of these responsibilities. This chapter reviews the guidelines and principles related to delegating and assignment-making, two very important roles of the nurse. Guidelines for time management are also reviewed because managing time efficiently is a key factor for completing activities and tasks within a definite time period.

Chapter 11 COMMUNICATION QUESTIONS:

In the NCLEX-RN test plan, the National Council of State Boards of Nursing identifies the concept of communication as a component of one of the Integrated Processes. Therefore you will be presented with questions that relate to the communication process. This chapter reviews the guidelines and techniques to use when answering questions that relate to the communication process.

Chapter 12 PHARMACOLOGY QUESTIONS:

Pharmacology is one of the most difficult nursing content areas to master and feel comfortable with. The NCLEX-RN test plan addresses pharmacological and parenteral therapies in the Physiological Integrity category and identifies 13% to 19% as the percentage of test questions relating to pharmacology that will appear on your examination. Therefore, it is important for you to spend ample time reviewing pharmacology in preparation for this examination. This chapter provides you with the guidelines and strategies to use to answer pharmacology questions correctly.

Chapter 13 ADDITIONAL PYRAMID STRATEGIES:

This chapter reviews additional helpful strategies that will assist in answering a test question correctly. Also included in this chapter are strategies that are useful for answering questions that relate to medication and intravenous calculations, questions that relate to laboratory values, and questions that relate to client positioning.

PART III: More Tips for Test-Takers

Chapter 14 TIPS FOR REPEAT TEST-TAKERS:

This chapter provides information about the tips and strategies that will help you prepare to retake the NCLEX-RN examination if necessary. Some of these tips and strategies address the procedure for self-assessment, developing a remediation plan, the steps in a remediation plan, and planning a retake date.

Chapter 15 TIPS FOR INTERNATIONAL NURSES:

This chapter is written specifically for the international or foreign-educated nurse who wants to take the NCLEX-RN examination. This chapter provides the information regarding the processes that will need to be pursued to become a registered nurse in the United States.

PART IV: Practice Test

Part IV includes a 265-question practice test that contains questions representative of the NCLEX-RN test plan. Multiple choice questions and questions in the alternate test question format are included in this test.

SPECIAL FEATURES OF THE BOOK

▲ PYRAMID POINTS

Pyramid Points are the bullets that are placed at specific areas throughout the chapters. The Pyramid Points provide you with immediate recognition of information that is important in preparation for the NCLEX-RN examination.

▲ PRACTICE TEST QUESTIONS

The chapters in this book contain several practice questions that illustrate specific test-taking strategies. In addition to the practice questions integrated into the chapters, there is a 265-question practice test in the book and software that accompanies the book and contains a total of 500 questions (265 questions from the practice test and 235 additional questions.)

▲ ALTERNATE FORMAT TEST QUESTIONS

In additional to multiple choice questions, alternate format test questions are included in both the practice test located in Part IV and on the accompanying software. The alternate format questions include fill in the blank, multiple response, prioritizing (ordered response), and questions that contain a figure or illustration.

▲ ANSWER SECTION FOR PRACTICE TEST QUESTIONS

The answer sections for each practice test question in Part IV and on the accompanying software include the correct answer, rationale, test-taking strategy, question categories, and reference source. The structure for the answer section is unique and provides the following information.

Rationale: The rationale provides you with the significant information regarding both correct and incorrect options.

Test-Taking Strategy: The test-taking strategy provides you with the logical path in selecting the correct option and assists you in selecting an answer to a question on which you must guess. Specific suggestions for review are identified in the test-taking strategy.

Question Categories: Each question is identified based on the categories used by the NCLEX-RN test plan. Additional content categories are provided with each question to assist you in identifying areas in need of review. The categories identified with each practice question include Level of Cognitive Ability, Client Needs, Integrated Process, and the specific nursing Content Area. All categories are identified by their full names so that you do not need to memorize codes or abbreviations.

Reference: A reference, including a page number, is provided so you can easily find the information that you need to review in your undergraduate nursing textbooks.

▲ SOFTWARE

Packaged with this book you will find a CD-ROM containing NCLEX-RN review software. This software contains 500 practice questions in the multiple choice format or in alternate question formats such as fill in the blank, multiple response, prioritizing (ordered response), and questions that contain figures or illustrations. This Windows- and Macintosh-compatible program offers two testing modes for review.

Study: All questions in a specific selected content area. The answer, rationale, test-taking strategy, question categories, and reference source appear after answering each question.

Examination: Seventy-five randomly chosen questions from the entire pool of 500 questions. The answer, rationale, test-taking strategy, question categories, reference source, and results appear after you answer all 75 questions.

▲ CONTENT AREAS ON THE SOFTWARE

When you use the software, you will be able to select practice questions based on a Client Needs area or a content area. The Client Needs areas include Safe, Effective Care Environment; Health Promotion and Maintenance; Psychosocial Integrity; and Physiological Integrity. The content areas are shown in the following box.

CONTENT AREAS

Fundamental Skills	Adult Health/Neurological
Maternity/Antepartum	Adult Health/Musculoskeletal
Maternity/Intrapartum	Adult Health/Immune
Maternity/Postpartum	Adult Health/Gastrointestinal
Child Health	Adult Health/Endocrine
Mental Health	Adult Health/Renal
Delegating/Prioritizing	Adult Health/Oncology
Leadership/Management	Adult Health/Respiratory
Pharmacology	Adult Health/Cardiovascular
Adult Health/Eye	Adult Health/Integumentary
Adult Health/Ear	

How to Use this Book

Saunders Strategies for Success for the NCLEX-RN Examination is especially designed to help you with your successful journey to the peak of the *Saunders Pyramid to Success*, becoming a registered nurse. This book focuses on test-taking strategies that will help you pass your nursing examinations and the NCLEX-RN examination. You should begin your process through the *Saunders Pyramid to Success* by reading all of the chapters in this book to learn the strategies that you can use to answer test questions. Next, answer the questions in the practice test located in Part IV. Finally, use the software that accompanies this book and answer these practice questions.

When using the software, it is best to begin by selecting the *Study* mode because you will receive immediate feedback regarding the answers, rationales, test-taking strategies, question codes, and reference source. Therefore, you are provided with immediate information about your strengths and weaknesses. Once you have answered the practice test question, read the rationale and the test-taking strategy. The rationale provides you with the significant information regarding both the correct and incorrect options. The test-taking strategy presents the logical path to selecting the correct option. The strategy also identifies content area that you need to review if you had difficulty with the question. Use the reference source listed to find the information that you need to review easily.

It is very important to identify your strengths and weaknesses with regard to nursing content areas. Additionally, it is important to strengthen any weak areas in order to be successful on the NCLEX-RN examination. There are several products in *Saunders Pyramid to Success* that can be used to strengthen any weak areas. These additional products, including the online specialty tests and the online review course, can be obtained by calling 1-800-426-4545 or visiting www.elsevierhealth.com. These products are described in the text that follows.

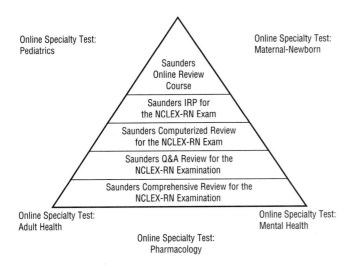

Saunders Comprehensive Review for the NCLEX-RN Examination

This is an excellent resource to use both while you are in nursing school and in preparation for the NCLEX-RN examination. This book contains 20 units and 76 chapters, and each chapter is designed to identify specific components of nursing content. The book and accompanying software contain over 4000 practice questions and include alternate format questions.

Saunders Q & A Review for the NCLEX-RN Examination

This book and accompanying software provide you with over 3500 practice questions based on the NCLEX-RN test plan. The chapters in this book are uniquely designed and are based on the NCLEX-RN examination test plan framework, including Client Needs and Integrated Processes. Alternate format questions are included. With practice questions uniquely focused on the Client Needs and the Integrated Processes, you can assess your level of competence.

Saunders Computerized Review for the NCLEX-RN Examination

This product is a computer disk program that contains over 2000 NCLEX-RN-style practice questions that will help you determine your readiness for the NCLEX-RN examination. The questions in this program are written to address the higher levels of cognitive ability. All questions are either application or analysis questions. The software provides a detailed analysis similar to that provided with standardized nursing examinations.

Online Specialty Tests: Adult Health, Mental Health, Maternal-Newborn, Pediatrics, Pharmacology

Additional resources to assist you in preparing for this examination include the online specialty tests titled *Adult Health, Mental Health, Maternal-Newborn, Pediatrics,* and *Pharmacology.* Each specialty test provides you with 100 practice test questions in NCLEX format and a printout that provides a detailed analysis of your performance.

Online Review Course: Saunders Online Review Course for the NCLEX-RN Examination

The online NCLEX-RN review course addresses all areas of the test plan identified by the National Council of State Boards of Nursing, Inc. The course provides you with a systematic and individualized method for preparing to take the NCLEX examination. It contains a pretest that provides feedback regarding your strengths and weaknesses and generates an individualized study schedule in a calendar format. Content review with practice questions and case studies, figures and illustrations, a glossary, and animations and videos are included. A cumulative examination and a computerized adaptive exam (CAT) are also key components of the online review course. There are thousands of questions in this program and the types of practice questions in this course include multiple choice, fill in the blank, multiple response, those that require you to prioritize (ordered response), and questions containing figures that may require you to use the computer mouse to answer.

Saunders Instructor's Resource Package for the NCLEX-RN Examination.

A final component of the *Saunders Pyramid to Success* is the *Saunders Instructor's Resource Package for the NCLEX-RN Examination.* This manual and CD-ROM accompany the Saunders program of NCLEX-RN review products. Be sure to ask your nursing program director and nursing faculty about this CD-ROM and its use for a review course or a self-paced review in your school's computer laboratory.

Good Luck with your journey through the *Saunders Pyramid to Success*. I wish you continued success throughout your nursing program and in your new career as a Registered Nurse!

— **Linda Anne Silvestri, MSN, RN**

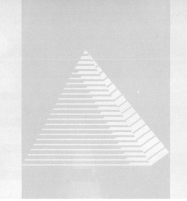

To All Nursing Students and Graduates,

Taking a nursing examination can be a very anxiety-provoking situation because you must pass your nursing examinations in order to pass nursing courses and ultimately become a graduate nurse. Taking the NCLEX-RN examination is just as anxiety provoking because you must pass the NCLEX examination in order to become a registered nurse and begin your career.

It is critically important that you learn how to take an examination. You must use your nursing knowledge and what you learned from your clinical experiences to help you with testing. However, you also need to become skillful with test-taking strategies to pass examinations. Becoming skillful with testing takes time and practice; that's why it is important to develop, refine, and master these skills early on, when you begin your nursing education. Mastering these test-taking skills will bring you success!

I am excited and pleased to be able to provide you with the *Saunders Pyramid to Success* products that will prepare you for taking tests during your nursing program and prepare you for the NCLEX-RN examination. I want to thank all of my former nursing students that I have assisted in preparing for the NCLEX-RN examination for their willingness to offer ideas regarding their needs in preparing for licensure. Student ideas have certainly added a special uniqueness to all of the products available in *Saunders Pyramid to Success*.

This publication provides you with all of the test-taking strategies that will help you with testing. Once you have practiced these strategies and mastered the skill of successful test-taking, the examination experience will be a more comfortable one.

So, let's get started and begin our journey through the *Pyramid to Success* and let's master the skill of test-taking!

Sincerely,

Linda Anne Silvestri MSN, RN

Linda Anne Silvestri, MSN, RN

Acknowledgments

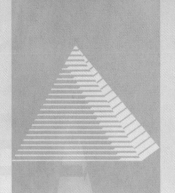

Sincere appreciation and warmest thanks are extended to the many individuals who in their own ways have contributed to the publication of this book.

First, I want to thank the faculty and student reviewers of this book and all of my nursing students at the Community College of Rhode Island in Warwick, who approached me in 1991 and persuaded me to assist them in preparing to take the NCLEX-RN examination. Their enthusiasm and inspiration led to the commencement of my professional endeavors in conducting NCLEX-RN review courses for nursing students. I also thank the numerous nursing students who have attended my review courses for their willingness to share their needs and ideas. Their input has certainly added a special uniqueness to this publication.

I wish to acknowledge all of the nursing faculty who taught in my NCLEX-RN review courses. Their commitment, dedication, and expertise have certainly assisted nursing students in achieving success with the NCLEX-RN. Additionally, I want to acknowledge Laurent W. Valliere for his commitment and dedication in assisting my nursing students to prepare for NCLEX-RN from a nonacademic point of view.

I would like to sincerely acknowledge and thank four very important individuals from Elsevier Health Sciences. I thank Loren Wilson, Director of Review and Testing, for all of her assistance and ideas with creating this publication. I also thank Shelly Hayden, Managing Editor, for her continuous assistance, enthusiasm, and support as I prepared this publication. And I thank Nancy O'Brien, Managing Editor of Review and Testing, and Charlene Ketchum, Associate Developmental Editor, for all of their assistance in maintaining organization and assisting me in completing this publication.

I also want to acknowledge all of the staff at Elsevier Health Sciences for their tremendous assistance throughout the preparation and production of this publication. A special thank you to all of them.

I thank all of the special people in the production department: Melissa Lastarria, Publishing Services Manager; Kelly Steinmann, Project Manager; and Jyotika Schroff, Designer, whose consistent editing assisted in finalizing this publication.

I sincerely thank Bob Boehringher, Director of Nursing Marketing, and Andrew Eilers, Marketing Manager, whose support, hard work, and special creativity assisted with this publication.

I would also like to acknowledge Patricia Mieg, Educational Sales Representative, who encouraged me to submit my ideas about the *Pyramid to Success* to the W.B. Saunders Company.

I sincerely want to acknowledge and thank Mike Ederer and Kate Mannix at Graphic World Publishing Services in St. Louis, Missouri, for their attention to detail and their support and assistance in the production of this book.

I want to acknowledge my parents who opened my door of opportunity in education. I thank my mother, Frances Mary, for all of her love, support, and assistance as I continuously worked to achieve my professional goals. I thank my father, Arnold Lawrence, who always provided insightful words of encouragement. My memories of his love and support will always remain in my heart.

I also thank my sister, Dianne Elodia, my brother, Lawrence Peter, and my niece, Gina Marie, who were continuously supportive, giving, and helpful during my research and preparation of this publication.

I sincerely thank Mary Ann Hogan, MSN, RN, from the University of Massachusetts in Amherst, Massachusetts, and Dr. JoAnn Mullaney from Salve Regina University in Newport, Rhode Island. These colleagues and friends have always encouraged and supported me through my professional endeavors.

I also need to thank Salve Regina University for the opportunity to educate nursing students in the baccalaureate nursing program and for its support during my research and writing of this publication. I would like to especially acknowledge my colleagues, Dr. Sandra Solem, Dr. Ellen McCarty, Dr. JoAnn Mullaney, Dr. Jane McCool, Dr. Peggy Matteson, and Dr. Bethany Sykes for all of their support and encouragement.

I wish to acknowledge the Community College of Rhode Island, which provided me the opportunity to educate nursing students in the Associate Degree of Nursing Program; and a special thank you to Patricia Miller, MSN, RN, and Michelina McClellan, MS, RN, from Baystate Medical Center, School of Nursing, in Springfield, Massachusetts who were my very first mentors in nursing education.

Lastly, a very special thank you to all my nursing students, past, present and future. You light up my life! Your curiosity, enthusiasm to learn, and desire to become successful is so inspiring.

Linda Anne Silvestri, MSN, RN

Contents

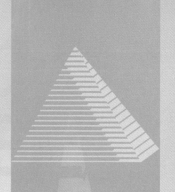

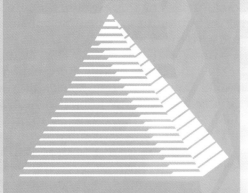

"If you are easily distracted by noises, you should request earplugs. There will be various noises in the room. Who wants to worry about blocking out noises when you are trying to concentrate on the test?"

—Anissa, Piedmont Technical College, Greenwood, South Carolina

"Keep several NCLEX review books scattered throughout the house. I had one in the kitchen for "quizzing while cooking," one in the living room in front of the television for quizzing during commercials, and one next to my bed so I could do my "obligatory 100 questions per night." I also had a set of NCLEX review cards that I split up into several stacks and stashed in various bags/purses, so I would always have them with me when out and about."

—Charlene, University of Southern Indiana, Evansville, Indiana

Part I

The NCLEX-RN® Examination

Chapter

The Test Plan

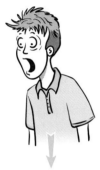

Awareness of what the test is all about!

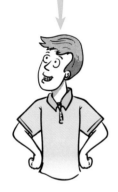

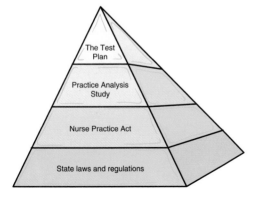

An important strategy for success for the National Council Licensure Examination for Registered Nurses (NCLEX-RN) is to become as familiar as possible with the NCLEX-RN Test Plan. A significant amount of anxiety can occur in a candidate (test-taker) facing the challenge of passing this examination. Knowing the format and general content of the examination will assist in alleviating your fear and anxiety.

This chapter focuses on how the test is developed and the components of the Test Plan. Some of this information was obtained from the National Council of State Boards of Nursing (NCSBN) Web site (www.ncsbn.org) and from the NCLEX-RN Test Plan (effective date: April 2004). Additional information regarding the test and its development can be obtained by accessing the NCSBN Web site or by writing to the NCSBN (see the box below for NCSBN contact information).

NATIONAL COUNCIL OF STATE BOARDS OF
NURSING CONTACT INFORMATION

National Council of State Boards of Nursing
111 E. Wacker Drive
Suite 2900
Chicago, IL 60601
Web site: www.ncsbn.org

HOW IS THE TEST PLAN DEVELOPED?

The Test Plan for the NCLEX-RN examination is developed by the NCSBN. As an initial step in the test development process, the NCSBN considers the legal scope of nursing practice as governed by state laws and regulations, including the nurse practice act, and uses these laws to define the areas on the examination that will assess the competence of a candidate (test-taker) for nurse licensure.

The NCSBN also conducts a Practice Analysis study to determine the framework for the Test Plan. The participants in this study include newly licensed registered nurses from all types of basic education programs. The participants are provided a list of nursing activities and are asked about the frequency of performing these specific activities, their impact on maintaining client safety, and the setting where the activities were performed. The results of the study are analyzed by a panel of experts at the NCSBN and decisions are made regarding the Test Plan framework.

WHO WRITES THE QUESTIONS?

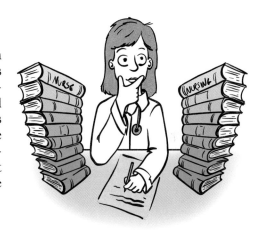

Question (item) writers are selected by the NCSBN after an extensive application process. The writers are registered nurses who hold a Master's degree or a higher degree. Many of the writers are nursing educators; however, a nurse currently employed in clinical nursing practice and working directly with nurses who have entered practice within the last 12 months may be selected to participate in this process. Question writers voluntarily submit an application to become a writer and must meet specific established criteria designated by the NCSBN to be accepted as a participant in the process.

WHAT ARE THE COMPONENTS OF THE TEST PLAN?

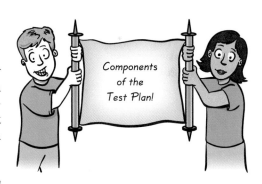

The content of NCLEX-RN reflects the activities that a newly licensed, entry-level, registered nurse must be able to perform to provide clients with safe and effective nursing care. The questions are written to address the Levels of Cognitive Ability, Client Needs, and Integrated Processes as identified in the Test Plan developed by the NCSBN (see the box below).

> **EXAMINATION QUESTIONS**
> **Each examination question addresses:**
> A Level of Cognitive Ability
> A Client Needs category
> An Integrated Process

Levels of Cognitive Ability

The examination for licensure as a registered nurse may include questions at the cognitive levels of knowledge, comprehension, application, and analysis. However, most questions are written at the application or higher Levels of Cognitive Ability, such as the analysis level, because the practice of nursing requires critical thinking in decision making. This means that you will be required to analyze and/or apply the information provided in the test question to answer the questions correctly. To understand the differences in the four cognitive levels, read the sample questions below.

LEVELS OF COGNITIVE ABILITY
Knowledge
Comprehension
Application
Analysis

Sample Question

Level of Cognitive Ability: Knowledge
A nurse reviews the laboratory results of a client's blood glucose level. The nurse knows that which of the following is a normal level?

1. 40 mg/dL
2. 100 mg/dL
3. 180 mg/dL
4. 220 mg/dL

Answer: 2

In a knowledge type of question, you need to simply recall data. In this sample question, recalling the normal blood glucose level is all that is needed to answer correctly. Remember, the normal blood glucose level ranges from 70 to 110 mg/dL.

Sample Question

Level of Cognitive Ability: Comprehension
A hospitalized client with type 1 diabetes mellitus reports hunger and nervousness, and the nurse notes that the client is diaphoretic. The nurse understands that the client is most likely experiencing:

1. Anxiety related to the hospitalization
2. Signs related to an infection
3. A hyperglycemic reaction
4. A hypoglycemic reaction

Answer: 4

In a comprehension type of question, you need to understand the basis for the information presented in the question and draw inferences from that information. In this question, you need to recognize that the client's signs and symptoms are a result of the diagnosis and treatment for type 1 diabetes mellitus and that the signs and symptoms relate to hypoglycemia. Remember, hunger, nervousness, and sweating are signs of hypoglycemia. Relate the "3 Ps"—polyuria, polydipsia, and polyphagia—to hyperglycemia.

Sample Question

Level of Cognitive Ability: Application

A client is experiencing a hypoglycemic reaction. The nurse should administer which of the following items to best treat the reaction?

1. Water
2. Diet soda
3. Milk
4. One sugar-free cookie

Answer: 3

In an application type of question, you will be asked about an intervention, a nursing action, a decision, or a problem that needs to be solved. In this sample question, you are asked to select the best item for treating a hypoglycemic reaction. Remember, if a hypoglycemic reaction occurs, the client should be given an item that contains 10 to 15 g carbohydrate.

Sample Question

Level of Cognitive Ability: Analysis

The nurse administers 10 units of Regular insulin at 7:00 AM to a client with type 1 diabetes mellitus. The nurse monitors the client most closely for a hypoglycemic reaction during which time frame?

1. 9:00 AM to 10:00 AM
2. 1:00 PM to 7:00 PM
3. 9:00 AM to 3:00 PM
4. 11:00 AM to 12:00 PM

Answer: 1

In an analysis type of question, you are required to consider and examine possibly several concepts in the question to answer it correctly. In this question, it is necessary to know that Regular insulin is short-acting insulin (i.e., it peaks in 2 to 3 hours) and that a hypoglycemic reaction is most likely to occur during peak time. Remember, the peak time of the insulin is the most likely time for a hypoglycemic reaction to occur.

Client Needs

The NCSBN identifies a Test Plan framework based on Client Needs. The NCSBN identifies four major categories of Client Needs and some of these categories are further divided into subcategories. The Client Needs categories include: Safe, Effective Care Environment; Health Promotion and Maintenance; Psychosocial Integrity; and Physiological Integrity. Table 1-1 identifies these Client Needs categories, any subcategories, and the associated percentage of test questions. Chapter 3 explains each Client Need category, lists the content most likely to be addressed on the examination, and provides sample questions for each category or subcategory.

Table 1-1

CLIENT NEEDS CATEGORIES, SUBCATEGORIES, AND PERCENTAGE (%) OF QUESTIONS	
Categories/Subcategories	Questions(%)
Safe, Effective Care Environment	
Management of Care	13%-19%
Safety and Infection Control	8%-14%
Health Promotion and Maintenance	6%-12%
Psychosocial Integrity	6%-12%
Physiological Integrity	
Basic Care and Comfort	6%-12%
Pharmacological and Parenteral Therapies	13%-19%
Reduction of Risk Potential	13%-19%
Physiological Adaptation	11%-17%

 Integrated Processes

The NCSBN identifies four processes that are fundamental to the practice of nursing. These processes are a component of the Test Plan and are integrated throughout the four categories of Client Needs: Safe Effective Care Environment; Health Promotion and Maintenance; Psychosocial Integrity; and Physiological Integrity. The Integrated Processes identified by the NCSBN include: Caring; Communication and Documentation; Nursing Process (assessment, analysis, planning, implementation, and evaluation); and Teaching/Learning. Chapter 4 explains each Integrated Process and provides sample questions for each.

> **INTEGRATED PROCESSES**
> Caring
> Communication and Documentation
> Nursing Process
> Teaching/Learning

REFERENCES

Ignatavicius D, Workman, M: *Medical surgical nursing: critical thinking for collaborative care*, ed 4, Philadelphia, 2002, WB Saunders.

Lewis S, Heitkemper M, Dirksen S: *Medical-surgical nursing: assessment and management of clinical problems*, ed 6, St Louis, 2004 Mosby.

National Council of State Boards of Nursing: Test Plan for the National Council Licensure Examination for Registered Nurses (effective date: April 2004). Chicago, 2003, National Council of State Boards of Nursing.

National Council of State Boards of Nursing on line: Available at www.ncsbn.org

Phipps W, Monahan F, Sands J, Marek J, Neighbors M: *Medical-surgical nursing: health and illness perspectives*, ed 7, St Louis, 2003, Mosby.

2 Chapter

The Examination Process

A significant amount of anxiety can occur in a candidate (test-taker) taking the National Council Licensure Examination for Registered Nurses (NCLEX-RN) examination. Knowing what you will encounter during the process of testing will assist in alleviating your fear and anxiety.

COMPUTERIZED ADAPTIVE TESTING: HOW DOES IT WORK?

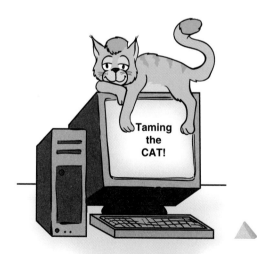

The abbreviation CAT stands for "computerized adaptive testing." This means that the examination is created as you answer each question. All of the test questions are categorized on the basis of the test plan structure and the level of difficulty of the question. As you answer a question, the computer will determine your competency on the basis of the answer that you selected. If you selected a correct answer, the computer scans the question bank and selects a more difficult question for your next question; if you selected an incorrect answer, the computer scans the question bank and selects an easier question for your next question. Table 2-1 illustrates how this process works. This process continues until the test plan requirements, based on the test plan structure, are met and a reliable pass or fail decision is made.

When a test question is presented on the computer screen, it must be answered or the test will not move on. This means that you will not be able to skip questions, go back and review questions, or go back and change answers. Remember, in a CAT examination, once an answer is recorded, all subsequent questions administered depend, to an extent, on the answer selected for that question. Skipping and then returning to earlier questions is not compatible with the logical methodology of a CAT examination. The inability to skip questions or go back to change previous answers will not be a disadvantage to you. Actually, you will not fall into that "trap" of changing a correct answer to an incorrect one with CAT.

Table 2-1

COMPUTER SELECTION OF TEST QUESTIONS

Question	Level of Difficulty	Test-Taker Response
1	Easy	Correct
2	Difficult	Correct
3	Most difficult	Correct
4	Most difficult	Incorrect
5	Difficult	Incorrect
6	Easy	Correct
7	Difficult	Incorrect
8	Easy	Correct
9	Difficult	Correct
10	Most difficult	Correct

The test questions will continue to be selected in this way until a reliable pass or fail decision is made.

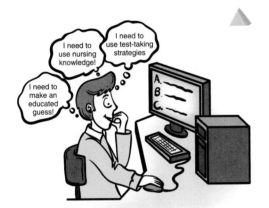

If you are faced with a question that contains unfamiliar content, you may need to make an educated guess to answer. There is no penalty for guessing on this examination. Remember, with most questions, the answer will be right there in front of you. If you need to guess, use your nursing knowledge to its fullest extent, as well as all of the test-taking strategies that you have learned in this book.

You do not need any computer experience to take this examination. You will be provided with a keyboard tutorial at the start of the examination that will instruct you on the use of the on-screen optional calculator, the use of the mouse, and how to record an answer. In addition to the traditional four-option, multiple-choice question, the tutorial also provides instructions on how to respond to different question formats. A proctor always is present to assist in explaining the use of the computer to ensure your full understanding of how to proceed.

KEYBOARD TUTORIAL
How to use the computer
How to use the on-screen optional calculator
How to use the mouse
How to record an answer
How to respond to different question formats

REGISTERING FOR THE EXAMINATION: WHAT DO YOU NEED TO DO?

The initial step in the registration process is to submit an application to the state board of nursing for the state in which you intend to obtain licensure. You need to obtain information from the board of nursing regarding the specific registration process because the process may vary from state to state. In most states, you may register for the examination through the Internet, by mail, or by telephone. The NCLEX candidate Web site provides information regarding what you will need to register to take this examination.

> **NCLEX CANDIDATE WEB SITE**
> www.vue.com/nclex

It is important that you follow the registration instructions and complete the registration forms precisely and accurately. Registration forms that are not properly completed, or not accompanied by the proper fees in the required method of payment, will be returned to you and will delay testing dates.

There is a fee for taking the examination, and you may also have to pay additional fees to the board of nursing in the state in which you are applying. You will be sent a confirmation indicating that your registration was received. If you do not receive a confirmation within 4 weeks of submitting your registration, you should contact the candidate services.

AUTHORIZATION TO TEST FORM: WHAT DO YOU NEED IT FOR?

Once your eligibility to test has been determined by the board of nursing in the state in which licensure is requested, your registration form is processed and an Authorization to Test (ATT) form will be sent to you. You cannot make an appointment until the board of nursing declares your eligibility and you receive an ATT form.

The ATT form contains important information including your test authorization number, candidate identification number, and an expiration date. Note the expiration date on the form, because you must take the test by this date. You also need to take your ATT form to the test center on the day of your examination. You will not be admitted to the examination without it.

HOW DO YOU SCHEDULE A TESTING DATE?

The examination will take place at a Pearson Professional Center; an appointment can be made through the Web site or by telephone. First-time test-takers will be offered an appointment within 30 days of making contact to schedule an appointment, and repeat test-takers will be offered an appointment within 45 days. You can schedule an appointment at any Pearson Professional Center; a confirmation of your appointment will be sent to you. You do not have to take the examination in the same state in which you are seeking licensure.

If for any reason you need to cancel or reschedule your testing appointment, you can make the change on the candidate Web site (www.vue.com/nclex) or by calling candidate services. The change needs to be made one full business day (24 hours) before your scheduled appointment.

If you fail to arrive for the examination or do not cancel or reschedule your testing appointment without providing appropriate notice, you will forfeit your examination fee and your ATT will be invalidated. This information will be reported to the board of nursing in the state in which you have applied for licensure, and you will be required to register and pay the testing fees again.

It is important that you arrive at the testing center at least 30 minutes before the time the test is scheduled to begin. If you arrive late for the scheduled testing appointment, you may be required to forfeit your examination appointment. If it is necessary for the appointment to be forfeited, you will need to re-register for the examination and pay an additional fee. The board of nursing will be notified that you did not take the test.

> Arrive at the test center at least 30 minutes before the test is scheduled!

A few days before your scheduled date of testing, take the time to drive to the testing center to determine its exact location, the length of time required to arrive at that location, and any potential obstacles that may delay you, such as road construction, traffic, or parking sites.

WHAT DO YOU DO IF YOU NEED SPECIAL TESTING ACCOMMODATIONS?

A test-taker with needs who requires special testing accommodations should contact the board of nursing before submitting a registration form. The board of nursing will provide the procedures for the request. The board of nursing must authorize special testing accommodations. After board of nursing approval, the National Council of State Boards of Nursing reviews the requested accommodations and must also approve the request. If the request is approved, the testing appointment must be made by the NCLEX Program Coordinator, who can be contacted by calling NCLEX candidate services. Canceling or rescheduling an appointment must be done through the NCLEX Program Coordinator.

THE TESTING CENTER: WHAT CAN YOU EXPECT?

The testing center is designed to ensure complete security of the testing process. Strict candidate identification requirements have been established. To be admitted to the testing center, you must bring the ATT form and two forms of identification (ID). Both forms of ID must be signed and current or nonexpired, and one must contain a recent photograph of you. The name on the photograph ID must be the same as the name on the ATT form.

WHAT YOU MUST BRING TO THE TESTING CENTER
The ATT form
Two forms of ID that are signed and current or
    nonexpired

A digital fingerprint, signature, and photograph will be taken at the test center and accompany the NCLEX results to confirm your identity. If you leave the testing room for any reason, you will be required to have your fingerprint taken again to be readmitted to the room.

Personal belongings are not allowed in the testing room. Secure storage will be provided for you; however, storage space is limited, so you must plan accordingly. In addition, the testing center will not assume responsibility for your personal belongings. The test center waiting areas are generally small; therefore, friends or family members who accompany you are not permitted to wait in the testing center while you are taking the examination.

Once you have completed the admission process and a brief orientation, the proctor will escort you to your assigned computer. You will be seated at an individual table area with an appropriate work space that includes computer equipment, appropriate lighting, an erasable note board, and a marker. No items, including unauthorized scratch paper, are allowed into the testing room. Electronic devices such as watches, pagers, or cell phones are not allowed in the testing room. Eating, drinking, and the use of tobacco are not allowed in the testing room.

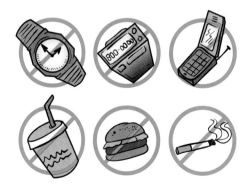

You will be observed at all times by the test proctor while taking the examination. In addition, video and audio recording of all test sessions occurs. Pearson Professional Centers has no control over the sounds made by typing on the computer. If these sounds are distracting, raise your hand to summon the proctor. Earplugs are available on request.

You must follow the directions given by the test center staff and must remain seated during the test, except when authorized to leave. If you feel that you have a problem with the computer, need an additional note board, need to take a break, or need the test proctor for any reason, you must raise your hand.

HOW MUCH TESTING TIME DO YOU HAVE?

The maximum testing time is 6 hours, and this time period includes the tutorial, two preprogrammed optional breaks, and any unscheduled breaks that you may take. The first preprogrammed optional break takes place after 2 hours of testing; the second preprogrammed optional break is after 3.5 hours of testing. The computer screen will notify you of the time for these breaks. You must leave the testing room during breaks; when you return, you will be required to provide a fingerprint to be readmitted to the testing room.

Maximum testing time: six hours!

HOW MANY QUESTIONS ARE IN THE EXAMINATION?

The minimum number of questions that you will need to answer is 75. Of these 75 questions, 60 will be operational (scored) questions and 15 will be pretest (unscored) questions. The maximum number of questions in the test is 265. Fifteen of the total number of questions that you need to answer will be pretest (unscored) questions.

The pretest questions are questions that may be presented as scored questions on future examinations. These pretest questions are not identified as such; that is, you will not know which questions are the pretest (unscored) questions. Therefore, it is important to answer every question as if it were being scored.

> The minimum number of questions in the test is 75.
> The maximum number of questions in the test is 265.

WHAT HAPPENS WHEN THE EXAMINATION IS COMPLETED?

Once the test is completed, you will complete a brief, computer-delivered questionnaire about your testing experience. After this questionnaire is completed, you need to raise your hand to summon the test proctor. The test proctor will collect and inventory all note boards and then will permit you to leave.

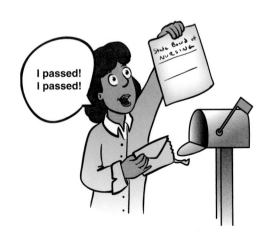

I passed! I passed!

HOW ARE THE RESULTS PROCESSED?

Every computerized examination is scored twice: once by the computer at the testing center, and then again after the examination is transmitted to Pearson Professional Centers. No results are released at the test center. The board of nursing will mail your results to you approximately 1 month after you take the examination.

You should not telephone Pearson Professional Centers, the National Council of State Boards of Nursing, candidate services, or the state board of nursing for results.

HOW IS A PASS OR FAIL DECISION MADE?

All of the examination questions are categorized by test plan area and level of difficulty. This is an important point to keep in mind when considering how a pass or fail decision is made by the computer because a pass or fail decision is not based on a percentage of correctly answered questions. After the minimum number of questions have been answered (75 questions), the computer compares the test-taker's ability level to the standard required for passing. The standard required for passing is set based on the expert judgment of several individuals appointed by the National Council of State Boards of Nursing. If the test-taker is clearly above the passing standard, then the test-taker passes the examination. If the test-taker is clearly below the passing standard, then the test-taker fails the examination. If the computer is not able to clearly determine whether the test-taker has passed or failed because the test-taker's ability is close to the passing standard, then the computer continues asking questions. After each question, the test-taker's ability is determined, and when it becomes clear on which side of the passing standard that the test-taker falls (above or below the standard), the examination ends. If the test-taker is administered the maximum number of questions (265 questions), the computer will make a pass or fail decision by recomputing the test-taker's final ability level, on the basis of every question answered, and comparing it with the passing standard. If the ability level is above the passing standard, the test-taker passes (Fig. 2-1); if it is not above the passing standard, the test-taker fails (Fig. 2-2).

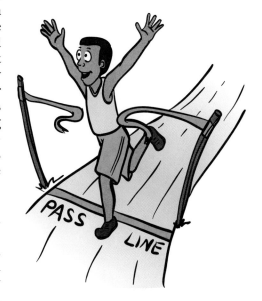

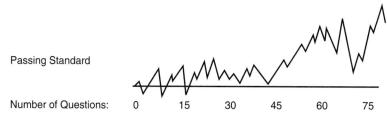

Fig. 2-1 A test-taker who has passed. The test-taker is clearly above the passing standard.

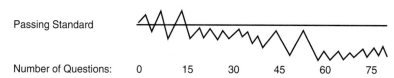

Fig. 2-2 A test-taker who has failed. The test-taker is clearly below the passing standard.

HOW IS A PASS OR FAIL DECISION MADE IF YOU RUN OUT OF TIME?

If the examination ends because you have run out of time, the computer may not have enough information to make a clear pass or fail decision. If this is the situation, the computer will review the test-taker's performance during testing. If the test-taker's ability was consistently above the passing standard, the test-taker passes.

WHO RECEIVES A CANDIDATE PERFORMANCE REPORT?

A candidate performance report is provided to a test-taker who failed the examination. This report provides the test-taker with information about his or her strengths and weaknesses in relation to the test plan and provides a guide for studying and retaking the examination. The test-taker must wait a period of 45 or 91 days (based on board of nursing policy) before retaking the examination.

WHAT IS INTERSTATE ENDORSEMENT?

Because the NCLEX-RN examination is a national examination, you can apply to take the examination in any state. Once licensure is received, you can apply for Interstate Endorsement, which is obtaining another license in another state to practice nursing in that state. The procedures and requirements for Interstate Endorsement may vary from state to state, and these procedures can be obtained from the State Board of Nursing in the state in which endorsement is sought. You may also be allowed to practice nursing in another state if the state has enacted the Nurse Licensure Compact.

WHAT IS NURSE LICENSURE COMPACT?

It may be possible to hold one license from the state of residency and practice nursing in another state under the mutual recognition model of nursing licensure, if the state has enacted the Nurse Licensure Compact. Visit the National Council of State Boards of Nursing's website for more information."

REFERENCES

National Council of State Boards of Nursing: Test Plan for the National Council Licensure Examination for Registered Nurses (effective date: April 2004). Chicago, 2003, National Council of State Boards of Nursing.

National Council of State Boards of Nursing on line: Available at www.ncsbn.org

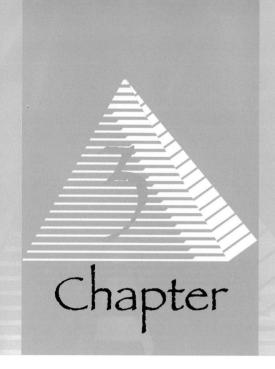

Chapter

Client Needs

In the Test Plan implemented in April 2004, the National Council of State Boards of Nursing (NCSBN) has identified a test plan framework based on Client Needs.

The NCSBN identifies four major categories of Client Needs, and some of these categories are further divided into subcategories. The Client Needs categories include: Safe, Effective Care Environment; Health Promotion and Maintenance; Psychosocial Integrity; and Physiological Integrity.

> **CLIENT NEEDS CATEGORIES**
> Safe, Effective Care Environment
> Health Promotion and Maintenance
> Psychosocial Integrity
> Physiological Integrity

Some of the information contained in this chapter was obtained from the NCSBN Test Plan for the National Council Licensure Examination for Registered Nurses and the NCSBN Web site (www.ncsbn.org).

SAFE, EFFECTIVE CARE ENVIRONMENT

The Safe, Effective Care Environment category includes two subcategories: Management of Care and Safety and Infection Control. Management of Care (13% to 19%) addresses content that tests the knowledge, skills, and abilities required to enhance the care delivery setting to protect clients, families, significant others, visitors, and health care personnel. Safety and Infection Control (8% to 14%) addresses content that tests the knowledge, skills, and abilities required to protect clients, families, significant others, visitors, and health care personnel from health and environmental hazards.

Management of Care

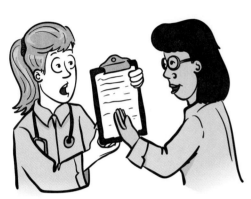

In the Management of Care subcategory, content may include the following*:

- Advance directives
- Case management
- Client advocacy
- Client rights, including confidentiality and informed consent
- Collaboration and consultation with other health care team members
- Continuity of care
- Delegating and supervising
- Educating staff
- Ethical and legal issues

Question: Management of Care

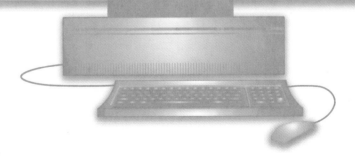

A client scheduled for surgery tells the nurse that he signed an informed consent but was never told about the risks of the surgery. The nurse serves as the client's advocate by:

1. Writing a note on the front of the client's record so that the surgeon will see it when the client arrives in the operating room
2. Documenting in the client's record that the client was not told about the risks of the surgery
3. Contacting the surgeon and asking the surgeon to explain the surgical risks to the client
4. Reassuring the client that the risks are minimal and unlikely to occur

*Portions copyright by the National Council of State Boards of Nursing, Inc. All rights reserved.

Answer: 3

Test-Taking Strategy:

Use therapeutic communication techniques to eliminate option 4. From the remaining options, focus on the words "never told about the risks of the surgery." A nurse serves as a client advocate by protecting the rights of clients to be informed and to participate in decisions regarding their own care. The only option that ensures that the client will be informed of the surgical risks is option 3.

SAFE, EFFECTIVE CARE ENVIRONMENT

Management of Care = 13% to 19% of the questions

Safety and Infection Control = 8% to 14% of the questions

Management concepts

Performance improvement

Prioritizing

Referrals and resource management

An example of a question that addresses this subcategory is provided on the previous page.

Safety and Infection Control

In the Safety and Infection Control subcategory, content may include the following*:

Disaster planning and an emergency response plan

Handling hazardous and infectious material

Medical and surgical asepsis

Preventing accidents and preventing errors

Preventing injuries and home safety

Reporting accidents or errors and documenting on Incident Reports

Restraints and safety devices

Safe use of equipment

Security plan

Standard, transmission-based, and other precautions

An example of a question that addresses this subcategory follows.

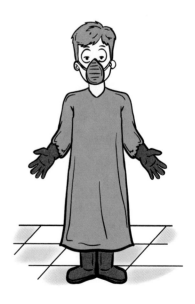

---

*Portions copyright by the National Council of State Boards of Nursing, Inc. All rights reserved.

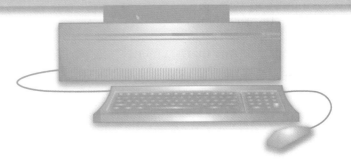

Question: Safety and Infection Control

An emergency department nurse receives a telephone call from the police department and is told that several victims involved in a train accident will be brought to the emergency department. The nurse's immediate action is to:

1. Call as many nurses as possible at home to have them come to the hospital to care for the victims
2. Follow the directions outlined in the hospital's disaster preparedness plan (emergency response plan)
3. Ask the housekeeping and laundry department to deliver an extra cart of linen that contains several blankets
4. Call the operating room and inform the staff that they may be receiving numerous victims that require surgery

Answer: 2

Test-Taking Strategy:
If the emergency department nurse is notified that several victims of a disaster will be arriving to the emergency department, the nurse would immediately activate the emergency response plan by notifying the supervisor and by following the directions in the plan. Also, note that option 2 is the umbrella (global) option and once this action is implemented, the others will follow.

HEALTH PROMOTION AND MAINTENANCE

The Health Promotion and Maintenance category (6% to 12%) addresses the principles related to growth and development. This Client Needs category also addresses content that tests the knowledge, skills, and abilities required to assist the client, family members, and/or significant others in preventing health problems, recognizing alterations in health, and developing health practices that promote and support wellness.

In the Health Promotion and Maintenance category, content may include the following*:

Disease prevention

Family planning, family systems, and human sexuality

Growth and development, developmental stages and transitions, and the aging process

Maternity (antepartum, intrapartum, postpartum) and newborn care

Expected body image changes

Health and wellness, health screening, and health promotion programs

High-risk behaviors

Immunizations

Lifestyle choices

Physical assessment techniques

Principles of teaching/learning

Self-care

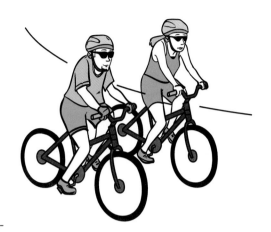

An example of a question that addresses the Health Promotion and Maintenance category is provided below.

Question: Health Promotion and Maintenance

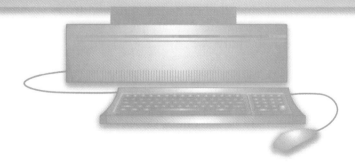

A nurse is preparing to care for a hospitalized female teenager who is in skeletal traction. The nurse plans care knowing that the most likely primary concern of the teenager is:

1. Obtaining adequate nutrition
2. Body image
3. Keeping up with school work
4. Obtaining adequate rest and sleep

Answer: 2

Test-Taking Strategy:

Note the keyword "primary" and focus on the client, a teenager. Thinking about the psychosocial development of the teenager (adolescent) will direct you to option 2. Remember, body image is of particular importance to adolescents and teenagers.

HEALTH PROMOTION AND MAINTENANCE
Health Promotion and Maintenance = 6% to 12% of the questions

---

PSYCHOSOCIAL INTEGRITY

The Psychosocial Integrity category (6% to 12%) addresses content that tests the knowledge, skills, and abilities required to promote and support the client, family, and/or significant others' ability to cope, adapt, and problem solve during stressful events. This Client Needs category also addresses the emotional, mental, and social well-being of the client, family, or significant other, and the knowledge, skills, and abilities required to care for the client with an acute or chronic mental illness.

PSYCHOSOCIAL INTEGRITY
Psychosocial Integrity = 6% to 12% of the questions

In the Psychosocial Integrity category, content may include the following*:

Abuse or neglect
Behavioral interventions
Chemical dependency
Coping mechanisms
Crisis intervention
Cultural diversity
End-of-life issues
Family dynamics
Grief and loss
Mental health concepts
Religious and spiritual influences on health
Sensory and perceptual alterations
Situational role changes
Stress management
Support systems
Therapeutic communication techniques
Therapeutic environment
Unexpected body image changes

An example of a question that addresses the Psychosocial Integrity category is provided on the following page.

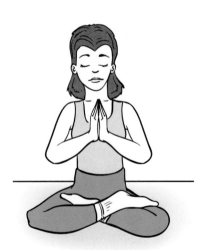

---

*Portions copyright by the National Council of State Boards of Nursing, Inc. All rights reserved.

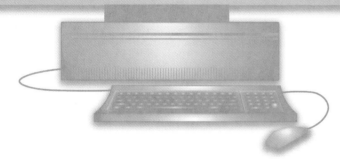

Question: Psychosocial Integrity

A boy is brought to the school nurse's office with reports of abdominal pain. On assessment, the nurse notes the presence of several bruises on the child's abdomen and back and several cigarette burn marks. The nurse suspects child abuse and plans for which priority action?

1. Calling the parents to ask them how the child's bruises and burn marks occurred

2. Removing the child from the abusive situation to prevent further injury

3. Documenting about the bruises noted on the child

4. Asking the child how long his parents have been abusing him

Answer: 2

Test-Taking Strategy:

Use Maslow's Hierarchy of Needs theory. Remember that physiological needs are the priority, and if a physiological need does not exist, then safety is the priority. This will direct you to option 2. In the case of suspected child abuse, the priority is to remove the child from the abusive situation to prevent further injury. In addition, all cases of suspected child abuse must be reported to local authorities.

PHYSIOLOGICAL INTEGRITY

The Physiological Integrity category includes four subcategories: Basic Care and Comfort, Pharmacological and Parenteral Therapies, Reduction of Risk Potential, and Physiological Adaptation. Basic Care and Comfort (6% to 12%) addresses content that tests the knowledge, skills, and abilities required to provide comfort and assistance to the client in the performance of activities of daily living. Pharmacological and Parenteral Therapies (13% to 19%) addresses content that tests the knowledge, skills, and abilities required to administer medications and parenteral therapies. Reduction of Risk Potential (13% to 19%)

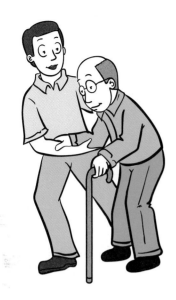

addresses content that tests the knowledge, skills, and abilities required to prevent complications or health problems related to the client's condition or any prescribed treatments or procedures. Physiological Adaptation (11% to 17%) addresses content that tests the knowledge, skills, and abilities required to provide care to clients with acute, chronic, or life-threatening conditions.

Basic Care and Comfort

In the Basic Care and Comfort subcategory, content may include the following*:

  Alternative and complementary therapies
  Assistive devices
  Elimination
  Hygiene
  Mobility and immobility
  Nonpharmacological comfort interventions
  Nutrition and oral hydration
  Rest and sleep

An example of a question that addresses this subcategory is provided below.

Question: Basic Care and Comfort

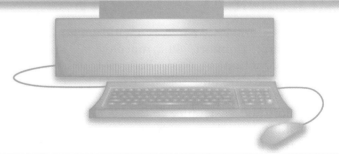

A nurse has provided information to a client about measures that will promote normal urination patterns and prevent urinary tract infections. Which statement by the client indicates a need for further information?

1. "I should eat foods that will make my urine acidic."
2. "I should try to hold my urine as long as I can rather than expelling it when I feel the urge."
3. "I should drink plenty of fluids during the day."
4. "I should take my furosemide (Lasix) in the morning."

---

*Portions copyright by the National Council of State Boards of Nursing, Inc. All rights reserved.

Answer: 2

Test-Taking Strategy:
Use the process of elimination and note the words "a need for further information." Focusing on the issue (prevent urinary tract infections) and recalling that urinary stasis can lead to infection will direct you to option 2. Remember, the client should be instructed to urinate at regular intervals and when the urge to void is felt.

PHYSIOLOGICAL INTEGRITY

Basic Care and Comfort = 6% to 12% of the questions

Pharmacological and Parenteral Therapies = 13% to 19% of the questions

Reduction of Risk Potential = 13% to 19% of the questions

Physiological Adaptation = 11% to 17% of the questions

Pharmacological and Parenteral Therapies

In the Pharmacological and Parenteral Therapies subcategory, content may include the following*:

Blood products

Central venous access devices

Dosage calculations

Expected outcome and effects

Intravenous therapy and parenteral fluids

Medication administration

Pharmacological agents, actions, contraindications, interactions, side effects, and adverse effects

Pharmacological pain management

Total parenteral nutrition

An example of a question that addresses this subcategory is provided on the following page.

---

*Portions copyright by the National Council of State Boards of Nursing, Inc. All rights reserved.

Question: Pharmacological and Parenteral Therapies

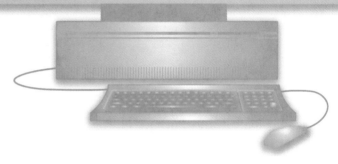

Cyclosporine (Sandimmune) oral solution is prescribed for a client who had a kidney transplant. The nurse provides information to the client about the medication and tells the client that which of the following is most important to monitor?

1. Apical heart rate
2. Peripheral pulses
3. Platelet count
4. Temperature

Answer: 4

Test-Taking Strategy:

Use the process of elimination. Eliminate options 1 and 2 first because they are similar. From the remaining options, note the keywords "most important". Recalling that infection is an adverse effect will direct you to option 4. Remember, the most common adverse effects of cyclosporine are nephrotoxicity, infection, hypertension, tremor, and hirsutism.

Reduction of Risk Potential

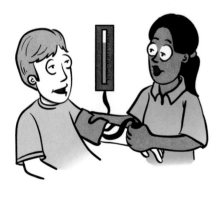

In the Reduction of Risk Potential subcategory, content may include the following*:

> Diagnostic tests and laboratory values
> Monitoring conscious sedation
> Potential for alterations in body systems
> Potential for complications of diagnostic tests and surgical and nonsurgical treatments and procedures
> System specific assessments
> Therapeutic procedures
> Vital signs

*Portions copyright by the National Council of State Boards of Nursing, Inc. All rights reserved.

An example of a question that addresses this subcategory follows.

Question: Reduction of Risk Potential

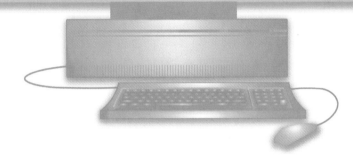

The nurse assists a physician in performing a liver biopsy on a client. After the procedure, the nurse assists the client to which position?

1. Prone

2. On the right side

3. On the left side

4. Left Sims' position

Answer: 2

Test-Taking Strategy:

Use knowledge regarding anatomy and the anatomic location of the liver to answer the question. Recalling that the liver is located on the right side of the upper abdomen will direct you to option 2. Remember, after a liver biopsy, the client is positioned on the right side for a minimum of 2 hours to splint the puncture site and prevent bleeding.

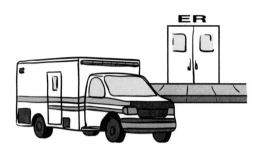

Physiological Adaptation

In the Physiological Adaptation subcategory, content may include the following*:

Alterations in body systems
Fluid and electrolyte imbalances
Hemodynamics and illness management
Infectious diseases
Medical emergencies
Pathophysiology
Radiation therapy
Unexpected responses to therapy

An example of a question that addresses this subcategory follows.

Question: Physiological Adaptation

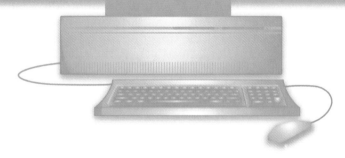

A nurse is reviewing the medical records of the four clients she will be caring for. The nurse determines that which client is at risk for a fluid volume deficit?

1. The client receiving long-term corticosteroid therapy
2. The client with congestive heart failure
3. The client with syndrome of inappropriate antidiuretic hormone
4. The client with a nasogastric tube attached to suction

Answer: 4

Test-Taking Strategy:

Focus on the issue—the client at risk for fluid volume deficit. Think about the pathophysiology associated with each condition identified in the options. The only client that loses fluid is the client with a nasogastric tube attached to suction.

---

*Portions copyright by the National Council of State Boards of Nursing, Inc. All rights reserved.

REFERENCES

Harkreader H, Hogan MA: *Fundamentals of nursing: caring and clinical judgment,* ed 2, Philadelphia, 2004, WB Saunders.

Hodgson B, Kizior R: *Saunders nursing drug handbook 2005,* Philadelphia, 2005, WB Saunders.

Ignatavicius D, Workman M: *Medical surgical nursing: critical thinking for collaborative care,* ed 4, Philadelphia, 2002, WB Saunders.

Lewis S, Heitkemper M, Dirksen S: *Medical-surgical nursing: assessment and management of clinical problems,* ed 6, St Louis, 2004, Mosby.

National Council of State Boards of Nursing: Test Plan for the National Council Licensure Examination for Registered Nurses (effective date: April 2004), Chicago, 2003, National Council of State Boards of Nursing.

National Council of State Boards of Nursing on line: Available at www.ncsbn.org

Phipps W, Monahan F, Sands J, et al: *Medical-surgical nursing: health and illness perspectives,* ed 7, St Louis, 2003, Mosby.

Potter P, Perry A: *Fundamentals of nursing,* ed 6, St Louis, 2005, Mosby.

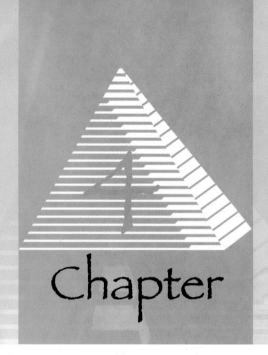

Chapter 4

Integrated Processes

The National Council of State Boards of Nursing identifies four processes that are fundamental to the practice of nursing. These processes are a component of the Test Plan and are integrated throughout the four categories of Client Needs: Safe, Effective Care Environment; Health Promotion and Maintenance; Psychosocial Integrity; and Physiological Integrity. The Integrated Processes are Caring, Communication and Documentation, Nursing Process (assessment, analysis, planning, implementation, and evaluation), and Teaching/Learning.

INTEGRATED PROCESSES
Caring
Communication and Documentation
Nursing Process
Teaching/Learning

CARING

Caring is the essence of nursing and is basic to any helping relationship. Caring is central to every encounter that a nurse may have with a client. Through caring, the nurse humanizes the client. Treating the client with respect and dignity is a true expression of caring. In the technological environment of health care, emphasizing the client's individuality counteracts any potential process of depersonalization. Caring is an Integrated Process of the Test Plan for the National Council Licensure Examination for Registered Nurses (NCLEX-RN). This means that this concept is central to all Client Needs components of the Test Plan.

On the NCLEX-RN, the concept of caring is primary. It is easy for you to become involved with looking at a question from a technological viewpoint, but you also need to think about the concept of caring when reading a test question and when selecting an option. Remember that this examination is all about nursing, and that nursing is caring!

Integrated Process: Caring

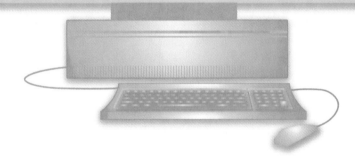

An infant is brought to the emergency department by emergency medical services (EMS) with suspected sudden infant death syndrome (SIDS). The infant's parents have accompanied EMS and are present when the infant is pronounced dead. The most important aspect of compassionate care for the parents is to:

1. Explain to the parents that the death was not their fault
2. Allow the parents to say goodbye to the infant
3. Gather data about the events that occurred before the infant was found
4. Encourage the parents to attend a support group

Answer: 2

Test-Taking Strategy:

Focus on the issue: compassionate care. This will direct you to option 2, because it is the only option that addresses this issue. The nurse would gather data about the events that occurred before the infant was found, would ask factual questions that avoid placing guilt on the parents, and would encourage the parents to attend a support group; however, these interventions are not specifically related to the aspect of compassionate care. Remember that the concept of caring is primary, and that nursing is caring!

COMMUNICATION AND DOCUMENTATION

Communication

The process of communication occurs as the nurse interacts with a client or the client's family member or significant others.

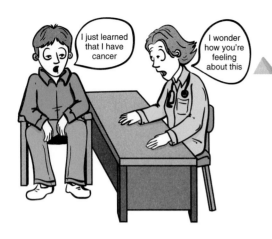

Communication-type test questions are integrated throughout the NCLEX-RN Test Plan and may address a situation in any health care setting.

Use of therapeutic communication techniques is key to an effective nurse–client relationship. When answering a test question, select the option that identifies use of a therapeutic communication technique and avoid selecting an option that identifies use of a nontherapeutic communication technique. Always select the option that focuses on the client's feelings, concerns, anxieties, or fears.

Therapeutic communication techniques indicate a correct option.

Nontherapeutic communication techniques indicate an incorrect option.

If an option reflects the client's feelings, anxieties, or concerns, select that option.

Integrated Process: Communication

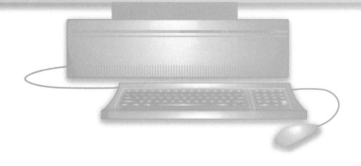

A client says to a nurse, "I'm scared about my surgery that I am having tomorrow." The nurse should make which appropriate response to the client?

1. "There is no reason to be scared."

2. "You have plenty of reasons to be scared. Surgery is a scary thing."

3. "Scared?"

4. "Most people who have to have surgery are scared."

Answer: 3

Test-Taking Strategy:

Use therapeutic communication techniques to direct you to option 3. In option 3, the nurse uses the therapeutic technique of reflection to encourage the client to further discuss his or her feelings of being scared. Options 1, 2, and 4 are examples of nontherapeutic communication techniques. Option 1 uses false reassurance. Option 2 will escalate the client's fear about surgery. Option 4 belittles the client's expressed feelings. Remember, therapeutic communication techniques indicate a correct option!

Documentation

Documentation is a critical component of a nurse's responsibility. The process of documentation serves many purposes and provides a comprehensive representation of the client's health status and the care given by all members of the health care team. There are many methods of documentation, but the responsibilities surrounding this practice remain the same.

The ethical and legal responsibilities related to documentation and the specific guidelines and principles related to both narrative and computerized documentation systems are important areas to review.

Integrated Process: Documentation

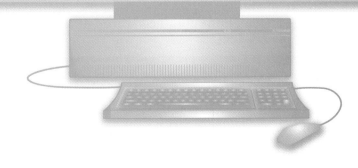

A nurse discovers that she needs to make a correction to a written entry in a client's chart. Which of the following is the appropriate action?

1. Contact the nursing supervisor to cosign the correction.
2. Remove the page, recopy the data to a new page, and add the correct entry.
3. Draw a single line through the entry that needs correction followed by his or her (the nurse's) initials.
4. Erase the entry that needs correction and add the correct entry.

Answer: 3

Test-Taking Strategy:

Use guidelines and principles related to documentation to answer this question. This will direct you to option 3. There are no useful reasons for options 1 and 2. The nurse would never erase an entry made in a client's chart. Remember to review the guidelines and principles related to both narrative and computerized documentation systems!

NURSING PROCESS

The steps of the Nursing Process include assessment, analysis, planning, implementation, and evaluation. These steps are extremely useful when answering questions that require you to prioritize. Following the steps of the Nursing Process will guide you to the correct option.

Assessment

Assessment is the first step of the Nursing Process. It involves a systematic method of collecting data about a client for the purpose of identifying actual and risk for (potential) health problems and establishing a database. The database provides the foundation for the remaining steps of the Nursing Process. Therefore, a thorough and adequate database is essential.

Data collection begins with the first contact with the client. During all successive contacts, the nurse continues to collect information significant to the needs of the client. During the assessment process, the nurse collects data about the client from a variety of sources, primarily the client. Family members or significant others are secondary sources of assessment data, and these sources may supplement or verify information provided by the client. Data may also be obtained from the client's record through the medical history, laboratory results, and diagnostic reports. Medical records from previous admissions may also provide additional client data. The nurse may also consult with other health care team members who had contact with the client. A thorough database is obtained through a health history and physical assessment and contains both subjective and objective data. Subjective data include the information given by the client. Objective data are the observable, measurable pieces of information about the client. Objective data include measurements such as vital signs or laboratory findings and information obtained using the senses. Objective data also include clinical manifestations such as the signs and symptoms of an illness or disease. The process of assessment also consists of confirming and verifying the client data, communicating information obtained through the assessment

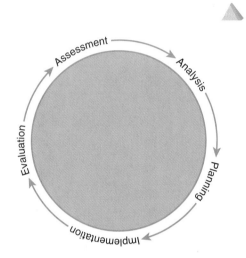

Subjective data include the information given by the client. Objective data are the observable, measurable pieces of information about the client.

process, and documenting assessment findings in a thorough and accurate manner.

When answering a test question, if the question requires you to prioritize, remember that assessment is the first step of the nursing process. If an assessment action is presented as one of the options, that option is most likely the correct answer. However, a possible exception to this guideline is if the question presents an emergency situation. In this case, read the information carefully. In an emergency situation, an intervention rather than an assessment may be the priority!

ASSESSMENT

Assessment is the first step of the Nursing Process.

If you are asked to identify the initial or first action, follow the steps of the nursing process; if an assessment action is presented as one of the options, that option is most likely correct.

If the question addresses an emergency situation, read carefully; an intervention may be the priority!

Integrated Process: Nursing Process/Assessment

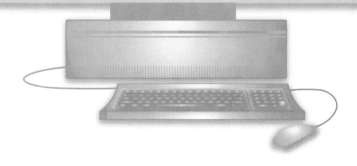

A postoperative client asks the nurse for pain medication. The nurse would take which action first?

1. Ask the client how long it has been since the last dose of pain medication was administered.
2. Gather data from the client about the pain.
3. Prepare the prescribed dose of pain medication.
4. Ask the client if the last dose of the medication was effective.

Answer: 2

Test-Taking Strategy:

Use the steps of the Nursing Process and remember that assessment is the first step. This will assist in eliminating option 3, because this option relates to implementing rather than assessing. From the remaining options, focus on the word "first." Option 1 can be eliminated because the nurse would not ask the client how long it has been since the last dose of pain medication; the nurse would check the client's medication record for these data. Although option 4 is an appropriate action, it does not focus on the issue of the question that the client asks for pain medication. Also, note the relationship between the issue and option 2.

Analysis

Analysis is the second step of the Nursing Process. In this step, the nurse focuses on the data gathered during the assessment process and identifies actual, risk for (potential), or wellness nursing diagnoses. Collaborative health care needs, problems, or both, requiring the interventions of more than one member of the health care team, may also be identified. During this process, the nurse summarizes and interprets the assessment data, organizes and validates the data, and determines the need for additional data. Client assessment data are compared with the normal expected findings and behaviors for the client's age, education, and cultural background. The nurse then draws conclusions regarding the client's unique needs, health care risks, and problems. Client health problems are categorized as actual problems requiring management or interventions, potential or at-risk problems requiring prevention, wellness indicating that the client is functioning effectively but desires a greater level of wellness, or collaborative requiring the assistance of other health care team members to resolve a problem. The nurse reports the results of analysis to appropriate members of the health care team and documents the client's unique health care problems, needs, or both.

Questions that address the process of analysis are the most difficult because they require an understanding of the principles of physiological responses and require interpreting the data on the basis of the assessment findings. Analysis questions may address formulating nursing diagnoses, critical thinking, and determining the rationale for therapeutic interventions related to the specific issue addressed in the question.

ANALYSIS

Analysis is the second step of the Nursing Process.

Analysis involves summarizing and interpreting the assessment data, organizing and validating the data, and determining the need for additional data.

During the process of analysis, the nurse draws conclusions regarding the client's unique needs, health care risks, and problems.

Integrated Process: Nursing Process/Analysis

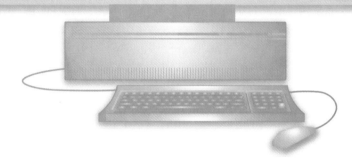

A nurse is caring for a client after a craniotomy (supratentorial surgery) involving the pituitary gland. Which finding indicates a complication of the surgical procedure and the need to notify the physician?
1. Periorbital edema
2. 30 mL fluid in the Jackson–Pratt drain
3. Urine specific gravity of 1.001
4. Client reports of mouth dryness

Answer: 3

Test-Taking Strategy:
To answer this question correctly, it is necessary to understand several concepts and know that after craniotomy the client is at risk for complications, one of which is diabetes insipidus. Recalling the expected and unexpected findings after craniotomy and the signs of diabetes insipidus will assist in answering the question. Options 1, 2, and 4 are expected findings after craniotomy. A urine specific gravity of 1.001 is low and may be an indication of diabetes insipidus.

Planning

Planning is the third step of the Nursing Process. This step involves the functions of setting priorities, determining goals and outcome criteria for goals of care, developing the plan of care, collaborating with other health care team members, and communicating the plan of care. Setting priorities assist the nurse in organizing and planning care that solves the most urgent problems. Priorities may change as the client's level of wellness changes. Both actual and risk for (potential) problems should be considered when establishing priorities.

> **PLANNING**
> Planning is the third step of the Nursing Process.
> Planning involves setting priorities, determining goals
> and outcome criteria for goals of care, developing the
> plan of care, collaborating with other health care
> team members, and communicating the plan of care.

Once priorities are established, the client and nurse mutually decide on the expected goals. The goals serve as a guide in the selection of nursing interventions and in determining the criteria for evaluation. Before implementing nursing actions, the nurse should establish mechanisms to determine goal achievement and the effectiveness of nursing interventions. Unless criteria have been predetermined, it is difficult to know whether the goal is achieved and the problem is resolved. It is important for the nurse to identify health or social resources available to the client and to collaborate with other health care team members when planning the delivery of care. The nurse needs to communicate the plan of care, review the plan of care with the client, and document the plan of care thoroughly and accurately.

When answering a test question, keep in mind that actual problems usually are more important than risk for (potential) problems. However, read the question carefully because, at times, risk for (potential) problems may take precedence over actual problems. Also, remember that the examination you will be taking is a nursing examination, not a medical examination. Therefore, the answer to the question most likely involves something that is included in the nursing care plan rather than the medical plan, unless the question specifically asks you what prescription (medical order) is anticipated. A sample question is provided on the following page.

Implementation

Implementation is the fourth step of the Nursing Process and includes initiating and completing nursing actions required to accomplish the defined goals. This step is the action phase that involves counseling, teaching, organizing, and managing client care; providing care to achieve established goals; supervising and coordinating the delivery of client care; and communicating and documenting the nursing interventions and client responses.

During implementation, the nurse uses intellectual skills, interpersonal skills, and technical skills. Intellectual skills involve critical thinking, problem solving, and making judgments. Interpersonal skills involve the ability to communicate, listen, and convey compassion. Technical skills relate to the performance of treatments and procedures and the use of necessary equipment when providing care to the client.

The nurse implements actions independently, including activities that do not require a physician's order. The nurse also implements actions collaboratively based on the physician's orders. Sound nursing judgment and working with other health

Integrated Process: Nursing Process/Planning

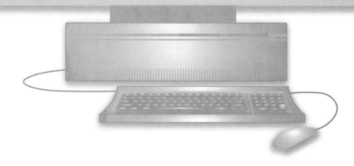

A nurse is reviewing the nursing diagnoses written in a nursing care plan for a client with chronic obstructive pulmonary disease. The nurse determines that which nursing diagnosis is the priority?

1. Altered role performance related to role loss
2. Altered thought processes related to sleep deprivation
3. Anxiety related to loss of control during dyspneic episodes
4. Imbalanced nutrition, less than body requirements, related to dyspnea and fatigue

Answer: 4

Test-Taking Strategy:

Note the keyword "priority". Maslow's Hierarchy of Needs theory can be used as a guide to answer this question. According to Maslow's theory, physiological needs are the priority. This will direct you to option 4. Options 1, 2, and 3 are psychosocial needs and are a lesser priority than physiological needs. Remember, physiological needs are the priority.

INTELLECTUAL SKILLS
   Critical thinking
   Problem solving
   Making judgments
INTERPERSONAL SKILLS
   Ability to communicate
   Ability to listen
   Ability to convey
      compassion
TECHNICAL SKILLS
   Performing treatments
      and procedures
   Using the necessary equipment when providing
      care to the client

care team members is incorporated in the process of implementation.

The implementation step concludes when the nurse's actions are completed and these actions, including their effects and the client's response, are communicated and documented.

The client presented in the test question is your only assigned client. When you are selecting an option, remember that you are caring for one and only one client, unless the question indicates that you are caring for multiple clients. For example, if a question asks for the best nursing action for a client who is anxious about surgery, which is scheduled later that day, do not be reluctant to select the option that addresses staying with the client until the time of surgery. Remember, this is your only assigned client, so implement what is best for the client!

You need to answer the question from a textbook, and ideal perspective rather than a reality perspective. Remember, always follow textbook guidelines and principles when carrying out procedures and performing interventions!

Answer the question remembering that you have all the time that you need and that the necessary resources and supplies are readily available at the client's bedside. For example, if a question addresses a client with cardiac disease who experiences chest pain, remember that you have all of the supplies needed for that client (such as oxygen, nitroglycerin, and an electrocardiogram machine) readily available and that you will not need to waste time obtaining these supplies from other hospital areas. A sample question is provided on the following page.

IMPLEMENTATION

Implementation is the fourth step of the Nursing Process.
The client in the test question is your only assigned client.
The client in the test question is the only client that requires your concern.
Answer the question from a textbook and ideal perspective rather than a reality perspective.
Answer the question remembering that you have all the time that you need and that the necessary resources and supplies are readily available at the client's bedside.

Evaluation

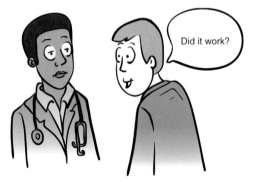

Did it work?

Evaluation is the fifth and final step of the Nursing Process. The process of evaluation identifies the degree to which the nursing diagnoses, plans for care, and interventions have been successful.

Although evaluation is the final step of the Nursing Process, it is an ongoing and integral component of each step. The process of data collection and assessment is reviewed to determine whether sufficient information was obtained, and if the information obtained was specific and appropriate. The nursing

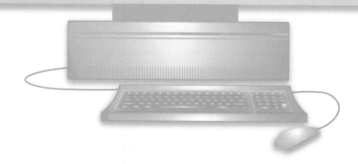

Integrated Process: Nursing Process/Implementation

A nurse is monitoring a client after a cardiac catheterization procedure. The client suddenly reports a feeling of wetness at the injection site. The nurse quickly assesses the site and discovers that the client is bleeding. The best initial nursing action is to:

1. Apply firm pressure to the site using a sterile gauze pad
2. Apply firm pressure to the site using a bath towel
3. Call the physician
4. Check the client's blood pressure

Answer: 1

Test-Taking Strategy:

Note the keywords "best initial nursing action." These words may indicate that more than one or all of the options are correct and that you need to prioritize the actions. Although options 3 and 4 are correct, they are not the initial actions. From the remaining options, select option 1 because using a sterile gauze pad to apply pressure is the best action to prevent an infection. Remember that all of your needed supplies are readily available at the client's bedside.

diagnoses are evaluated for accuracy and completeness on the basis of the specific needs of the client. The plan and expected outcomes are examined to determine whether they are realistic, achievable, measurable, and effective. Interventions are examined to determine their effectiveness in achieving the expected outcomes. Because evaluation is an ongoing process, it is vital to all steps of the Nursing Process. It is the continuous process of comparing actual outcomes with expected ones, and it provides the means for determining the need to modify the plan of care. Inherent in this step of the Nursing Process are the communication of evaluation findings and the process of documenting the client's response to treatment, care, and/or teaching.

> **EVALUATION**
>
> Evaluation is the fifth step of the Nursing Process.
>
> Evaluation is a continuous process of comparing actual outcomes with expected ones.
>
> Evaluation provides the means for determining the need to modify the plan of care.

Evaluation questions may be written to address the comparison of actual outcomes of care with the expected outcomes, to examine how the nurse should monitor or make a judgment concerning a client's response to therapy or to a nursing action, or to determine a client's understanding of the prescribed treatment measures. Evaluation questions frequently are written in a false response format. For example, the question may ask for a client statement that indicates inaccurate information related to the issue of the question.

Integrated Process: Nursing Process/Evaluation

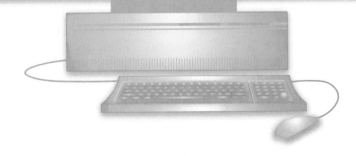

Ibuprofen (Motrin) has been prescribed for a client. On a follow-up physician's visit, the nurse determines that the medication is effective if the client states relief of:

1. Abdominal bloating
2. Constipation
3. Joint stiffness
4. Heartburn

Answer: 3

Test-Taking Strategy:

Medication questions can be difficult to answer correctly if you are unfamiliar with the medication. Knowing that ibuprofen is a non-steroidal anti-inflammatory medication used to treat osteoarthritis and rheumatoid arthritis will assist in answering this question. If you did not know this, use the process of elimination, noting that options 1, 2, and 4 are similar in that they all relate to the gastrointestinal system. Options that are similar are incorrect!

TEACHING/LEARNING

Client and family education is a primary professional nursing responsibility. However, remember that assessment of the client's readiness and the client's motivation to learn is the initial step in the teaching/learning process. Always use the principles related to teaching/learning theory to answer this type of question. Frequently, these types of questions ask what the nurse would teach the client or what observation by the nurse indicates that the client needs instruction.

Teaching/Learning Principles

There are many teaching/learning principles that nursing professionals should use including the following:

- The nurse needs to determine the client's readiness and motivation to learn as well as the client's learning needs.

> If a test question addresses client teaching, remember that client motivation and client readiness to learn is the FIRST priority.

- The nurse needs to assess the client's existing knowledge of the information to be presented and plan to teach by building on that existing knowledge.
- The nurse needs to understand that the client's ability to learn depends on his or her physical and cognitive abilities.
- The nurse needs to consider the client's health beliefs and how they will influence the client's willingness to learn.
- The nurse needs to consider the client's age, developmental level, and educational level, and design teaching strategies on the basis of these factors.
- The nurse needs to remember that learning objectives facilitate the teaching process and identify what the client is to be taught.
- The client should be an active participant in the teaching/learning process.
- The nurse should include the client's spouse, significant other, or another family member in the learning process, if appropriate.

- The nurse should use a combination of teaching methods (cognitive, affective, and psychomotor) and teaching tools to improve the client's attentiveness and involvement.

> **TEACHING TOOLS**
> Pamphlets, booklets, brochures
> Diagrams, graphs, charts, pictures
> Slides, audiotapes, videotapes, television
> Physical objects
> Programmed instruction
> Computer instruction

- The nurse should allow ample time for the client to understand the material being taught.

The nurse should evaluate a client's learning by observing the client's performance of the behavior.

Integrated Process: Teaching/Learning

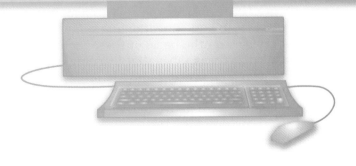

A nurse has taught a client's spouse how to change the client's colostomy bag. The nurse would best determine that the spouse understands the procedure by:

1. Asking the spouse if she has any questions about the procedure
2. Asking the spouse if she understands what items are needed to perform the procedure
3. Asking the spouse to perform the procedure and observe her performing it
4. Asking the spouse if she feels comfortable performing the procedure

Answer: 3

Test-Taking Strategy:
Note the keyword "best" in the stem of the question and focus on the issue: the spouse's ability to perform a procedure. The nurse would best evaluate learning by observing the performance of the behavior. Although options 1, 2, and 4 are questions that the nurse would ask, they do not evaluate the spouse's ability to perform the procedure. Remember, use teaching/learning principles when answering this question.

REFERENCES

Harkreader H, Hogan MA: *Fundamentals of nursing: caring and clinical judgment*, ed 2, Philadelphia, 2004, WB Saunders.

Hodgson B, Kizior R: *Saunders nursing drug handbook 2005*, Philadelphia, 2005, WB Saunders.

Ignatavicius D, Workman M: *Medical surgical nursing: critical thinking for collaborative care*, ed 4, Philadelphia, 2002, WB Saunders.

Lewis S, Heitkemper M, Dirksen S: *Medical-surgical nursing: assessment and management of clinical problems*, ed 6, St Louis, 2004, Mosby.

National Council of State Boards of Nursing: Test Plan for the National Council Licensure Examination for Registered Nurses (effective date: April 2004), Chicago, 2003, National Council of State Boards of Nursing.

National Council of State Boards of Nursing on line: Available at www.ncsbn.org

Phipps W, Monahan F, Sands J, et al: *Medical-surgical nursing: health and illness perspectives*, ed 7, St Louis, 2003, Mosby.

Potter P, Perry A: *Fundamentals of nursing*, ed 6 St Louis, 2005, Mosby.

Chapter 5

Types of Questions on the Examination

The types of questions that may be administered to you when you take this examination include multiple choice, fill in the blank, chart/exhibit, multiple response, prioritizing (ordered response), and questions that contain a figure or illustration.

> **TYPES OF QUESTIONS ON THE EXAMINATION**
> Multiple choice
> Fill in the blank
> Chart/Exhibit
> Multiple response
> Prioritizing (ordered response)
> Figure or illustration

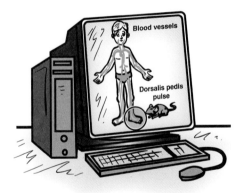

Some questions, such as those that present a figure or illustration, may require you to use the mouse component of the computer system. For example, you may be presented with a figure that displays the arterial vessels of an adult client. In this figure, you may be asked to "point and click" (using the mouse) on the area (represented by a circle and also known as the "hot spot") where the dorsalis pedis pulse could be felt.

The National Council of State Boards of Nursing provides specific directions for you to follow when answering these questions to guide you in your process of testing. Be sure to read these directions as they appear on the computer screen.

> Carefully follow the directions that appear with a question!

MULTIPLE CHOICE QUESTIONS

Most of the questions that you will be asked to answer will be in the multiple choice format. These questions will provide you with data about a particular client situation, together with four answers or options. You are probably very familiar with this type of question.

> Most questions will be in a multiple choice format!

Types of Questions: Multiple Choice

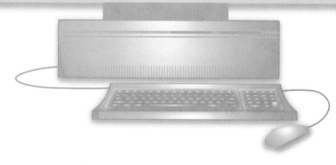

The nurse is preparing a client for a right thoracentesis and places the client in which position to perform this procedure?
1. Supine on the right side
2. Prone
3. Sitting on the side of the bed
4. Semi-Fowler's

Answer: 3

Test-Taking Strategy:

First, think about what this procedure entails. If you are not sure, use medical terminology skills recalling that *thora-* relates to the lung and *-centesis* relates to removal of fluid. Visualize this procedure and note that the client will have a right thoracentesis. Also, recall that gravity allows fluid to accumulate in the lower thoracic cavity. This will help you to eliminate options 1, 2, and 4.

FILL IN THE BLANK QUESTIONS

The fill in the blank questions will ask you to perform a medication calculation, calculate an intravenous flow rate, or calculate an intake or output record on a client. You will need to type in your answer. When answering these types of questions, three things are very important. First, follow the directions on the computer screen. In a medication calculation question, the directions may indicate to type in only the numeric component of the answer if the question requires a calculation. In other words, if the answer to a question is 2.5 mL, type only 2.5 if the directions indicate to do so. In an intravenous flow rate question, the directions may indicate to round the answer to the nearest whole number. For example, if the answer is 21.4 drops per minute, type the answer as 21. Second, use the on-screen calculator for your calculations; then use the erasable note board provided to you for testing to recalculate and verify your answer. Third, in a medication calculation question it is important to remember to place a zero before a decimal point in the answer and to avoid placing trailing zero(s) in the answer. For example, if the answer is two tenths, type in 0.2 NOT .2 and NOT 0.20 or .20.

FILL IN THE BLANK QUESTIONS

Follow directions!

Use the on-screen calculator and verify calculations!

Type in only the numeric component of the answer if directed to do so!

Round the answer to the nearest whole number if directed to do so!

Place a zero before a decimal point in the answer and avoid placing trailing zero(s) in the answer!

On the following pages are examples of fill in the blank questions.

Types of Questions: Fill in the Blank

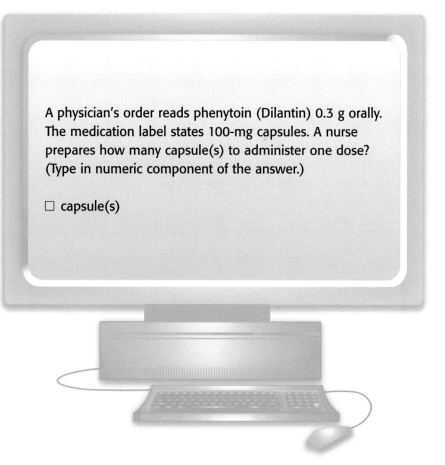

A physician's order reads phenytoin (Dilantin) 0.3 g orally. The medication label states 100-mg capsules. A nurse prepares how many capsule(s) to administer one dose? (Type in numeric component of the answer.)

☐ capsule(s)

Answer: 3

Test-Taking Strategy:

Read the information in the question and the directions and note that it is necessary to convert 0.3 g to milligrams. In the metric system, to convert grams (larger unit) to milligrams (smaller unit), multiply by 1000 or move the decimal three places to the right. Therefore, 0.3 g = 300 mg. The nurse would prepare three capsules. Remember to use the on-screen calculator and verify your answer. As directed, type in only the numeric component of the answer.

Types of Questions: Fill in the Blank

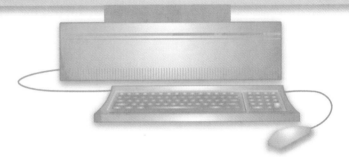

A physician orders 1000 mL of one-half normal saline to infuse over 8 hours. The drop factor is 15 drops per 1 mL. The nurse sets the flow rate at how many drops per minute? (Round answer to the nearest whole number and type in numeric component of the answer.)

☐ drops

Answer: 31

Test-Taking Strategy:

Read the information in the question and the directions. Using the IV flow rate formula yields a result of 31.2 drops per minute. Rounding to the nearest whole number yields 31. Remember to use the on-screen calculator and verify your answer. As directed, type in only the numeric component of the answer.

Types of Questions: Fill in the Blank

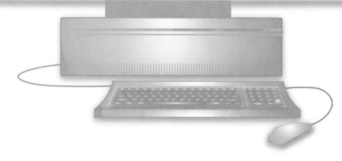

A nurse notes that the client consumed 4 oz orange juice, 6 oz water, and 8 oz tea with breakfast. The client also consumed 6 oz diet soda and 8 oz coffee at lunchtime and drank 4 oz water at 10:00 AM and at 2:00 PM with his medications. The nurse documents that the client consumed how many milliliters of fluid? (Type in numeric component of the answer.)

☐ mL

Answer: 1200

Test-Taking Strategy:

Focus on the information in the question and note that the client consumed a total of 40 oz. Next, note that the question requires determining the amount of milliliters consumed. Recall that 1 oz equals 30 mL and multiply 40 oz by 30 mL to yield 1200 mL. Remember to use the on-screen calculator and verify your answer. As directed, type in only the numeric component of the answer.

▲ CHART/EXHIBIT

In this type of question, you will be presented with a question and a chart/exhibit. you will need to refer to the information in the chart/exhibit in order to answer the question. A sample question is presented below.

Types of Questions: Chart/Exhibit

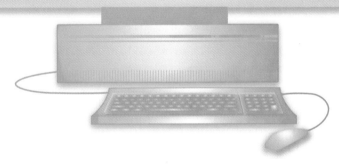

The nurse reviews the client's laboratory results for electrolyte levels. the nurse reports which abnormal results?

1. Sodium
2. Potassium
3. Chloride
4. Bicarbonate

CLIENT'S CHART

LABS	MEDS	NOTES
Sodium 150 mEq/L		
Potassium 4 mE/L		
Chloride 102 mEq/L		
Bicarbonate 26 mEq/L		

Answer: 1

Test-Taking Strategy:

In this question you are provided with the client's chart and laboratory results. you need to refer to the laboratory results in order to answer the question. On the NCLEX-PN examination, you will need to use the computer mouse and click on the appropriate tab noted on the client's chart. in this question you would click on the Laboratory tab. The normal sodium level is 135 to 145 mEq/L; normal potassium is 3.5 to 5.1 mEq/L; chloride 98 to 107 mEq/L; and bicarbonate 22 to 29 mEq/L.

MULTIPLE RESPONSE QUESTIONS

In multiple response questions, you must select or check all of the options, such as nursing interventions, that relate to the information in the question. There is no partial credit given for correct selections. You must select ALL that apply.

MULTIPLE RESPONSE QUESTIONS

All correct options ONLY must be selected for the answer to be correct!

If not all of the correct options are selected, the answer is incorrect!

If any incorrect options are selected, the answer is incorrect!

Types of Questions: Multiple Response

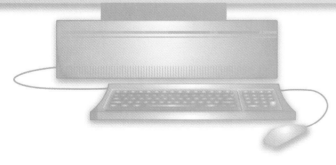

The nurse is performing an assessment on a client with a diagnosis of hypothyroidism. The nurse expects to note which of the following when obtaining subjective and objective data?

____ Client complaints of fatigue
____ Slurred speech
____ Client complaints of heat intolerance
____ Family member statements that the client has experienced personality and mental status changes
____ Client reports of increased appetite and weight loss
____ Presence of exophthalmos

Answer:

  X   Client complaints of fatigue
  X   Slurred speech
 ____ Client complaints of heat intolerance
  X   Family member statements that the client has experienced personality and mental status changes
 ____ Client reports of increased appetite and weight loss
 ____ Presence of exophthalmos

Test-Taking Strategy:

Focus on the issue: assessment findings in a client with a diagnosis of hypothyroidism (insufficient circulating thyroid hormone). Recalling the action of thyroid hormone and that hypothyroidism has systemic effects that slow bodily processes will assist in selecting the correct options.

PRIORITIZING (ORDERED RESPONSE) QUESTIONS

Prioritizing (ordered response) questions may ask you to number or use the computer mouse to drag and drop your nursing actions in order of priority. Information will be presented in a question, and based on the data, you need to determine what you would do first, second, third, and so forth.

Types of Questions: Prioritizing

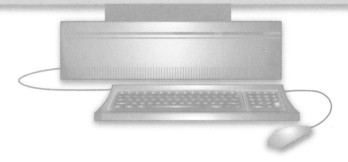

List in order of priority the steps that the nurse would take to perform adult one-rescuer cardiopulmonary resuscitation (CPR) on a hospitalized client. (Number 1 is the first priority and 5 is the last priority.)

____ Assess for signs of circulation
____ Determine unresponsiveness
____ Open the airway
____ Assess for cessation of breathing
____ Provide rescue breathing if necessary

Answer: 5, 1, 2, 3, 4

Test-Taking Strategy:

First, remember that determining unresponsiveness is a component of assessment and is the first step. From this point, use the ABCs—airway, breathing, and circulation—to determine the order of the remaining options.

FIGURE OR ILLUSTRATION

A figure or illustration question will ask you to answer the question based on the accompanying figure or illustration. The question could contain a chart, table, or a figure or illustration. In this type of question, you may also be asked to use the computer mouse and "point and click" on a specific area (circle or "hot spot") in the visual. Remember, a figure or illustration may appear in any type of question, including a multiple choice question.

Types of Questions: Figure or Illustration

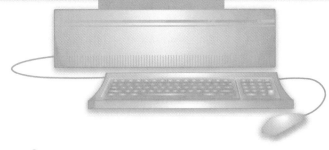

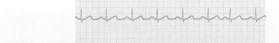

A nurse employed in a cardiac telemetry unit notes this rhythm displayed on a client's cardiac monitor. The nurse takes which appropriate action?

1. Asks the client to perform a Valsalva maneuver
2. Documents the rhythm in the client's medical record
3. Contacts the physician
4. Prepares to administer atropine sulfate

(Illustration from Phipps W, Monahan F, Sands J et al: *Medical-surgical nursing: health and illness perspectives*, ed 7, St Louis, 2003, Mosby, p 676.)

Answer: 2

Test-Taking Strategy:

Focus on the rhythm identified in the question. Noting that the rhythm identifies normal sinus rhythm will direct you to the correct option. Also, note that all of the incorrect options identify nursing actions that indicate that the rhythm is an abnormal one.

REFERENCES

Ignatavicius D, Workman M: *Medical surgical nursing: critical thinking for collaborative care*, ed 4, Philadelphia, 2002, WB Saunders.

Lewis S, Heitkemper M, Dirksen S: *Medical-surgical nursing: assessment and management of clinical problems*, ed 6, St Louis, 2004, Mosby.

National Council of State Boards of Nursing: Test Plan for the National Council Licensure Examination for Registered Nurses (effective date: April 2004), Chicago, 2003, National Council of State Boards of Nursing.

National Council of State Boards of Nursing online: Available at www.ncsbn.org

Phipps W, Monahan F, Sands J et al: *Medical-surgical nursing: health and illness perspectives*, ed 7, St Louis, 2003, Mosby.

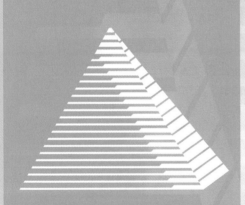

"A lot of my classmates thought I was crazy to start at the end of the first year, but I found using NCLEX CD-ROM disks to be the most helpful. The more time I spent getting comfortable with the question format and learning how to "break it down," the higher my scores became. Finally, because I had spent time using those disks, when I sat down in front of that computer to actually take those boards, I felt comfortable and secure, not afraid like a lot of my other classmates reported feeling. I passed the boards with 80 questions, but more importantly, I left the testing site confident"
—Trish, Hopkinsville Community College, Hopkinsville, Kentucky

"My first tip would be to do as many NCLEX review questions as possible. I did thousands and found that as I reviewed the material, not only did I become familiar with the content that was not covered in school, I began to see patterns in the material. I also suggest a comprehensive review book to prepare for tests while in school. I purchased Saunders Comprehensive Review for the NCLEX-RN Examination by Linda Silvestri early in my program, and I used it until I took the NCLEX exam. The content is also very well organized and I found it very comparable to the nursing textbooks from which we were studying—but easier to understand."
—Lori, Valencia Community College, Orlando, Florida

Part II

Strategies for Success

Chapter 6

Nonacademic Preparation: Your Path to Success

The National Council Licensure Examination for Registered Nurses (NCLEX-RN) examination is an important examination because receiving your nursing license means that you can begin your career as a registered nurse.

A positive attitude, a structured study plan for preparation, and control over test anxiety will ensure achievement in reaching the peak of the Pyramid to Success.

> **REACHING THE PEAK OF THE PYRAMID**
> A positive attitude
> A structured study plan for preparation
> Control over test anxiety

HOW CAN YOU MAINTAIN A POSITIVE ATTITUDE?

The first step in maintaining a positive attitude is to think about the accomplishments that you have achieved. You have been successful in your nursing program, and you have become a graduate nurse. It is also important to avoid any negative thoughts about yourself and your ability to pass the NCLEX-RN examination. Confidence in yourself and your ability is critical. So keep thinking about accomplishments.

Whenever you begin to doubt yourself and your ability to pass the NCLEX-RN examination, change those negative feelings into positive ones. You may be asking yourself, "How can I do this?" Always remember that you can accomplish anything if you believe in yourself. Whenever you feel doubt about your abilities, stop whatever you are doing, stand up, brush yourself off with your hands, and repeat to yourself, "I am getting rid of these negative feelings! I am confident in myself and, YES, I can do this!"

Another way to maintain a positive attitude is with the use of visuals. Draw a picture of yourself and below the picture write your name and the letters R.N. after it. Make several copies of the picture and post them in several places that you frequent, such as on your mirror, on your refrigerator, in your car, and in your other special places. Remember to place a copy in front of you when you study for this examination. Smile whenever you look at your picture, because smiling will keep you happy and help to make you feel good about yourself.

Remember, you can accomplish anything if you have confidence and believe in yourself!

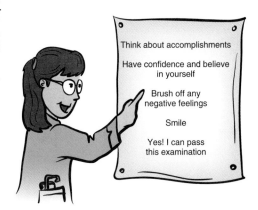

Think about accomplishments

Have confidence and believe in yourself

Brush off any negative feelings

Smile

Yes! I can pass this examination

HOW DO YOU DEVELOP A STRUCTURED STUDY PLAN FOR PREPARATION?
When Should You Schedule a Date for the Examination?

An important decision to make is when to take the NCLEX-RN examination. Once you have a date in mind or planned, you can develop your structured study plan. You may be asking yourself, "When should I schedule my date? How do I know when I will be ready?" Readiness to take this examination is highly individual. Your readiness may be very different from someone else's readiness. What you need to remember is that your nursing education has focused on preparing you for this examination. Now what you need to do is to review nursing content in a structured and focused way in preparation for this examination. There are two things to keep in mind as you are trying to decide on a date for taking the NCLEX-RN examination. First, remember that review and preparation are necessary. Second, you want to take the examination soon after graduation while all of the nursing knowledge is still fresh in your mind. Focus on your needs and your strengths and weaknesses, and plan to take this examination within 1 and no later than 2 months after graduation.

SCHEDULING A DATE FOR THE EXAM

SCHEDULING A DATE FOR THE EXAMINATION
Review and prepare.
Focus on your strengths and weaknesses.
Schedule an examination date within 1 to 2 months
    of graduation.

How Do You Start to Develop a Study Plan?

The first task in developing a study plan is to decide what study patterns worked best for you in the past, and then remain with these patterns. In other words, if you have always studied alone and this has always been successful, continue with this pattern and avoid joining a study group. If you have been most successful with studying in a group, then plan to prepare for this examination with the study partners you have always prepared with previously. Remember, it is best not to plan study sessions that are different from what has brought you success in the past.

The next step is to get yourself a calendar and name it, for example, "My Special NCLEX Calendar." On the calendar, mark your long-term goal, which should be the date of your examination. On all of the days preceding the date of your examination, mark your short-term goals, which will be your daily study times. Now, there may be days that you will not be able to devote to study time because of personal and other commitments. On these days, place an *X*. On all of the remaining days, write in your study times and plan to schedule at least five study days each week. Remember, you need some days for rest, relaxation, and fun!

How Long and When Should You Schedule Each Study Session?

The length of the study session will depend on you and your ability to focus and concentrate. What you need to think about is quality rather than quantity when you are deciding on a realistic amount of time for each session. Plan to schedule, at the very least, 2 hours of quality study time daily. If you can spend more than 2 hours, then by all means do so.

You may be asking yourself, "What do you mean by quality time?" Quality time means spending uninterrupted quiet time at your study session. This may mean that you will have to isolate yourself for these study sessions. Think about what has worked for you during nursing school when you studied for examinations, and again select a study place that has also worked for you in the past. If you have a special study room at home that you have always used, then plan your study sessions in that special room. If you have always studied at a library, then plan your study sessions at the library. If you plan to study at home, make the time spent studying an uninterrupted and quiet time. Sometimes it is difficult to balance your study time with your family obligations and possibly a work schedule, but if possible, plan your study time for when you know that you will be at home alone. Try to eliminate anything that may be distracting during your study time. For example, unplug your telephone so that you will not be disturbed. If you have small children, plan your study time during their nap time or during their school hours.

Another consideration in planning your study session is the time of the session. Some individuals find that they are more alert and will retain more if they study in the morning, whereas others may find that afternoon or evening hours are best for retaining information. So plan your sessions according to your individual needs. Remember, this examination is all about YOU, so plan to meet YOUR needs and stick to YOUR plan!

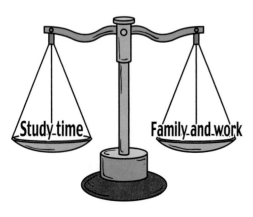

What Do You Use to Study?

Remember that this examination consists entirely of questions that you need to answer. Therefore, the best way to prepare for this examination is to study from a question and answer perspective. Also, remember that this examination is administered on a computer, therefore use of a computer to study is extremely beneficial. Obtain a notebook, name it, for example, "My Special NCLEX Notes," and keep it next to your computer when you are studying. As you are studying, write down the specific topics with which you may have difficulty. These are the areas that you may need to review further. There are several resources available to you depending on your needs. The *Saunders Comprehensive Review for the NCLEX-RN Examination* is one valuable tool that contains both content and practice questions. Its accompanying CD-ROM contains 4000 practice questions, and therefore provides you with questions on a computer. The questions are presented in multiple choice format and also in the alternate test questions format that is used in the NCLEX-RN examination. When using this CD-ROM, it is best to access the Study Mode because it provides important information immediately after answering the question. This information includes the correct answer, rationale for the correct and incorrect options, the test-taking strategy for answering the question, content area to review if you answered the question incorrectly, and the reference source. As you are studying, if you have difficulty with a specific topic, write it in your "Special NCLEX Notes" and be sure to review the topic. Do not attempt to prepare for this examination by studying all of the class notes that you have from nursing school, because they are much too detailed and you will become overwhelmed. Also, do not prepare for this examination by planning to read all of your nursing textbooks. You have already read them, and you need to use them together with your review book as a resource if necessary for difficult information.

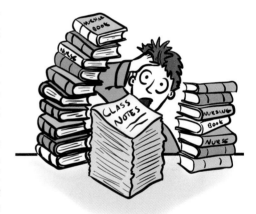

Additional resources to use for studying include the *Saunders Q & A Review for the NCLEX-RN Examination*, which provides you with more than 3500 practice questions on its CD-ROM that are different from those in the *Saunders Comprehensive Review for the NCLEX-RN Examination*, and the *Saunders Computerized Review for NCLEX-RN*, a computer disk program that contains more than 2000 NCLEX-RN–style questions to help you determine your readiness for the NCLEX-RN. Also available are online specialty tests titled Adult Health, Mental Health, Maternal-Newborn, Pediatrics, and Pharmacology and the on-line NCLEX-RN review course.

The Saunders Online Review Course for the NCLEX-RN contains a pretest that provides feedback regarding your strengths and weaknesses and generates an individualized study schedule in a calendar format. Therefore, if you need assistance with developing a study schedule, this program will do it for you. Content review with practice questions and case studies, figures and illustrations, a glossary, and animations and videos are included in this resource, together with a cumulative examination and a computerized adaptive exam. These additional resources, including the online specialty tests and the online review course, can be obtained online at the Elsevier Health Web site (www.elsevierhealth.com).

Review books and online resources can be obtained at the Elsevier Health Web site in the Nursing Review and Testing Section: www.elsevierhealth.com

HOW CAN YOU CONTROL TEST ANXIETY?

How Will Anxiety Affect You?

Preparing to take the NCLEX-RN examination can produce a great deal of anxiety. You may be thinking that the NCLEX-RN is the most important examination you will ever have to take, and that it reflects the culmination of everything you have worked so hard to achieve. NCLEX-RN is an important examination because receiving your nursing license means that you can begin your career as a registered nurse. Some anxiety about the examination can be helpful because it keeps your senses and thinking processes alert and sharp. However, a great deal of anxiety can be detrimental because it can block your thinking processes.

What Will Eliminate Some of the Anxiety?

An important component to eliminate some of the anxiety is to be as prepared as possible for this examination. Maintaining a positive attitude and discipline, together with following your structured study plan, will certainly help.

Another way to eliminate some anxiety is to be comfortable with where the testing center is located. A test drive to the testing center a few days before the examination is beneficial. Note the time of your examination and drive to the testing center as if you were planning to take the examination. Time the drive and note the amount of traffic, road construction, parking facilities, or whatever else that may delay you. You will most likely have some anxiety on the day of your examination, and the last thing that you need is traffic delays or other situations that may delay you and increase your anxiety. On the test drive, when you arrive at the test facility, you may want to walk into the center and become familiar with the lobby and the surroundings. This may help to alleviate some of the peripheral nervousness associated with entering an unknown building. Remember, do whatever it takes to keep your anxiety under control.

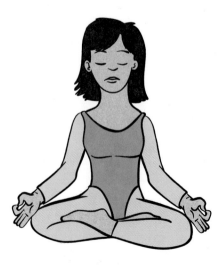

What Can You Do to Relax When You Become Anxious?

Breathing exercises are extremely helpful in alleviating anxiety and can be used at any time, including during your testing. These exercises will not only help to relax you, but will also help to oxygenate your body. During your clinical experience as a nursing student, you most likely cared for a client whose oxygenation level was being monitored by pulse oximetry. If the client's pulse oximetry was low, and you instructed the client to take slow, deep breaths, you would note that the oxygenation level increased. This same effect will occur if you take slow, deep breaths. Also, you want to decrease the anxiety, relax, and have your body and brain as oxygenated as possible on the day of the examination.

During the time before the examination, if you become anxious or are having difficulty sleeping at nighttime, sit or lie in a comfortable position, close your eyes, relax, inhale deeply, hold your breath to a count of four, exhale slowly, and, again, relax. Repeat this breathing exercise several times until you begin to feel relaxed and free from anxiety. During the examination, if you find that you are becoming anxious and/or distracted and are having difficulty focusing, sit back, close your eyes, and perform your breathing exercises to help relax and get the oxygen moving through your body. Remember, you want oxygen in your brain on the day of the examination!

What Is Positive Pampering and Why Is It Important?

Positive pampering means that you will take care of yourself from a holistic perspective. It will help to maintain an academic and nonacademic balance as you prepare for this examination, and it also will help to alleviate some anxiety. You need to care for yourself by including physical activity, a balanced diet, and fun and relaxation in your preparation plan.

POSITIVE PAMPERING
Physical activity
Balanced diet
Fun
Relaxation

Just as you have developed a schedule for study, you need a schedule that includes some fun and a form of physical activity. It is your choice, but some suggestions are aerobics, running, weight lifting, bowling, a movie, a massage, going to the beach, or whatever makes you feel good about yourself. Time spent away from the hard study schedule and devoted to some form of fun and physical exercise pays its rewards 100-fold. You will feel more energetic with a schedule that includes these activities.

Establish healthy eating habits if you have not already done so. Eat lighter and well-balanced meals and eat more frequently. Include complex carbohydrates in your diet for energy. Avoid caffeine, because it will make you jittery and anxious, and avoid eating fatty foods, because they will slow you down and make you feel sleepy.

Remember, pamper yourself to maintain balance!

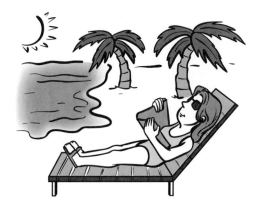

What Should You Do on the Day before the Examination?

On the day before the examination you may become anxious and immediately think, "I am not ready!" Stop whatever you are doing and reflect on all that you have accomplished. Smile, brush those negative feelings off of you, do your breathing exercises, and look at all of the pictures of yourself with your name and the letters R.N. after it.

Your goal on the day of the examination is to maintain your positive attitude and control any anxiety that you may experience. You need to rest your body and your mind. Remember that the mind is like a muscle: If it is overworked, it has no strength or stamina. Therefore, on the day before the examination, put your review books back in the bookshelf and spend the day doing activities that you enjoy and that you find relaxing. Positive pampering is important on the day before the examination, and you need to treat yourself to what you enjoy the most. At bedtime do the breathing exercises and listen to soothing music to help you relax and fall asleep and remember that you have prepared yourself well for the challenge of tomorrow.

What Should You Do on the Day of the Examination?

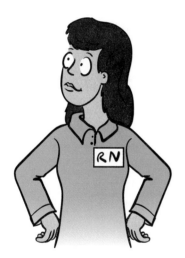

On the day of the examination, think positive! When you wake up and get out of bed, say, "Yes!" Brush any negative feelings off of you and look at your picture with your name and R.N. after it. Remember that you are absolutely ready to succeed, and that all you have accomplished is about to propel you to the professional level of registered nurse. Allow yourself plenty of time, eat a healthy breakfast, and groom yourself for success. Remain confident and believe in yourself that you are ready to meet the challenges of the day and overcome any obstacle that may face you. Remember that soon, today will be history, and in the very near future you will receive the envelope on which your name with the words "Registered Nurse" after it will be written.

> **ON THE DAY OF THE EXAMINATION**
> Think positive.
> Groom yourself for success.
> Maintain confidence and belief in yourself.
> Meet the challenges of the day.
> Become a Registered Nurse.
> YES!

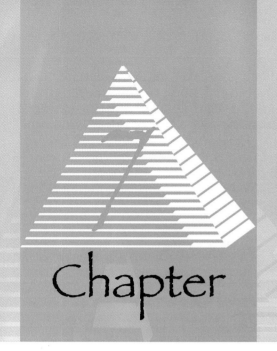

How to Avoid "Reading into the Question"

Chapter

One of the pitfalls that can cause a problem when trying to answer a question correctly is "reading into the question." What this means is that you are considering issues beyond the information presented in the question. There are some strategies that you can use to prevent this from happening when answering a question. Some of these include identifying the parts of a question, reading carefully and looking for keywords or key phrases, identifying the issue of the question and what the question is asking, using the process of elimination, and avoiding the "What If?" syndrome.

> Identify the parts of a question.
> Read carefully.
> Look for keywords or key phrases.
> Identify the issue.
> Use the process of elimination.
> Avoid asking yourself "What if?"

▲ PARTS OF A QUESTION
What Are the Parts of a Question?

With the exception of fill in the blank questions and the prioritizing (ordered response) questions, the question will contain a case situation, a question stem, and the options. Fill in the blank questions will contain a case situation and a question stem but will not contain options. Remember, fill in the blank questions will require you to perform a medication calculation, calculate an intravenous (IV) flow rate, or calculate an intake and output. Because you need to type in the answer for these type of questions, it makes sense that options will not be provided.

In a prioritizing (ordered response) question, several items will be presented, such as nursing interventions. In this type of question, you will not need to select options; rather, you will be required to list the items presented, such as nursing interventions, in order of priority. Remember, in a prioritizing (ordered response) question, all of the items listed will be correct.

It is important for you to identify the parts of a question as you read it because this will help you sort out the facts and determine what the question is asking.

QUESTION PARTS
Case situation
Question stem
Options

What Is the Case Situation?

The case situation is the "heart" of the question. It provides you with the information that you need to think about to answer the question.

What Is a Question Stem?

The question stem is a statement that generally follows the case situation and asks you something very specific about the information in the case situation.

What Are the Options?

The options are all of the answers presented with the question. In a multiple choice question, there will be four options, and you must select one. In a multiple response question, there will be several options, and you must select all options that apply to the case situation and the question stem.

A figure or illustration question may be presented in a multiple choice format. For example, you may be given a question with a figure of a rhythm strip, a case situation and question stem related to the rhythm strip, and four options of which only one will be correct. Or you may be given a question with a figure or illustration, and you will be asked to use the computer mouse to click on the correct option. For example, the question may contain a figure of the human body, a case situation, and a question stem. On the figure you may note small circles, sometimes called "hot spots," and will be asked to click on the circle that indicates the correct answer to the question.

Examples of the various types of questions that may appear in the examination and the specific parts of the questions are provided below. The answers to these example questions and the test-taking strategy also are provided.

Parts of a Question: Multiple Choice

Case Situation:
The nurse is reviewing the laboratory results of a client who is receiving magnesium sulfate by IV infusion and notes that the magnesium level is 7 mEq/L. **Question Stem:** Based on this laboratory result, the nurse would most likely expect to note which of the following in the client?

Options:
1. No specific signs or symptoms because this value is a normal level
2. Tremors
3. Respiratory depression
4. Hyperactive reflexes

Answer: 3

Test-Taking Strategy:
Read each option carefully. Use the process of elimination and note the keywords *most likely*. Knowing that the level identified in the question is elevated will assist in eliminating option 1. Next, eliminate options 2 and 4 because they are similar. Remember, use nursing knowledge, focus on the information in the case situation, identify what the question is asking (the issue), note the keywords, read carefully, and use the process of elimination.

Parts of a Question: Fill in the Blank

Case Situation:
The physician prescribes an IV antibiotic to be administered in 50 mL 0.9% normal saline and to infuse in 30 minutes. The drop factor for the IV tubing is 15 drops/mL. **Question Stem:** The nurse sets the flow rate of the infusion at how many drops per minute?

Answer: 25

Test-Taking Strategy:
Note the keywords *sets the flow rate*. Focus on the information in the question and that 50 mL fluid is to infuse in 30 minutes and the drop factor is 15. Use the computer on-screen calculator and the formula for calculating an IV infusion to answer the question. Verify your answer. Remember, use nursing knowledge, focus on the information in the case situation, identify what the question is asking (the issue), and note the keywords.

Parts of a Question: Multiple Response

Case Situation:
The nurse enters a hospitalized client's room and discovers that the client is having a tonic-clonic seizure. **Question Stem:** Select all actions that the nurse should implement?

Options:
____   Check airway patency.
____   Restrain the client's extremities loosely.
____   Call a code.

_____ Protect the client from injury.
_____ Establish an IV access.

Answer:
  X   Check airway patency.
_____ Restrain the client's extremities loosely.
_____ Call a code.
  X   Protect the client from injury.
  X   Establish an IV access.

Test-Taking Strategy:

Read each option carefully. Use the process of elimination and note the keywords *all actions*. In this type of question, it is helpful to visualize the situation to assist in determining the nurse's actions. Remember, use nursing knowledge, focus on the information in the case situation, identify what the question is asking (the issue), note the keywords, read carefully, and use the process of elimination.

Parts of a Question: Prioritizing (Ordered Response)

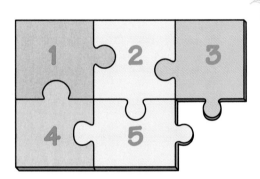

Case Situation:

A nurse is preparing to change an abdominal dressing using sterile technique. **Question Stem:** List in order of priority the actions that the nurse would take to perform this procedure. (Number 1 indicates the first action and 5 indicates the last action.)

  Options:
_____ Don clean gloves and remove the old dressing.
_____ Set up a sterile field.
_____ Explain the procedure to the client.
_____ Don sterile gloves.
_____ Wash hands.

Answer: 4, 3, 1, 5, 2

Test-Taking Strategy:

Read each option carefully and note the keywords *order of priority*. In this type of question, it is helpful to visualize the situation to assist in determining the nurse's order of actions. Remember, use nursing knowledge, read carefully, focus on the information in the case situation, identify what the question is asking (the issue), and note the keywords.

Parts of a Question: Figure or Illustration

Case Situation:

The nurse is checking the arterial pulses on an adult client. **Question Stem:** Using the computer mouse, click on the area where the nurse would palpate the carotid pulse (See Fig. 7-1 on page 67).

Answer: Answer is indicated by the circle containing the X

Test-Taking Strategy:

Note the keywords *carotid pulse*. In this type of question, it is helpful to visualize the pulse points for assessment of arterial

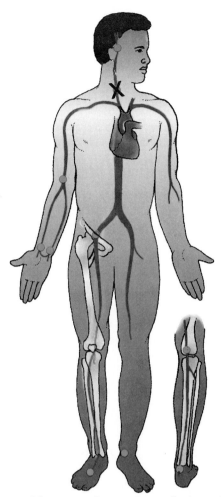

Fig. 7-1   From Ignatavicius D, Workman M: *Medical-surgical nursing: critical thinking for collaborative care,* ed 4, Philadelphia, 2002, WB Saunders, p 637, with permission.

pulses to identify the correct answer. Remember, use nursing knowledge, read carefully, focus on the information in the case situation, identify what the question is asking (the issue), and note the keywords.

KEYWORDS OR KEY PHRASES

Always read every word in the question carefully. As you read, look for keywords or key phrases in the case situation and stem of the question. Keywords or key phrases will focus your attention on specific or critical points that you need to consider when answering the question.

Some keywords or key phrases may indicate that all of the options are correct and that it will be necessary to prioritize to select the correct option. Remember, as you read the question, look for the keywords or key phrases; they will make a difference with regard to how you will answer the question.

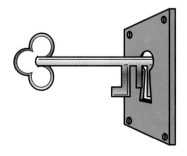

> **KEYWORDS OR KEY PHRASES**
> Focus your attention on critical and specific points
> May indicate that there is only one option
> May indicate that you need to prioritize
> May indicate a true response question
> May indicate a false response question

What Are the Commonly Used Keywords or Key Phrases to Look for?

Common Keywords or Key Phrases That Indicate There Is Only One Correct Option

Some of the keywords or key phrases used in a question will indicate that there is only one correct option. Some of these words and phrases include the following:

Early sign
Late sign
Understands
Goal has been achieved
Adequately tolerating
Avoid
Needs reinforcement of the instructions
Lack of understanding
Goals have not yet been fully met
Has not met the outcome criteria
Ineffective
Inadequate
Unable to tolerate

Common Keywords or Key Phrases That Indicate the Need to Prioritize

There are also keywords or key phrases that may indicate that all of the options are correct, and that it will be necessary to prioritize to select the correct option. Some of these words and phrases include the following:

Best
First
Initial
Immediately
Most likely or least likely
Most appropriate or least appropriate
Highest or lowest priority
Order of priority
At highest risk
At lowest risk
Best understanding

Common Keywords or Key Phrases That Indicate a True or False Response Question

Finally, there are keywords or key phrases that indicate that the question is a true response or a false response question. Keywords or key phrases used in these types of questions may indicate that there is only one correct option or may indicate the need to prioritize to select the correct option. (Additional information about true and false response questions can be found in Chapter 8.)

Common words or phrases that indicate a true response question include the following:

Early sign
Late sign
Best
First
Initial
Immediately
Most likely
Most appropriate
Highest priority
Order of priority
All nursing interventions that apply
Goal has been achieved
Adequately tolerating

Common words or phrases that indicate a false response question include the following:

Least likely
Least appropriate
Least priority
Least helpful
At lowest risk
Avoid
Needs reinforcement of the instructions
Needs additional teaching
Lack of understanding
Goals have not yet been fully met
Has not met the outcome criteria
Ineffective
Inadequate
Unable to tolerate

Use of Keywords or Key Phrases in a Question

You may be asking yourself: How are these keywords or key phrases used in a question? Following are some examples of question stems that contain keywords:

Select all nursing interventions that apply in the care of the client.
Which statement by a client indicates an understanding of the instructions?
What is the initial nursing action?
Which of the following is an early sign of hypoxia?
List in order of priority the actions that the nurse would take.

Which of the following individuals is least likely to develop hypertension?

Which nursing diagnosis is of least priority?

The nurse would avoid which of the following actions?

The nurse determines that the client needs additional teaching if the client stated which of the following?

The nurse determines that the treatment is ineffective if which if the following is noted?

THE ISSUE OF THE QUESTION
What Is the Issue of the Question?

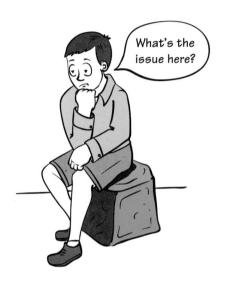

What's the issue here?

The issue of the question is the specific subject content that the question is asking about. It is important to read every word in the question. As you read and note the keywords or key phrases, determine what the question is asking. Identifying the issue of the question will assist in eliminating the incorrect options and direct you to selecting the correct option.

What Are Some Examples of Question Issues?

There are hundreds of issues that you could be asked about when you take this examination. This is understandable, especially when you think about all of the information that you needed to learn in nursing school. A test question may ask about any Client Needs area of the Test Plan for the National Council Licensure Examination for Registered Nurses (NCLEX-RN), any content area of nursing, or anything that has to do with the role and responsibilities of the nurse. Therefore, the list of issues that could be tested is never ending. It may be helpful to obtain a copy of the Test Plan for the NCLEX-RN, which is published by the National Council of State Boards of Nursing (NCSBN). This Test Plan identifies some of the content that will be tested in this examination and can be obtained at the NCSBN Web site (www.ncsbn.org).

Examples of issues that may be used in a test question are identified below. These examples are based on the Client Needs components of the Test Plan for the NCLEX-RN. (Refer to Chapter 3 for additional information about content in the Client Needs components of the Test Plan.)

> **"WILL IT EVER END?"**
> **Test Question Issues***
> **Physiological Integrity**
> *Basic Care and Comfort*
> Implementing alternative and complementary therapies
> Using canes, walkers, crutches, or other assistive devices
> Promoting and monitoring elimination patterns
> Addressing complications of immobility
> Promoting nutrition and therapeutic diets
>
> *(Continued)*

Using measures that promote comfort
Recognizing personal hygiene issues
Pharmacological and Parenteral Therapies
Action of a medication
Side effect of a medication
Toxic or adverse effect of a medication
Contraindications of a medication
Interactions associated with a medication
Client teaching related to a medication or other health
   care area
Administration of IV therapy
Insertion of an IV
Complications of an IV
Administration of blood
Complications of a blood transfusion
Complications of total parenteral nutrition
Care for a central venous access device
Reduction of Risk Potential
Preparation for a diagnostic test, treatment, or procedure
Complications of a diagnostic test, treatment, or procedure
Preprocedure and postprocedure care of a diagnostic
   test, treatment, or procedure
Care to the client requiring surgery
Procedures for taking vital signs
Recognition of alterations in the client
Analysis of laboratory results
Physiological Adaptation
Assessment of the client for a fluid or electrolyte imbalance
Interventions if a fluid and electrolyte imbalance exists
Interventions in the care of a client with an infectious
   disease
Response to a medical emergency
Care for the client receiving radiation therapy
Safe, Effective Care Environment
Management of Care
Acting as a client advocate
Knowing and understanding types of advance directives
Prioritizing nursing actions
Upholding client rights
Maintaining confidentiality
Adhering to components of informed consent
Understanding the components of case management
Collaborating and consulting with other members of
   the health care team
Accepting the roles of the nurse as leader and/or manager
Acting with regard to ethical practice and legal rights
   and responsibilities

(Continued)

Delegating, assignment-making, and providing
  continuity of care
Supervising care and teaching staff
Using resources appropriately
Participating in Performance Improvement
  (Quality Assurance) Programs
Safety and Infection Control
Measures to prevent accidents and injuries
Measures to prevent an error
Interventions if a disaster occurs
Familiarity with an Emergency Response Plan
Knowledge of implementation of a security plan
Handling of hazardous and infectious materials
Maintenance of a safe environment in the client's home
Medical and surgical asepsis techniques
Implementation of standard, transmission-based,
  and other precautions
Safe use of restraints and other safety devices
Safe use of medical equipment
Completion of incident and other reports

Health Promotion and Maintenance

Stages of growth and development
Expected body image changes that occur with the
  aging process
Measures to promote health and wellness and
  prevent disease
Physical assessment techniques
Health screening and health promotion programs
Immunization schedules
High-risk behaviors and lifestyle choices that require
  intervention
Promoting self-care measures
Teaching and learning principles
Human sexuality and the family
Antepartum, intrapartum, and postpartum care
Care to the newborn infant

Psychosocial Integrity

Communication techniques
Cultural, religious, and spiritual considerations of care
Client abuse and neglect and nursing responsibilities
Substance abuse and addictions
Coping mechanisms
Intervention in a crisis
Grief or loss and end-of-life issues
Stress management and support systems
Care to the client with a mental health disorder

Sample Question: The Issue of the Question

A client with metastatic cancer is receiving a continuous IV infusion of morphine sulfate to alleviate pain. The nurse monitors the client for which adverse or toxic effect of the medication?

Issue:

In this question, note that the client is receiving morphine sulfate and that the question asks about an adverse or toxic effect of the medication. Therefore, the issue of this question is an adverse or toxic effect of morphine sulfate.

1. Dizziness
2. Sedation
3. Skeletal muscle flaccidity
4. Nausea

Answer: 3

Test-Taking Strategy:

Read every word in the question and specifically determine what the question is asking. The question is asking about the adverse or toxic effect of morphine sulfate. Dizziness, sedation, and nausea are side effects of morphine sulfate that the client may experience, but they are not adverse or toxic effects. Remember, focus on the information in the question and what the question is asking!

USING NURSING KNOWLEDGE AND THE PROCESS OF ELIMINATION
Why Nursing Knowledge Is So Important

Nursing knowledge is needed to assist in answering test questions because the knowledge provides you with information that you need to process and think about critically to answer the question. If you can use your nursing knowledge to answer the question, then by all means do so!

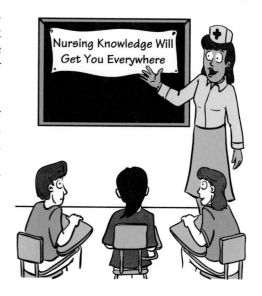

On the NCLEX-RN, do not be surprised if you are given questions that contain content with which you are totally unfamiliar or are only vaguely familiar. This happens to many individuals who take this examination. When you are given a question that contains unfamiliar content, read the question carefully and focus on the issue. Sometimes you do not even need to know much about the content to answer the question. In addition, with some of these unfamiliar questions, you may be able to use nursing knowledge from a different content area to answer the question. The important thing is not to become alarmed and anxious if you receive a question with unfamiliar content. Sit back, take a deep breath, read carefully, focus on the issue, and use nursing knowledge from a different content area to answer the question.

What Do You Mean by Using the Process of Elimination?

The process of elimination is a course of action that involves reading each option presented with a question and removing the options that are incorrect and do not address the issue of the question. Using the process of elimination is extremely important when you are reading the options to a question and trying to determine the correct answer. Do not just hastily select an option because it sounds good. Always read every option carefully before selecting an answer.

Some students will read a question, and before looking at the options they are able to determine a correct answer. This is a helpful strategy to use when answering a test question, because you are using nursing knowledge to assist in answering the question correctly. The problem with this strategy is that you may have an answer to the question in mind, but when you look at the options your answer is not there. This can be very frustrating and anxiety provoking. Let's look at the following example:

A client who has type 1 diabetes mellitus describes shakiness and hunger 2 hours after receiving a dose of regular insulin. The nurse determines that the client is having a hypoglycemic reaction and prepares to give the client which best item from the dietary kitchen to treat the reaction?

After you read this question, you will immediately think, "Orange juice! Yes, orange juice is the best item! I know the answer to this question." Then, you look at the options and find the following:

1. Milk
2. Diet soda
3. Sugar-free cookies
4. Sugar-free gelatin

Your answer, orange juice, is not there! So now what do you do? You need to use your nursing knowledge and think about what thought processes led you to identifying orange juice as the answer to the question. Remember that a food item that contains 10 to 15 g carbohydrate is used to treat a hypoglycemic reaction. Now, look at your options and use the process of elimination. In this question, you can eliminate options 2, 3, and 4 because these items do not contain carbohydrates.

What Do You Do if You Eliminate Two of the Options and Are Unsure of the Final Two?

As you use the process of elimination to rule out the incorrect options, it is likely that you will be able to easily eliminate two of the four options in a multiple choice question. Now what do you do with the last two options, and how do you proceed to select the correct one? Follow these helpful steps when you are trying to decide which of the last two options is correct.

1. Read the question again.
2. Identify the case situation from the stem of the question.
3. Look for the keywords or key phrases.
4. Identify the issue of the question.
5. Ask yourself, "What is the question asking?"

6. Read the options again.
7. Make your final choice by focusing on what the question is asking, using nursing knowledge, and implementing test-taking strategies.

What Is the "What If?" Syndrome?

The "What if?" syndrome occurs when you read a test question and, instead of simply focusing on the information in the question, you start asking yourself, "Well, what if?" You need to avoid asking yourself this question because this leads you right into the dreaded pitfall of "reading into the question." Read the question carefully, identify keywords or key phrases, and focus on the issue of the question. You may need to think critically to answer the question but stay on track! Asking yourself, "What if?" moves you off track with regard to what the question is asking. Let's look at two questions and then examine the ways to avoid reading into them.

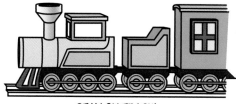

STAY ON TRACK!

Question Number 1

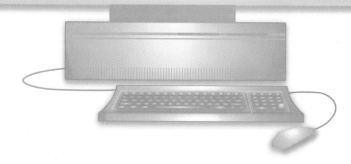

A nurse is changing the tapes on a tracheostomy tube. The client coughs and the tube is dislodged. The initial nursing action is to:

1. Cover the tracheostomy site with a sterile dressing to prevent infection.
2. Call the physician to reinsert the tube.
3. Grasp the retention sutures to spread the opening.
4. Call the respiratory therapy department to reinsert the tracheotomy.

Now you may immediately think, "The tube is dislodged and I need the physician!" Read the question carefully. Note the keyword *initial* and focus on the issue: the client's tube is dislodged. The question is asking you for a nursing action, so that is what you need to look for as you eliminate the incorrect options. Use nursing knowledge and test-taking strategies to assist in answering the question.

Answer: 3

Test-Taking Strategy:

Use the process of elimination and focus on the issue. Eliminate options 2 and 4 first because they are similar and will delay the immediate intervention needed. Eliminate option 1 because this action will block the airway. If the tube is accidentally dislodged, the initial nursing action is to grasp the retention sutures and spread the opening. In addition, use of the ABCs—airway, breathing, and circulation—will direct you to the correct option.

Question Number 2

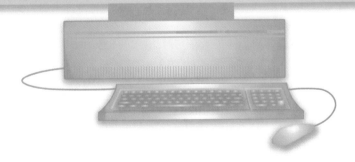

A nurse is caring for a hospitalized client with a diagnosis of congestive heart failure who suddenly reports shortness of breath and dyspnea. The nurse takes which immediate action?

1. Prepares to administer furosemide (Lasix)
2. Calls the physician
3. Administers oxygen to the client
4. Elevates the head of the client's bed

Now you may immediately think that the client has developed pulmonary edema, a complication of congestive heart failure, and needs a diuretic. Although pulmonary edema is a complication of congestive heart failure, there is no information in the question indicating the presence of pulmonary edema. The question simply states that the client suddenly reports shortness of breath and dyspnea. Read the question carefully. Note the keyword *immediate* and focus on the issue: the client's symptoms. The question is asking you for a nursing action, so that is what you need to look for as you eliminate the incorrect options. Use nursing knowledge and test-taking strategies to assist in answering the question.

Answer: 4

Test-Taking Strategy:
Use the process of elimination and focus on the information in the question and on the issue. Note the keyword *immediate*. Think about the client's symptoms and look for the immediate nursing action. Although the physician may need to be notified, this is not the immediate action. A physician's order is needed to administer oxygen. Furosemide is a diuretic and may or may not be prescribed for the client. Because there are no data in the question that indicate the presence of pulmonary edema, option 4 is correct.

REFERENCES

Hodgson B, Kizior R: *Saunders nursing drug handbook 2005,* Philadelphia, 2004, WB Saunders.

Lewis S, Heitkemper M, Dirksen S: *Medical-surgical nursing: assessment and management of clinical problems,* ed 6, St Louis, 2005, Mosby.

National Council of State Boards of Nursing: Test Plan for the National Council Licensure Examination for Registered Nurses (effective date: April 2004), Chicago, 2003, National Council of State Boards of Nursing.

True or False Response Questions

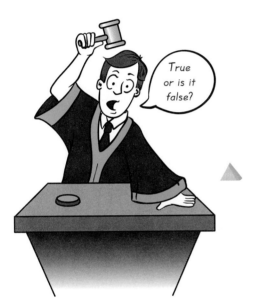

Chapter 8

True or is it false?

The questions presented on the National Council Licensure Examination for Registered Nurses (NCLEX-RN), including multiple choice, fill in the blank, multiple response, figure or illustration, and prioritizing (ordered responses) questions, will be written as either a true response or a false response question. The questions primarily will be written as a true response question; however, you need to be prepared for either type.

▲ TRUE RESPONSE QUESTIONS
What Is a True Response Question?

A true response question asks you to make a decision and select the option that is accurate or correct with regard to the data presented in the question. True response questions are primarily used on the NCLEX-RN. How will you know that the question is a true response one? Read the question carefully and focus on the stem of the question. The stem of the question will contain keywords or key phrases that will indicate that the question is a true response question.

> True Response Question: Select an option that is true or correct!

What Are the Keywords and Key Phrases Commonly Used in True Response Questions?

Remember to read the question carefully and focus on the stem of the question, because the stem of the question will contain keywords or key phrases that will indicate that the question is a true response question. Several examples of question stems and sample questions that indicate that the question is a true response question are listed below.

TRUE RESPONSE QUESTIONS: KEYWORDS

Early	First	Understands
Late	Immediately	Has been
Most likely	Most appropriate	achieved
Highest	Order of priority	Adequately
Best	All nursing inter-	tolerating
Initial	ventions that apply	

True Response Questions: Example Question Stems

What is the earliest sign of a change in level of consciousness?

Which of the following is a late sign of shock?

The nurse would most likely expect to note:

Which of the following individuals is at the greatest risk for committing suicide?

The nurse palpates the carotid pulse at which anatomic location?

The nurse would plan to order what type of diet for the evening meal before the test?

The nurse plans to administer how many milliliters of medication?

What best action will the nurse implement?

Which action will the nurse do first?

What is the initial nursing action?

Based on these findings, the nurse immediately:

Which nursing action is most appropriate?

List in order of priority the actions that the nurse takes.

The most appropriate response to the client is:

Which intervention would be of highest priority in the preoperative teaching plan?

Select all nursing interventions that apply in the care of the client.

Which statement made by a nursing assistant indicates to the registered nurse that the assistant understands the concepts related to suicide?

Which statement made by the client indicates the best understanding of how to prevent transmission of the disease?

Which of the following outcomes would indicate that the most important goal has been achieved for this client?

The nurse determines that the client is adequately tolerating the procedure if which of the following observations is made?

True Response Question: Multiple Choice

A client with suspected active tuberculosis is being scheduled for diagnostic tests. The nurse anticipates that which of the following diagnostic tests will most likely be prescribed to confirm the diagnosis?

1. Chest x-ray
2. Skin testing
3. White blood cell count
4. Sputum smear

Answer: 4

Test-Taking Strategy:

This question identifies an example of a true response question. Note the keywords *most likely*. Additional key words are *active* and *confirm*. Focus on the diagnosis presented in the question and the associated pathophysiology to assist in directing you to option 4. Remember, tuberculosis is an infectious disease caused by *Mycobacterium tuberculosis,* and the demonstration of tubercle bacilli bacteriologically is essential for establishing a diagnosis. It is not possible to make a diagnosis solely on the basis of a chest x-ray, and a positive reaction to a skin test indicates the presence of tuberculosis infection but does not show whether the infection is active or dormant. A white blood cell count may be increased, but it is not specifically related to the presence of tuberculosis. Remember, focus on the keywords!

True Response Question: Fill in the Blank

The nurse is preparing to administer digoxin (Lanoxin) 0.25 mg orally. The label on the medication bottle reads, "digoxin (Lanoxin) 0.125 mg per tablet." How many tablet(s) will the nurse plan to administer to the client?

Answer: 2

Test-Taking Strategy:

Note the keywords *plan to administer*. Focus on the information in the question and that a dose of 0.25 mg is prescribed. Use the computer on-screen calculator and the formula for calculating a medication dose to answer the question. Remember, focus on the keywords!

True Response Question: Multiple Response

Select all nursing interventions that apply in the care of an infant after a cleft lip repair (cheiloplasty).

____ Position the child on the abdomen.
____ Cleanse the suture line gently after feeding the infant.
____ Keep elbow restraints on the infant at all times.
____ Institute measures that will prevent vigorous and sustained crying.
____ Observe for bleeding at the operative site.
____ Assist the mother with breast-feeding if this is the feeding method of choice.

Answer:

____ Position the child on the abdomen.
_X_ Cleanse the suture line gently after feeding the infant.

_____ Keep elbow restraints on the infant at all times.

__X__ Institute measures that will prevent vigorous and sustained crying.

__X__ Observe for bleeding at the operative site.

__X__ Assist the mother with breast-feeding if this is the feeding method of choice.

Test-Taking Strategy:

Note the keywords *all nursing interventions that apply* and focus on the surgical procedure: a cleft lip repair. Visualize each intervention and think about its effect on the surgical repair to assist in selecting the correct interventions. Remember, focus on the keywords!

True Response Question: Using a Figure

The nurse is performing cardiopulmonary resuscitation on a 6-month-old infant. Using the computer mouse, click on the anatomic area that the nurse would palpate to assess circulation.

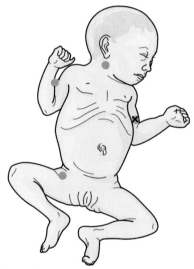

Fig. 8-1 From Lowdermilk D, Perry A: *Maternity & women's health care,* ed 8, St Louis, 2004, Mosby, p 1113, with permission.

Answer: Answer is indicated by the circle containing the X

Test-Taking Strategy:

Focus on the keywords *6-month-old infant* and *assess circulation*. Visualize the body structure of a 6-month old infant and recall that the very short and fat neck of the infant makes the carotid pulse difficult to palpate. In an infant younger than 12 months, the brachial pulse is used to assess circulation. Remember, focus on the keywords!

True Response Question: Prioritizing (Ordered Response)

List in order of priority the interventions that the nurse would take in the care of a client in whom acute pulmonary edema develops. (Number 1 indicates the first action and 4 indicates the last action.)

_____ Place the client on a cardiac monitor and pulse oximetry.

_____ Place the client in high-Fowler's position.

_____ Prepare the client for endotracheal intubation and mechanical ventilation.

_____ Prepare to administer furosemide (Lasix).

Answer: 2, 1, 4, 3

Test-Taking Strategy:

Focus on the keywords *order of priority*. Think about the pathophysiology associated with acute pulmonary edema. This will assist in determining that positioning the client in high-Fowler's would be the first action. Next select placing the client on a cardiac monitor and pulse oximetry, because this action relates to assessment. From the remaining interventions, recall that endotracheal intubation and mechanical ventilation is performed if oxygen administration through mask or nasal cannula is ineffective, and therefore would be performed as a last intervention. Remember, focus on the keywords!

▲ FALSE RESPONSE QUESTIONS

What Is a False Response Question?

A false response question asks you to make a decision and select the option that is inaccurate or incorrect with regard to the data presented in the question. False response questions are used less frequently on the NCLEX-RN than the true response questions, but you need to be alert in noting these types of questions. It is unlikely that false response questions will be presented in alternate test question formats. You will most likely note false response questions presented in a multiple choice format. How will you know that the question is a false response one? Read the question carefully and focus on the stem of the question. The stem of the question will contain keywords or key phrases that will indicate that the question is a false response question. Generally, false response questions are used in evaluation type questions and evaluate the effectiveness of a treatment, procedure, medication, or teaching.

> False Response Question: Select the option that is inaccurate or incorrect with regard to the data presented in the case situation.

What Are the Keywords and Key Phrases Commonly Used in False Response Questions?

Remember to read the question carefully and focus on the stem of the question, because the stem of the question will contain key words or key phrases that will indicate that the question is a false response question. Examples of question stems and sample questions that indicate that the question is a false response question are listed below.

FALSE RESPONSE QUESTIONS: KEYWORDS

Least likely

Least priority

Least helpful

Avoid

Needs reinforcement of the discharge instructions

Have not yet been fully met

Ineffective

Needs reinforcement of the medication administration instructions

Has not met the outcome criteria

False Response Questions: Example Question Stems

Which of the following individuals is least likely to experience development of coronary artery disease?

Which nursing diagnosis is of least priority?

Which of the following approaches by the nurse would be least helpful in assisting this client?

The nurse would avoid which of the following actions?

The nurse determines that the family needs reinforcement of the discharge instructions if the nurse observed which of the following being done by the family?

Which of the following outcomes indicates to the nurse that the goals have not yet been fully met?

The nurse determines that the medication is ineffective if the client continues to experience which symptom?

The nurse determines that the client needs reinforcement of the medication administration instructions if the client made which of the following statements?

The nurse determines that the client has not met the outcome criteria by discharge if the client:

False Response Questions: Multiple Choice

The nurse is reviewing the nursing care plan of a client hospitalized with sickle cell crisis. Which nursing diagnosis written in the plan is the least priority?

1. Acute pain
2. Deficient fluid volume
3. Ineffective tissue perfusion
4. Ineffective coping

Answer: 4

Test-Taking Strategy:

Focus on the keywords *least priority*. According to Maslow's Hierarchy of Needs theory, physiological needs are the priority, followed by safety needs, and then psychosocial needs. Using Maslow's theory will direct you to option 4 because this is the only option that addresses a psychosocial need. Remember, focus on the key words!

False Response Questions: Multiple Choice

The nurse has collected assessment data from four clients examined in the health care clinic. Which client is least likely to develop coronary artery disease?
1. A client with a blood cholesterol level of 289 mg/dL
2. A client with hypertension whose blood pressure has been maintained at 118/78 mm Hg
3. A client who has been smoking two packs of cigarettes daily for the past 20 years
4. A client who is obese, inactive, and has a stressful lifestyle

Answer: 2
Test-Taking Strategy:
Focus on the keywords *least likely*. Recalling the risk factors associated with coronary artery disease will direct you to option 2. Option 2 is the only option that identifies a risk factor that has been modified and controlled. Remember, focus on the key words!

False Response Questions: Multiple Choice

The nurse would avoid which of the following actions when communicating with a client with aphasia?
1. Increase environmental stimuli
2. Ask questions that can be answered with a "yes" or "no"
3. Speak with a normal volume or tone
4. Present one thought or idea at a time

Answer: 1
Test-Taking Strategy:
Focus on the keyword *avoid*. Recalling that the client with aphasia may need extra time to comprehend and respond to communication will direct you to option 1. Increased environmental stimuli may be distracting and disrupting to communication efforts. Remember, focus on the keywords!

False Response Questions: Multiple Choice

The nurse is collecting assessment data from a client who has been taking omeprazole (Prilosec) as prescribed. The nurse determines that the medication is ineffective if the client continues to experience which symptom?
1. Headaches
2. Muscle pains
3. Heartburn
4. Dizziness

Answer: 3

Test-Taking Strategy:

Focus on the keyword *ineffective*. Recalling that omeprazole is a gastric acid pump inhibitor (most medication names that end with *-zole* are gastric acid pump inhibitors) will direct you to option 3. Remember, focus on the keywords!

False Response Questions: Multiple Choice

A client treated for an episode of hyperthermia is being discharged to home from the emergency department. The nurse determines that the client needs reinforcement of the discharge instructions if the client states intentions to:
1. Stay in a cool environment when possible
2. Increase fluid intake for the next 24 hours
3. Monitor voiding for adequacy of urine output
4. Resume full activity level immediately

Answer: 4

Test-Taking Strategy:

Focus on the keywords *needs reinforcement of the discharge instructions*. Select the client statement that indicates that the nurse needs to provide further instructions. Resumption of full activity immediately is not helpful; rather, rest periods are indicated. Remember, focus on the keywords!

False Response Questions: Multiple Choice

The nurse has formulated a nursing diagnosis of Imbalanced Nutrition: Less Than Body Requirements for the unconscious client. Which of the following outcomes indicates to the nurse that the goals have not yet been met?
1. Stable weight
2. Intake equaling output
3. Blood urea nitrogen (BUN) 12 mg/dL
4. Total protein 4.5 g/dL

Answer: 4

Test-Taking Strategy:

Focus on the keywords *has not yet been met*. Because stable weight and equal intake and output are satisfactory indicators and the BUN is normal, option 4 is the answer to the question. Remember, focus on the keywords!

REFERENCES

Gulanick M, Myers J, Klopp A et al: *Nursing care plans: nursing diagnosis and intervention,* ed 5, St Louis, 2003, Mosby.

Hodgson B, Kizior R: *Saunders nursing drug handbook 2005,* Philadelphia, 2004, WB Saunders.

Lewis S, Heitkemper M, Dirksen S: *Medical-surgical nursing: assessment and management of clinical problems,* ed 6, St Louis, 2005, Mosby.

Lowdermilk D, Perry A: *Maternity & woman's health care,* ed 8, St Louis, 2004, Mosby.

Phipps W, Monahan F, Sands J et al: *Medical-surgical nursing: health and illness perspectives,* ed 7, St Louis, 2003, Mosby.

Wong D, Hockenberry M: *Wong's nursing care of infants and children,* ed 7, St Louis, 2003, Mosby.

Chapter

Questions That Require Prioritizing

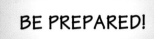

BE PREPARED!

Be prepared! Many of the test questions in the National Council Licensure Examination for Registered Nurses (NCLEX-RN) will require you to use the skill of prioritizing nursing actions. Most of the prioritizing questions will be presented in the multiple choice format; however, you may be presented with a question in the prioritizing (ordered response) format. Prioritizing questions will address content in any nursing area. These types of questions can be difficult, because when a question requires prioritization, all of the options may be correct, but you need to determine the correct order of action. There are some test-taking strategies that you can use to assist in answering these questions correctly. These strategies include noting the keywords or key phrases that indicate the need to prioritize; the ABCs (airway, breathing, and circulation); Maslow's Hierarchy of Needs theory; and the steps of the nursing process. Let us review the definition of prioritizing and these test-taking strategies.

> **GUIDES FOR PRIORITIZING**
> Keywords or key phrases
> The ABCs
> Maslow's Hierarchy of Needs theory
> The steps of the nursing process

▲ PRIORITIZING

What Does Prioritizing Mean?

Prioritizing means that you need to rank the client's problems in order of importance. It is important to read a question carefully and focus on the information in the question, because the order of importance may vary depending on the issue of the question, the clinical setting, the client's condition, and the client's needs. It also is important to consider what the client deems as a priority, which may be quite different from what the nurse may feel is most important. Remember to always consider what the client believes is the priority when planning care.

When you prioritize, you are deciding which client needs or problems require immediate action and which ones could be delayed until a later time because they are not urgent. As you read a question and are trying to determine which option identifies the nurse's priority, use the priority classification system. The priority classification system ranks nursing actions as either a high, intermediate (middle), or low priority. The description of these three types of classifications is listed below.

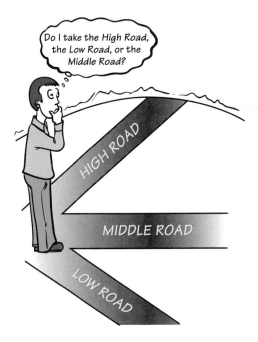

PRIORITY CLASSIFICATION SYSTEM

High Priority: a client need that is life-threatening, or if untreated could result in harm to the client

Intermediate (Middle) Priority: a nonemergency and non–life-threatening client need that does not require immediate attention

Low Priority: a client need that is not directly related to the client's illness or prognosis, is not urgent, and does not require immediate attention

When Do You Select the Option, "Call the Physician"?

An important point to remember is that the NCLEX-RN is testing you on your competence and ability to care for a client and to implement measures that are necessary in a particular situation. It is critically important to read the question carefully, note the information in the question, and read all of the available options. If the question does not describe a client situation that is life-threatening and there is an option that directly relates to a nursing action relevant to the situation, then it is best to select that option and not the option that indicates to "call the physician." Remember, there is usually an action that the nurse would take in a non–life-threatening situation before calling the physician.

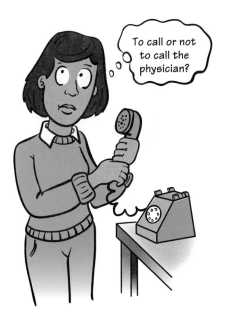

If the question presents a client situation that is life-threatening, then the correct option MAY be to call the physician. Unfortunately, this is not always clear-cut and can present a dilemma for you in your efforts to answer a question correctly. That is why it is so important to read carefully the question and all of the options. Let us review some sample questions that illustrate "when not" and "when to" select the option "call the physician."

When *Not* to Select the Option, "Call the Physician"

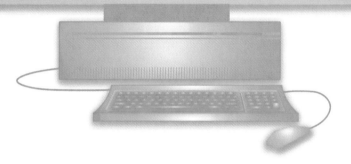

The nurse enters a client's room and finds the client slumped over in bed. The nurse quickly assesses the client and discovers that the client is not breathing. The nurse immediately:

1. Places oxygen via nasal cannula on the client
2. Sits the client upright in bed
3. Calls the physician
4. Begins cardiopulmonary resuscitation (CPR)

Answer: 4

Test-Taking Strategy:

Read the question carefully, note the keyword *immediately*, and focus on the issue: the client is not breathing. This information indicates a life-threatening situation, so read all of the options carefully. In this situation, the nurse needs to intervene immediately. Although the physician needs to be called, the immediate nursing action would be to administer CPR and provide breaths to the client. This option also represents the use of the ABCs as a strategy to answer the question. Options 1 and 2 are incorrect because neither of these options will assist this client.

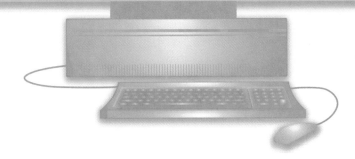

When *Not* to Select the Option: "Call the Physician"

A nurse is caring for a postoperative client who suddenly becomes restless. The nurse would most appropriately:
1. Check the client's vital signs
2. Notify the physician
3. Medicate the client for pain
4. Talk to the client in a calm voice

Answer: 1

Test-Taking Strategy:

Read the question carefully, note the keywords *most appropriately,* and focus on the issue: a postoperative client who becomes restless. There are no data in the question that indicate that the client has pain; therefore, eliminate option 3. Because option 4 is a psychosocial action rather than a physiological one (physiological needs are the priority), eliminate that option.

Recall that restlessness indicates an early sign of shock. However, there are no data in the question that indicate a life-threatening condition. Therefore, the nurse would gather more data about the client's condition and would most appropriately check the client's vital signs.

When *to* Select the Option: "Call the Physician"

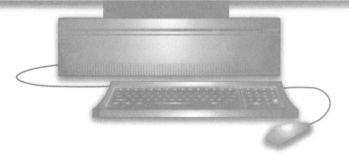

A nurse is caring for a client who just returned from the recovery room after a tonsillectomy and adenoidectomy. The client is restless and the pulse rate is increased. The nurse prepares to continue assessing the client, but the client begins to vomit large amounts of bright red blood. The immediate nursing action is to:

1. Call the surgeon
2. Continue with the assessment
3. Check the client's blood pressure
4. Obtain a flashlight and gauze

Answer: 1

Test-Taking Strategy:

Read the question carefully and note the keywords and the issue of the question. There are several keywords in this question that you need to note, including *restless, pulse rate is increased, large amounts, bright red blood,* and *immediate.* The issue of the question is that the client is actively bleeding and is exhibiting signs of shock. Remember to always read each option carefully. In this situation and from the options provided, the nurse would contact the surgeon. Options 2, 3, and 4 would delay necessary interventions needed in this life-threatening situation.

KEYWORDS OR KEY PHRASES
What Are the Keywords or Key Phrases That Indicate the Need to Prioritize Nursing Actions?

Remember, when a question requires prioritization, all options may be correct; therefore, you will need to determine the correct order of nursing action. Read the question carefully and look for the keywords or key phrases in the question that indicate the need to prioritize. Some of the common keywords or key phrases that indicate the need to prioritize are listed below and are followed by examples of how some of these words or phrases are used in a question.

Note the keywords that indicate the need to prioritize!

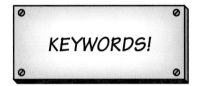

Common Keywords That Indicate the Need to Prioritize

Common keywords that indicate the need to prioritize include the following:

Best
Essential
First
Highest priority
Immediately
Initial
Most appropriate
Most effective
Most important
Most likely
Next
Order of priority
Priority
Primary
Vital

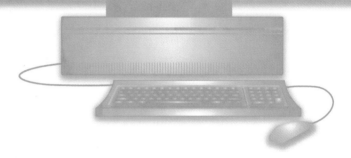

Sample Question: Keywords

A nurse is caring for a client with angina pectoris who begins to experience chest pain. The nurse administers a sublingual nitroglycerin (Nitrostat) tablet as prescribed, but the pain is unrelieved. Which action would the nurse take next?

1. Contact the physician
2. Call the client's family
3. Administer another nitroglycerin tablet
4. Reposition the client

Answer: 3

Test-Taking Strategy:

Note the keyword *next* and focus on the issue: the client is experiencing chest pain. Recalling that the nurse would administer three nitroglycerin tablets 5 minutes apart from each other to relieve chest pain will assist in directing you to option 3. Repositioning the client will not alleviate pain associated with angina pectoris. The nurse would call the physician if three nitroglycerin tablets administered 5 minutes apart from each other did not alleviate the pain. There is no useful reason to call the client's family.

Sample Question: Keywords

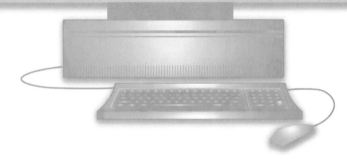

An infant with tetralogy of Fallot experiences a hypercyanotic spell during a blood draw. List in order of priority the actions that the nurse would take. (Number 1 is the highest priority and 4 is the lowest priority.)

____ Administer morphine subcutaneously as prescribed
____ Administer 100% oxygen by face mask as prescribed
____ Place the infant in a knee-chest position
____ Administer intravenous fluids as prescribed

Answer: 3, 2, 1, 4

Test-Taking Strategy:

Note the keywords *order of priority* and the issue of the question: a hypercyanotic spell. In questions that require you to determine the order of priority for nursing actions, if one of the options indicates client positioning, that option may be the first action. Positioning a client can relieve a symptom and is an intervention that takes only seconds to implement. Placing the infant in the knee-chest position reduces the venous return from the legs (which is desaturated) and increases systemic vascular resistance, which diverts more blood flow into the pulmonary artery. Note that the remaining options are all options that require a physician's order. Recalling that airway is a priority, the next action would be to administer oxygen to the infant. Remembering that morphine sulfate reduces spasm that occurs with these spells and that intravenous fluids are not always needed to treat these spells will assist in determining the order of priority for the remaining two interventions.

▲ THE ABCs
What are the ABCs and How Will They Help to Answer a Prioritizing Question?

The ABCs indicate *a*irway, *b*reathing, and *c*irculation, and direct the order of priority of nursing actions. Airway is always the first priority in caring for any client. When you are asked a question that requires prioritization, use the ABCs to assist in determining the correct option. If an option addresses maintenance of a patent airway, that will be the correct option. If none of the options address airway, move to B (breathing), followed by C (circulation). Some sample questions of how this strategy works are provided below.

> Use the ABCs to prioritize!

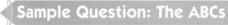 **Sample Question: The ABCs**

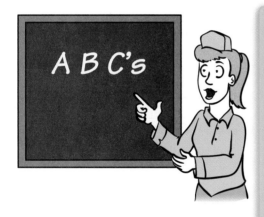

A client with a diagnosis of cancer is receiving morphine sulfate 10 mg subcutaneously every 3 to 4 hours for pain. When preparing the plan of care for the client, the nurse includes which priority action?
1. Monitor stools
2. Monitor the urine output
3. Encourage the client to cough and deep breathe
4. Encourage fluid intake

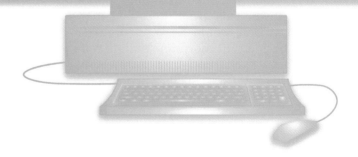

Answer: 3

Test-Taking Strategy:

Note the keyword *priority* and the issue: morphine sulfate. Use the ABCs as a guide directing you to the correct option. Recall that morphine sulfate suppresses the cough reflex and the respiratory reflex. Although options 1, 2, and 4 are components of the plan of care, the correct option addresses airway. Remember, use the ABCs to prioritize.

Sample Question: The ABCs

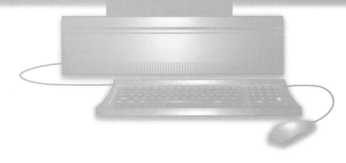

A nurse is assessing the client's condition after cardioversion. Which of the following observations would be of highest priority to the nurse?
1. Status of airway
2. Oxygen flow rate
3. Level of consciousness
4. Blood pressure

Answer: 1

Test-Taking Strategy:

Note the keywords *highest priority* and the issue: assessment after cardioversion. Nursing responsibilities after cardioversion include maintenance of a patent airway, oxygen administration, assessment of vital signs and level of consciousness, and dysrhythmia detection. Airway, however, is always the highest priority. Use the ABCs to direct you to option 1.

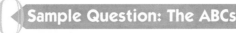

Sample Question: The ABCs

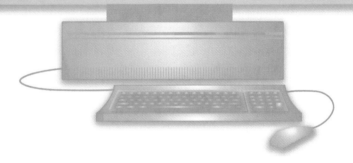

The nurse is providing preoperative teaching to a client scheduled for a cholecystectomy. Which intervention would be of highest priority in the preoperative teaching plan?
1. Teaching coughing and deep breathing exercises
2. Teaching leg exercises
3. Instructions regarding fluid restrictions
4. Assessing the client's understanding of the surgical procedure

Answer: 1

Test-Taking Strategy:

Note the keywords *highest priority* and note the issue: preoperative plan of care. Use the ABCs to answer the question. Option 1 relates to airway. After cholecystectomy, breathing tends to be shallow because deep breathing is painful as a result of the location of the incision. Teaching the importance of performing coughing and deep breathing exercises is the priority.

MASLOW'S HIERARCHY OF NEEDS THEORY

What Is Maslow's Hierarchy of Needs Theory and How Will It Help to Answer Prioritizing Questions?

Abraham Maslow theorized that human needs are satisfied in a particular order, and he arranged human needs in a pyramid or hierarchy. According to Maslow, basic physiological needs such as airway, breathing, circulation, water, food, and elimination needs are the priority. These basic physiological needs are followed by safety, and then the psychosocial needs, including security needs, love and belonging needs, self-esteem needs, and self-actualization needs, in that order.

Maslow's Hierarchy of Needs theory is a helpful guide when prioritizing client needs. When you are answering a question that requires you to prioritize, select an option that relates to a physiological need, remembering that physiological needs are the first priority.

If a physiological need is not addressed in the question or noted in one of the options, then continue to use Maslow's Hierarchy of Needs theory as a guide and look for the option that addresses safety. If neither physiological nor safety needs are addressed, then look for the option that addresses the client's psychosocial need. Figure 9-1 illustrates Maslow's Hierarchy of Needs theory. The sample questions below point out how Maslow's theory can be used as a guide when answering questions that require prioritizing.

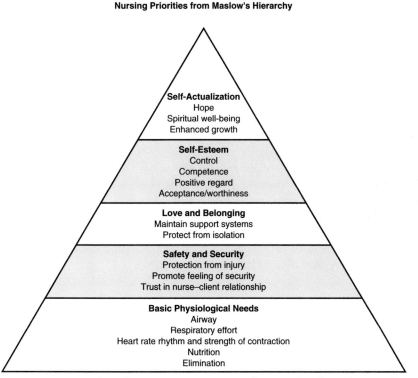

Fig. 9-1   From Harkreader H, Hogan MA: *Fundamentals of nursing: caring and clinical judgment,* ed 2, Philadelphia, 2004, WB Saunders, p 196, with permission.

Use Maslow's Hierarchy of Needs theory to prioritize!

Sample Question: Maslow's Hierarchy of Needs

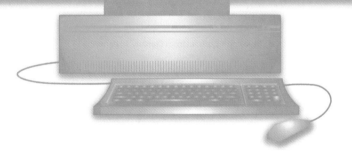

A nurse is admitting a client with a diagnosis of posttraumatic stress disorder to the mental health unit. The client is confused and disoriented. During the assessment, the nurse's primary goal for this client is to:
1. Stabilize the client's psychiatric needs
2. Orient the client to the unit
3. Explain the unit rules
4. Accept the client and make the client feel safe

Answer: 4

Test-Taking Strategy:

Note the keyword *primary* and focus on the issue: a client being admitted to the mental health unit. Use Maslow's Hierarchy of Needs theory and remember that when a physiological need does not exist, then safety needs take precedence. It is important to make a confused client feel safe. Stabilizing psychiatric needs is a long-term goal. Orientation and explaining the unit rules are part of any admission process.

Sample Question: Maslow's Hierarchy of Needs

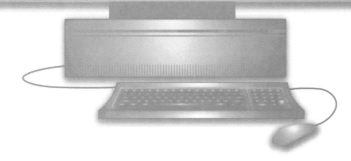

The nurse has developed a plan of care for a client diagnosed with anorexia nervosa. Which of the following nursing diagnoses would the nurse select as the priority in the plan of care?

1. Disturbed body image

2. Defensive coping

3. Deficient knowledge

4. Imbalanced nutrition: less than body requirements

Answer: 4

Test-Taking Strategy:

Note the keyword *priority* and focus on the issue: a nursing diagnosis. Use Maslow's Hierarchy of Needs theory, recalling that physiological needs are the priority. This will assist in directing you to option 4. Options 1, 2, and 3 are psychosocial needs and are of a lesser priority.

Sample Question: Maslow's Hierarchy of Needs

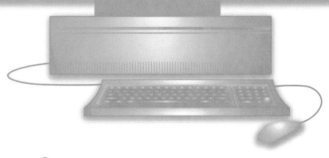

A nurse is preparing to teach a client how to use crutches. Before initiating the lesson, the nurse performs an assessment on the client. The priority nursing assessment should include which of the following?
1. The client's fear related to the use of the crutches
2. The client's understanding of the need for increased mobility
3. The client's muscle strength and previous activity level
4. The client's feelings about the restricted mobility

Answer: 3

Test-Taking Strategy:

Note the keyword *priority* and focus on the issue: teaching a client how to use crutches. Use Maslow's Hierarchy of Needs theory and remember that physiological needs take precedence over psychosocial needs. This should direct you to option 3. Assessing muscle strength will help determine whether the client has enough strength for crutch walking and if muscle-strengthening exercises are necessary. Previous activity level will provide information related to the tolerance of activity. Options 1, 2, and 4 are also a component of the assessment but relate to psychosocial needs.

 # NURSING PROCESS

How Will the Nursing Process Help to Answer Prioritizing Questions?

The Test Plan for the NCLEX-RN identifies nursing process as an Integrated Process. The nursing process provides a systematic method for providing care to a client. These steps include assessment, analysis, planning, implementation, and evaluation. These steps are usually followed in sequence with assessment being the first step and evaluation being the last step. However, once the nursing process begins, it becomes a cyclical process. The steps of the nursing process can be used as a guide to help you when answering questions that require prioritization. Remember that it is always important to read the question carefully to determine what the question is asking. When a question asks for the first or initial nursing action, use these steps and look for an assessment action in one of the options. If an assessment action is not addressed in one of the options, then continue to use the nursing process in a systematic order. Figure 9-2 illustrates the steps of the nursing process, and a description for each step is provided below.

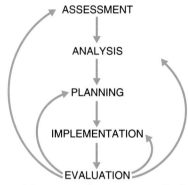

Fig. 9-2   From Ignatavicius D, Workman M: *Medical-surgical nursing: critical thinking for collaborative care,* ed 4, Philadelphia, 2002, WB Saunders, p 12, with permission.

Use the steps of the nursing process to prioritize!

Assessment

Assessment questions address the process of gathering subjective and objective data relative to the client, confirming that data, and communicating and documenting the data.

Remember that assessment is the first step in the nursing process. When you are asked to select your first and initial nursing action, look for an option that addresses assessment. If an option contains the concept of assessment or the collection of client data, it is best to select that option. There are some keywords to look for in the options that indicate an assessment action. Some of these keywords, as well as a sample question, are listed below.

Keywords in Options That Indicate Assessment

Keywords that indicate assessment include the following:
   Ascertain
   Assess

Check
Determine
Find out
Identify
Monitor
Observe
Obtain information

If an assessment action is not noted in one of the options, follow the steps of the nursing process as your guide in selecting your initial or first action. There is a possible exception to using the process of assessment as a guide to prioritize: If the question presents an emergency situation, read carefully; in an emergency situation, an intervention may be the priority!

Sample Question: Assessment

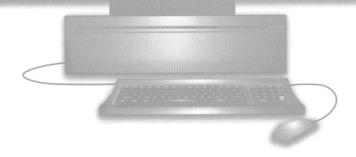

A nurse is teaching a client with coronary artery disease about dietary measures that should be followed. During the session, the client expresses frustration in learning the dietary regimen. The nurse would initially:
1. Identify the cause of the frustration
2. Continue with the dietary teaching
3. Notify the physician
4. Tell the client that the diet needs to be followed

Answer: 1

Test-Taking Strategy:

Note the keyword *initially* and focus on the issue: a nursing action. Use the steps of the nursing process. Of the four options presented, the only assessment action is option 1. Options 2, 3, and 4 identify the implementation step of the nursing process. The initial action is to identify the cause of the frustration. Remember, assessment in the first step of the nursing process.

Analysis

Beware! Analysis questions are the most difficult questions because they require understanding of the principles of physiological responses and require interpretation of the data on the basis of assessment. Analysis questions also require critical thinking and determining the rationale for therapeutic interventions that may be addressed in the question; therefore, many of the questions on the NCLEX-RN will be analysis type of questions. Questions that address this step of the nursing process may also address the formulation of a nursing diagnosis and the communication and documentation of the results of the process of analysis. Remember to read the question carefully, identify the keywords and the issue, and use the process of elimination to select the correct option. An example of an analysis-type question is provided below.

Sample Question: Analysis

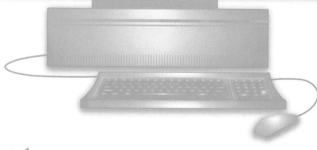

A nurse is reviewing the laboratory results of an infant suspected of having hypertrophic pyloric stenosis. Which of the following laboratory findings would the nurse most likely expect to note in this infant?

1. A blood pH of 7.50
2. A blood pH of 7.30
3. A blood bicarbonate of 22 mEq/L
4. A blood bicarbonate of 19 mEq/L

Answer: 1

Test-Taking Strategy:

Note the keywords *most likely* and focus on the issue: laboratory results. It is necessary to understand the physiology associated with hypertrophic pyloric stenosis and that metabolic alkalosis is likely to occur as a result of vomiting. Next, it is necessary to know which laboratory findings would be noted in this acid–base condition. Analysis of these data will direct you to the correct option. Remember, analysis is the second step of the nursing process.

Planning

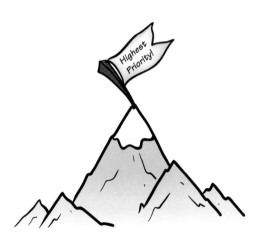

Planning questions frequently address nursing diagnoses. These questions require prioritizing nursing diagnoses, determining goals and outcome criteria for goals of care, developing the plan of care, and communicating and documenting the plan of care. With regard to questions that address the planning step of the nursing process, there are two important points to keep in mind. First, remember that this is a nursing examination and the answer to the question most likely involves something related to the nursing plan rather than to the medical plan, unless the question asks what you anticipate the physician will prescribe. The second point to remember relates to questions that contain options listing nursing diagnoses and require you to prioritize them or to select the nursing diagnosis of highest priority. In these questions, it is important to remember that actual client problems rather than potential or at-risk client problems will most likely be the priority. Read the information in the question carefully; this information will be your guide to selecting the correct option in this type of question. An example of a planning type of question is provided below.

Sample Question: Planning

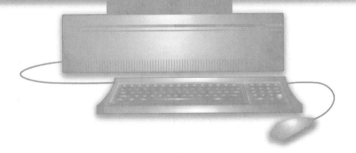

A nurse is reviewing the plan of care for a pregnant client with a diagnosis of sickle cell anemia. Which nursing diagnosis, if stated on the plan of care, would the nurse select as receiving the highest priority?

1. Anxiety
2. Ineffective coping
3. Disturbed body image
4. Deficient fluid volume

Answer: 4

Test-Taking Strategy:

Note the keywords *highest priority* and focus on the issue: a nursing diagnosis in the plan of care. To correctly answer this question, use Maslow's Hierarchy of Needs theory to prioritize, remembering that physiological needs come first. Using this guideline will direct you to option 4. Deficient fluid volume is a physiological need and is the priority nursing diagnosis. Options 1, 2, and 3 are psychosocial needs. Remember, physiological needs are the priority.

Implementation

Implementation questions address the process of organizing and managing care, counseling and teaching, providing care to achieve established goals, supervising and coordinating care, and communicating and documenting nursing interventions. Because the NCLEX-RN tests your competence and ability to function as a professional nurse, many of the questions on the examination will be implementation-type questions.

When you are presented with a question that requires you to determine what the nurse will do, there are two important points to keep in mind. The first point is that the only client that you need to be concerned about is the client in the question; remember, the client in the question is your only assigned client. This is an important point to bear in mind as you are trying to select the correct option.

> You have only one client to be concerned about!

The second important point to keep in mind when you are answering NCLEX-RN questions is that you need to answer the question from an ideal and textbook perspective not a reality perspective; you also need to answer the question as if the nurse has all the time available to care for the client and all the needed resources available at the client's bedside.

> Answer the question from an ideal and textbook perspective!

> Answer the question as if the nurse has all the time available to care for the client and all the needed resources available at the client's bedside!

To illustrate these important points, let us look at the following questions.

Sample Question: Implementation

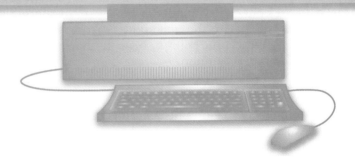

A nurse is caring for a preoperative client who verbalizes a great deal of anxiety about the surgical procedure scheduled in 2 hours. Which action by the nurse would best alleviate the client's anxiety?

1. Tell the client that you will spend some time answering his questions as soon as you get your other tasks completed.
2. Talk to the client for 15 minutes and return shortly thereafter to check on the client.
3. Call the client's wife and ask her to visit the client before surgery.
4. Stay with the client until he is brought to the operating room.

Answer: 4

Test-Taking Strategy:

Note the keyword *best* and focus on the issue: alleviating the client's anxiety. As you are reading the options, you may be hesitant to select option 4 and may say to yourself, "I could never stay with a client for 2 hours. I would never get any of my other client's taken care of." Stop right there and remember that on the NCLEX-RN, the only client that you are caring for is the client in the question. Therefore, option 4 is the best of the four options.

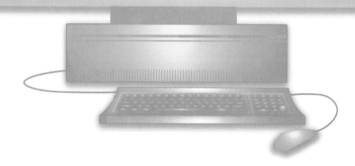

Sample Question: Implementation

A nurse is caring for a client after a cardiac catheterization. The client suddenly reports a feeling of wetness in the groin at the catheter insertion site. The nurse checks the site, notes that the client is actively bleeding, and takes which best action?

1. Dons a clean glove and places pressure on the insertion site with the gloved hand
2. Dons a sterile glove and places pressure on the insertion site using sterile gauze
3. Contacts the physician
4. Checks the client's peripheral pulse in the affected extremity

Answer: 2

Test-Taking Strategy:

Note the keyword *best* and focus on the issue: a nursing action. Active bleeding indicates the need for intervention and the application of pressure at the site of bleeding. This directs you to options 1 and 2 as the possible correct options. You may be hesitant to select option 2 because you may say to yourself, "I would not use the sterile gloves or gauze, because by the time I went to the treatment room, obtained these items, and returned to the room, the client would have lost a critically large amount of blood." Stop right there and remember that on the NCLEX-RN, you have all of the resources needed and readily available at the client's bedside. Because the catheter insertion site is an open area, the best option is to don a sterile glove and place pressure on the insertion site using sterile gauze.

Evaluation

Evaluation questions focus on comparing the actual outcomes of care with the expected outcomes and focus on how the nurse should monitor or make a judgment concerning a client's response to therapy or to a nursing action. These questions also address evaluating the client's ability to implement self-care, health care team members' ability to implement care, and the process of communicating and documenting evaluation findings.

In an evaluation question, it is important to note whether it is a true response or a false response question. Look for the words or phrases that indicate a false response question, because they are frequently used in evaluation type of questions and ask for inaccurate information related to the issue of the question. (Keywords or key phrases used in both true response questions and false response questions are listed in Chapter 8.) Following is an example of an evaluation type of question.

Sample Question: Evaluation

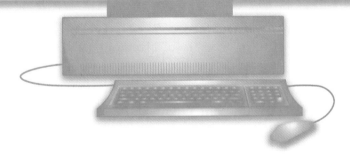

A client recovering from an exacerbation of left-sided heart failure has a nursing diagnosis of Activity Intolerance. The nurse determines that the client best tolerates mild exercise if the client exhibits which of the following changes in vital signs during activity?

1. Pulse rate increased from 80 to 104 beats/min
2. Respiratory rate increased from 16 to 19 breaths/min
3. Oxygen saturation decreased from 96% to 91%
4. Blood pressure decreased from 140/86 to 112/72 mm Hg

Answer: 2

Test-Taking Strategy:

Note the keyword *best* and focus on the issue: the client's ability to tolerate exercise. Use the process of elimination and nursing knowledge regarding normal vital sign values. Options 1 and 3 are incorrect because they represent changes from normal to abnormal values. Blood pressure decreases by more than 10 mm Hg are not a sign that indicates tolerance of activity. The only option that identifies values that remain within the normal range is option 2.

REFERENCES

Gulanick M, Myers J, Klopp A et al: *Nursing care plans: nursing diagnosis and intervention,* ed 5, St Louis, 2003, Mosby.

Harkreader H, Hogan MA: *Fundamentals of nursing: caring and clinical judgment,* ed 2, Philadelphia, 2004, WB Saunders.

Ignatavicius D, Workman M: *Medical-surgical nursing: critical thinking for collaborative care,* ed 4, Philadelphia, 2002, WB Saunders.

Potter P, Perry A: *Fundamentals of nursing,* ed 6, St Louis, 2005, Mosby.

Varcarolis E: *Foundations of psychiatric mental health nursing,* ed 4, Philadelphia, 2002, WB Saunders.

Wong D, Hockenberry M: *Nursing care of infants and children,* ed 7, St Louis, 2003, Mosby.

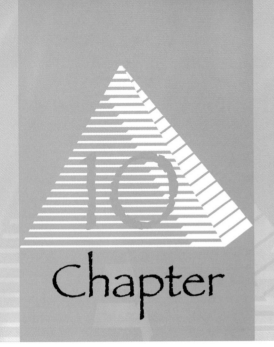

Leadership, Delegating, and Assignment-Making Questions

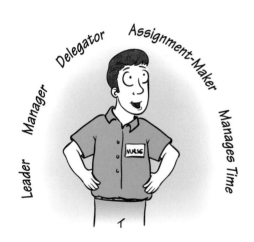

The professional nurse is both a leader and a manager. As a leader and a manager, there are many roles and responsibilities that the nurse needs to assume. The National Council Licensure Examination for Registered Nurses (NCLEX-RN) Test Plan, developed by the National Council of State Boards of Nursing, identifies the content related to these roles and responsibilities in the Management of Care subcategory, which is part of the Safe, Effective Care Environment category of Client Needs. This subcategory, which entails 13% to 19% of the Test Plan, addresses content that tests the nurse's knowledge, skills, and abilities required to enhance the care delivery setting to protect clients, families, significant others, visitors, and health care personnel. Chapter 3 lists some of the content in the Management of Care subcategory that will be tested in the NCLEX-RN. It is important to review information related to this subcategory to ensure that you are well prepared for questions regarding the role and responsibilities of the nurse as a leader and a manager.

Many of the test questions in the Management of Care subcategory relate to the nurse's responsibilities regarding delegating care and assignment making and the supervisory role of these responsibilities. You may also be presented with questions that require you to determine the priority of care for a group of clients. The questions in the Management of Care subcategory most likely will be in the multiple choice format; however, you may be presented with questions that address these responsibilities in the multiple response or the prioritizing (ordered response) format. This chapter reviews the guidelines and principles related to delegating and assignment making, which are two important roles of the nurse. Guidelines for time management also are reviewed because managing time efficiently is a key factor for completing activities and tasks within a definite time period.

DELEGATION AND ASSIGNMENT MAKING

What Is Delegation?

Delegation is the process of transferring a selected nursing task in a client situation to an individual who is competent to perform that specific task. It involves sharing activities and achieving outcomes with other individuals who have the competency to accomplish the task. The Nurse Practice Act and any other practice limitations such as agency policies and procedures define the aspects of care that can be delegated and the tasks and activities that need to be performed by the registered nurse, those that can be performed by the licensed practical nurse or licensed vocational nurse, and those that can be performed by an unlicensed individual such as a nursing assistant. When the nurse delegates an activity, the nurse needs to determine the degree of supervision that the delegatee may require and provide supervision as appropriate.

> Delegation: transferring a nursing task to an individual who is competent to perform the task

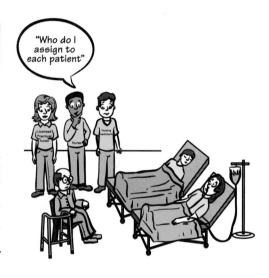

What Is Assignment Making?

Assignment making is a specific activity that involves planning care activities for a client or a group of clients and determining specifically who will provide the care or perform certain activities. As with delegating, the nurse practice act and any other practice limitations such as agency policies and procedures that define the aspects of care need to be used as a guide when planning assignments for activities and client care. Supervision of performance of the activity as appropriate also is important.

> Assignment Making: planning care activities for a client or a group of clients and determining who will provide the care or perform certain activities

What Are the Important Points to Keep in Mind When Delegating or Making Assignments?

When you are answering questions related to either delegating or assignment making there are two important points to keep in mind. First, even though a task or activity may be delegated to someone, the nurse who delegates the task or activity maintains

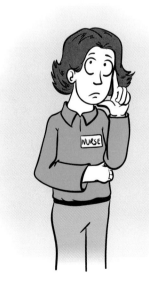

accountability for the overall nursing care of the client. Remember, only the task, not the ultimate accountability, may be delegated to another.

The second point to keep in mind is that this examination is a national examination. Therefore, use general guidelines, such as the Nurse Practice Act, regarding what a health care provider can competently and legally perform to answer the question correctly. Avoid using agency policies and procedures and agency position descriptions to answer the question, unless the question provides information to do so, because they are specific to the agency.

Let us review two sample questions: one that illustrates the use of general guidelines related to delegating and assignment making, and one that relates to specific agency policies and procedures.

Sample Question: General Guidelines

A registered nurse is planning client assignments for the day and has a licensed practical nurse and a nursing assistant on the nursing team. The nurse most appropriately assigns which client to the licensed practical nurse?

1. An older client recovering from pneumonia who requires ambulation every 3 hours
2. A client with a tracheostomy who requires frequent suctioning
3. An older client who requires turning and repositioning every 2 hours and range-of-motion exercises every 4 hours
4. A client who requires the collection of urine for a 24-hour period

Answer: 2

Test-Taking Strategy:

This question requires that you determine which client should most appropriately be assigned to the licensed practical nurse. There is no information in the question that indicates the need to use agency policies, procedures, or position descriptions to determine the most appropriate assignment; therefore, use general guidelines such as the Nurse Practice Act. As you read each option, think about and visualize the client's needs. The client described in option 2 has needs that cannot be met by the nursing assistant. Remember, the health care provider needs to be competent and skilled to perform the assigned task or client activity.

Sample Question: Specific Agency Policies and Procedures

A registered nurse employed in a hospital is assigning client care activities to a nursing assistant. The nursing assistant is a first-semester senior nursing student and works at the hospital as a nursing assistant part-time on weekends. The hospital position description for a nursing student who is employed as a nursing assistant indicates that he or she may perform procedures learned in nursing school if supervised by a registered nurse. Based on the hospital's position description, the registered nurse assigns which most appropriate activity to the nursing assistant?

1. Hang a unit of red blood cells on a client
2. Insert an intravenous catheter into an infant
3. Change a sterile abdominal dressing
4. Administer digoxin (Lanoxin) by intravenous push

Answer: 3

Test-Taking Strategy:

In this question, information is provided that directs you to use the hospital's description of the position to determine the most appropriate activity to assign to the nursing assistant. The keywords in the question are *most appropriate.* Based on the data provided in the question and in the options, it is best to select the least invasive activity. Also, recall that blood administration and medication administration must be performed by a licensed health care provider. Inserting an intravenous catheter into an infant is an invasive procedure that needs to be performed by a health care provider specially trained to perform it. Remember, the health care provider needs to be competent and skilled to perform the assigned task or client activity.

What Principles and Guidelines Can Be Used to Delegate and Make Assignments?

If you are presented with a question on the examination that requires you to delegate or plan assignments for a group of clients, there are principles and guidelines that can be used to assist in answering the question correctly. As you are using the process of elimination to determine the correct option, keep these principles and guidelines in mind. Also, read each option carefully. Think about and visualize the client's needs to determine which health care provider could best meet the client's needs. Following is a review of the principles and guidelines for delegating and assignment making:

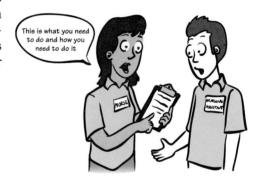

Always ensure client safety—never select an option that could potentially cause harm to the client.

Focus on the issue of the question and what the question is asking; for example, is the question asking you to delegate to another registered nurse, a licensed practical or vocational nurse, or a nursing assistant?

Determine which tasks or client care activities can be delegated and to whom and match the task to the delegatee on the basis of the Nurse Practice Act, agency policies and procedures, or position descriptions as appropriate; that is, think about the activities that the delegatee can safely and legally perform.

Think about individual variations in work abilities and determine the degree of supervision that may be required; for example, if the question asks to delegate or assign a client care activity to a new graduate, then you must think about the need for providing adequate supervision and the need to teach the new graduate about the assigned activity.

Always provide directions to the delegatee that are clear, concise, accurate, complete, and validate the person's understanding of the directions and expectations; that is, ask the delegatee to verbalize the procedure for performing the task and activity that was delegated.

Communicate a feeling of confidence to the delegatee and provide feedback promptly after the task or activity is performed regarding his or her performance; ensure that the delegatee completed the task and evaluate the outcome of the care provided.

Provide the delegatee with a timeline for completion of the task or activity; for example, if a client is scheduled for a diagnostic test and an activity or task needs to be completed before the test, it is important to identify this timeline to the delegatee.

Maintain continuity of care as much as possible when assigning client care; for example, it is best for the client to be cared for by a nurse with whom the client has developed a therapeutic relationship. However, it is also important to remember that there are some client situations in which maintaining continuity of care would be unfavorable with regard to ensuring a safe environment for a health care provider, such as with the client with an infectious disease or the client with a radiation implant.

Sample Question: Assignment-Making

A nurse is planning the client assignments for the day and is reviewing client data and the needs of the clients on the nursing team. To maintain continuity of care, the nurse would ensure that which client is cared for by the nurse who cared for the client on the previous day?

1. A client with a cervical radiation implant
2. A client with active tuberculosis
3. A client with herpes zoster (chickenpox)
4. A client recently diagnosed with inoperable cancer

Answer: 4

Test-Taking Strategy:

Focus on the issue of the question: to maintain continuity of care. Read each option carefully, keeping two points in mind: the client's needs and ensuring a safe environment for the health care provider. The clients described in options 1, 2, and 3 can potentially present a risk to the health care provider. The client in option 4 will likely have psychosocial needs that can best be met if the client is cared for by a health care provider with whom the client has developed a therapeutic relationship.

Who Can Do What?

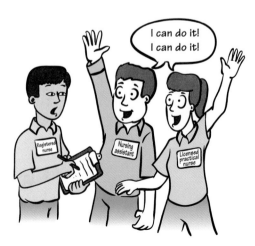

There are some general guidelines to follow when answering a question that requires determining what tasks and client care activities should be assigned to which health care provider. Remember, these are general guidelines, and the general guidelines are the ones that you need to follow when taking a national examination. These guidelines (listed below) are followed by sample questions in both multiple choice and multiple response formats.

Unlicensed Personnel

Generally, noninvasive tasks and basic client care activities can be assigned to an unlicensed individual, such as a nursing assistant. Some of these tasks and activities include the following:

Ambulation
Bathing
Client transport
Grooming
Hygiene measures
Positioning
Range-of-motion exercises
Skin care
Some specimen collections, such as urine or stool

Licensed Practical or Vocational Nurse

In addition to the tasks that the unlicensed personnel can perform, a licensed practical or vocational nurse can perform certain invasive tasks and client care activities. Some of these additional tasks include the following:

Administering oral medications
Administering intramuscular injections
Administering subcutaneous injections
Changing dressings
Irrigating wounds
Monitoring an intravenous flow rate
Suctioning
Teaching about basic hygienic and nutritional measures
Urinary catheterization
Using the nursing process: data collection, planning, implementing, and evaluating

Registered Nurse

The registered nurse is competent to perform many tasks and client care activities. In addition to the tasks and client care activities that a licensed practical or vocational nurse can perform, there are numerous procedures that the registered nurse can perform. To assist you in differentiating the role of the registered nurse and the licensed practical or vocational nurse, some of the tasks and client care activities that only the registered nurse can perform are as follows:

Administering intravenous medications
Leading others and managing the client care environment
Teaching
Using the nursing process: assessment, analyzing data, planning client care, implementing care, and evaluating care

Sample Question: Multiple Response

A registered nurse is planning the client assignments for the day and has a registered nurse, a licensed practical nurse, and a nursing assistant on the nursing team. Select all clients that could be safely assigned to the licensed practical nurse.

____ A client with a central intravenous line who requires the administration of intravenous antibiotics every 4 hours

____ A client with an open abdominal wound that requires wound irrigations every 3 hours

____ A client with a spinal cord injury who requires intermittent urinary catheterization every 4 hours

____ A client with pulmonary edema who was admitted to the hospital 2 hours ago and requires frequent respiratory assessments

____ A client newly diagnosed with diabetes mellitus who requires teaching about insulin administration

Answer:

____ A client with a central intravenous line who requires the administration of intravenous antibiotics every 4 hours

 X A client with an open abdominal wound that requires wound irrigations every 3 hours

 X A client with a spinal cord injury who requires intermittent urinary catheterization every 4 hours

____ A client with pulmonary edema who was admitted to the hospital 2 hours ago and requires frequent respiratory assessments

____ A client newly diagnosed with diabetes mellitus who requires teaching about insulin administration

Test-Taking Strategy:

Focus on the issue of the question: a client assignment to a licensed practical nurse. Use general principles and guidelines to assist in answering the question correctly. Think about and visualize the client's needs and determine whether the licensed practical nurse can competently and legally perform activities to meet these needs. The administration of intravenous medications needs to be done by a registered nurse. Client assessment is done by the registered nurse; however, the licensed practical nurse can collect data. Initial teaching about insulin administration needs to be done by a registered nurse. Remember, the health care provider needs to be competent and skilled to perform the assigned task or client activity.

Sample Question: Multiple Choice

A nurse is planning client assignments for the day and needs to assign four clients. There is a registered nurse, a licensed practical nurse, and two nursing assistants on the nursing team. Which client would the nurse most appropriately assign to the registered nurse?

1. A client with a right leg amputation who requires a dressing change
2. A client requiring a bed bath
3. A client who requires frequent ambulation
4. A client who was admitted to the hospital during the night after experiencing an acute asthma attack

Answer: 4

Test-Taking Strategy:

Note the keywords *most appropriately* and focus on the issue of the question: a client assignment to a registered nurse. Use general principles and guidelines to assist in answering the question correctly. Think about and visualize the client's needs. The client who was admitted to the hospital during the night after experiencing an acute asthma attack would most appropriately be assigned to the registered nurse because this client would require frequent respiratory assessments. The nursing assistant can most appropriately give a bed bath and ambulate a client. The licensed practical nurse can perform dressing changes. Remember, the health care provider needs to be competent and skilled to perform the assigned task or client activity.

Sample Question: Multiple Choice

A registered nurse is planning the client assignments for the day. Which of the following is the most appropriate assignment for the nursing assistant?
1. A client with difficulty swallowing food and fluids
2. A client who requires stool specimen collections
3. A client requiring colostomy irrigation
4. A client receiving continuous tube feedings

Answer: 2

Test-Taking Strategy:

Focus on the issue of the question: a client assignment to a nursing assistant. Use general principles and guidelines to assist in answering the question correctly. Think about and visualize the client's needs and determine whether the nursing assistant can competently and legally perform activities to meet these needs. In this situation, the most appropriate assignment for a nursing assistant would be to care for the client who requires stool specimen collections. The client with difficulty swallowing food and fluids is at risk for aspiration. Colostomy irrigations and tube feedings are not performed by unlicensed personnel. Remember, the health care provider needs to be competent and skilled to perform the assigned task or client activity.

Sample Question: Multiple Choice

A nurse on the day shift is assigned to care for four clients. Following report from the night shift, which client will the nurse plan to assess first?

1. Client scheduled for a cardiac catheterization at 10:00 AM
2. Client newly diagnosed with diabetes mellitus who is scheduled for discharge to home
3. Client with pulmonary edema who was treated with furosemide (Lasix) at 5:00 AM
4. Client scheduled to have an electrocardiogram (ECG) at 9:00 AM

Answer: 3

Test-Taking Strategy:

This question describes a situation in which the nurse needs to prioritize with regard to assigned clients. The keyword in the question is *first*.

Use the ABCs—airway, breathing, and circulation—to answer the question. Airway is always a high priority; therefore, the nurse would assess the client with pulmonary edema who was treated with furosemide (Lasix) at 5:00 AM first. The nurse would next assess the client scheduled for the cardiac catheterization, because this client will require preprocedure preparation. The client scheduled for discharge would be assessed next because there may be discharge needs that require attention. The client scheduled for an ECG can be assessed last.

TIME MANAGEMENT

What Is Time Management and Why Is It Important?

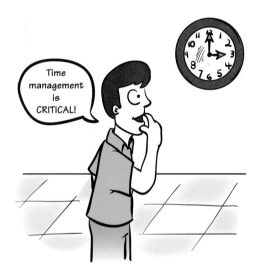

Time management is a technique used by the nurse to assist in completing tasks within a definite time period. It involves learning how, when, and where to use one's time and involves establishing personal goals and time frames. Time management requires an ability to anticipate the day's activities, to combine activities when possible, and to not be interrupted by nonessential activities. It also involves efficiency in completing tasks quickly and thoroughly, and effectiveness in deciding on the most important task to do and doing it correctly. The ability to manage time efficiently is important to complete tasks and client care activities within a reasonable time frame. In many client care situations, time management requires prioritizing. The registered nurse needs to be skilled in planning time resourcefully and needs to assist other health care providers with time management. Some of the principles and guidelines to use to assist in managing time efficiently are listed below.

> Time Management: the ability to manage time efficiently to complete tasks and client care activities within a reasonable time frame

Principles and Guidelines of Time Management

Following is a review of the principles and guidelines of time management:

Identify tasks, obligations, and client care activities, and write them down.

Organize the workday; identify which tasks and client care activities must be completed in specified time frames.

Prioritize client needs.

Anticipate the needs of the day and provide time for unexpected and unplanned tasks or client care activities that may arise.

Focus on beginning the daily tasks by working on the most important first, while keeping goals in mind; look at the final goal for the day, which will help to break down tasks into manageable parts.

Begin client rounds at the beginning of the shift, assessing and collecting data on each assigned client.

Delegate tasks when appropriate.

Keep a daily hour-by-hour log to assist in providing structure to the tasks that must be accomplished, and cross tasks off the list as they are accomplished.

Use hospital and agency resources efficiently, anticipating resource needs and gathering the necessary supplies before beginning the task.

Organize paperwork and continuously document task completion and necessary client data throughout the day.

At the end of the day, evaluate the effectiveness of time management.

TIME MANAGEMENT

Think!	Plan!
Organize!	Prioritize!

Sample Question: Prioritizing (Ordered Response)

A home care nurse is planning the home care visits for the day and plans to visit her first client at 8:00 AM. List in order of priority how the nurse will plan the home care visits for the day. All clients live within a 5-mile radius. (Number 1 is the first client that the nurse would visit and 4 is the last home care visit for the day.)

_____ A client with pneumonia who was discharged from the hospital 1 day ago; the client's spouse lives with the client, and the client will need to be admitted to home care

_____ A client who requires a daily dressing change on the foot

_____ A client who requires a fasting blood glucose draw before self-administering insulin

___   A client who will be cared for by a home health aide for the first time and is scheduled to arrive at the client's home at 9:00 AM

Answer: 4, 3, 1, 2

Test-Taking Strategy:

Use the principles and guidelines related to time management. Organize the workday and identify which tasks and client care activities must be completed in specified time frames. Because the client that requires the fasting blood glucose must remain NPO (nothing by mouth) until the blood is drawn, the nurse would visit this client first to draw the blood. The nurse would next visit the client who will be cared for by the home health aide. Because the home health aide is scheduled to visit the client at 9:00 AM, the nurse would visit this client next, so that the nurse could describe the client's plan of care to the home health aide. From the remaining two clients, it is best to visit the client requiring the daily dressing change next. The reason for this is that care to the client requiring admission to home care will take more time than it takes to perform a dressing change. The admission assessment and other admission procedures that will need to be done are time consuming.

REFERENCES

Harkreader H, Hogan MA: *Fundamentals of nursing: caring and clinical judgment,* ed 2, Philadelphia, 2004, WB Saunders.

National Council of State Boards of Nursing: Test Plan for the National Council Licensure Examination for Registered Nurses (effective date: April 2004), Chicago, 2003, National Council of State Boards of Nursing.

Potter P, Perry A: *Fundamentals of nursing,* ed 6, St Louis, 2005, Mosby.

Yoder-Wise P: *Leading and managing in nursing,* ed 3, St Louis, 2003, Mosby.

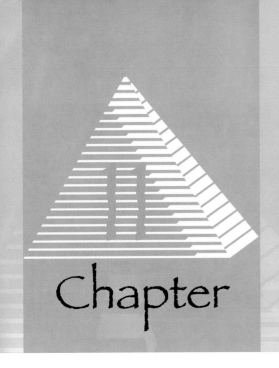

Chapter 11

Communication Questions

Communication is a process in which information is exchanged, either verbally or nonverbally, between two or more individuals (Fig. 11-1). According to the National Council of State Boards of Nursing (NCSBN), an Integrated Process of the Test Plan is a process that is fundamental to the practice of nursing and is incorporated throughout the Client Needs categories of the Test Plan. In the National Council Licensure Examination for Registered Nurses (NCLEX-RN) Test Plan, the NCSBN identifies the concept of communication as a component of one of the Integrated Processes. In addition, in the Psychosocial Integrity category of Client Needs (6% to 12% of test items), Therapeutic Communications is listed as content that is tested on the NCLEX-RN. Therefore, it is likely that you will be presented with questions that relate to the communication process. This chapter reviews the guidelines to follow when answering communication questions. Several sample questions are included to illustrate how these guidelines are used.

HOW ARE COMMUNICATION CONCEPTS TESTED IN A QUESTION?

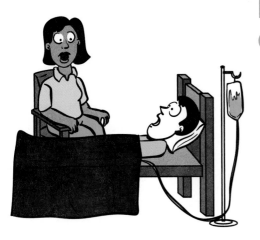

Communication is an important characteristic of the nurse–client relationship. Therefore, test questions that refer to the concept of communication may address a client situation in any clinical setting and any nursing care area. That is, communication questions may address client situations in the adult health area, the maternity area, the pediatric area, or the mental health area in settings such as the hospital, clinic, physician's office, or other health care setting.

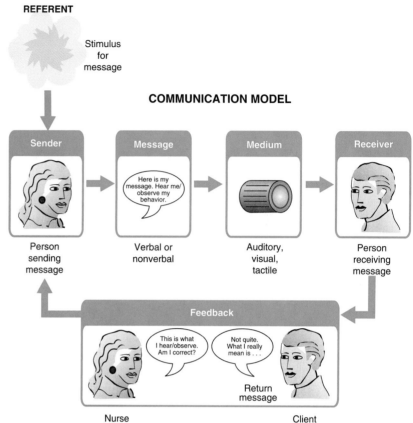

Fig. 11-1   Varcarolis EM: *Foundations of psychiatric mental health nursing,* ed 4, Philadelphia, 2002, WB Saunders, p 248.

Communication questions may address a client situation
in any clinical setting and any nursing care area!

   When we think about communication concepts and the nurse–client relationship, we usually visualize an interaction between the nurse and the client. Although this is an accurate visualization, it is important to broaden our thinking with regard to the communication process and the concepts that will be tested on the examination. Test questions not only will address the communication process between the nurse and the client, but also will address the process between the nurse and a client's family member or significant other, or the nurse and another member of the health care team such as another nurse, a nursing assistant, or a physician. For example, you may be asked about how you would respond to a staff member who makes an inappropriate statement, or how you would respond to a physician who is demanding. Most of the questions that test the concept of communication will be in the multiple choice format and will relate to how the nurse would respond to the person with whom he or she is communicating.

WHAT GUIDELINES CAN BE USED TO ANSWER COMMUNICATION QUESTIONS?

There are four primary guidelines to use when answering communication questions. These guidelines are as follows:

1. Use therapeutic communication techniques to answer communication questions because of their effectiveness in the communication process. As you read the question and each option, look for the option that indicates the use of a therapeutic communication technique.

2. Nontherapeutic communication techniques are ineffective and need to be avoided when responding to a client, a client's family member or significant other, or another member of the health care team. As you read the question and each option, eliminate the options that indicate the use of a nontherapeutic communication technique.

3. Focus on feelings, concerns, anxieties, or fears. As you read the question and each option, look for the option that indicates the use of a therapeutic communication technique and focuses on the feelings, concerns, anxieties, or fears of the client, the client's family member or significant other, or the health care team member.

4. Consider cultural differences as you answer the question. If you note that a question contains information that identifies a specific cultural group, you need to think about specific cultural characteristics to answer the question correctly. Remember that each culture is unique with regard to the characteristics related to the process of communication.

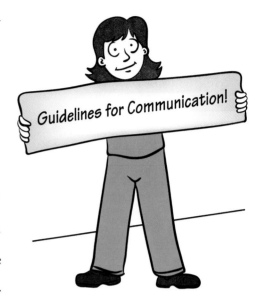

GUIDELINES FOR COMMUNICATION

Use therapeutic communication techniques.

Avoid nontherapeutic communication techniques.

Focus on the client's feelings, concerns, anxieties, or fears.

Consider cultural differences.

COMMUNICATION TECHNIQUES

What Are the Therapeutic Communication Techniques?

Using therapeutic communication techniques encourages the client, or other individual with whom the nurse is communicating, to express his or her thoughts and feelings. There are many therapeutic communication techniques that can be used to promote verbalization. You are probably quite familiar with these techniques from your first nursing course in nursing school; however, the following section provides a brief review of these techniques.

Therapeutic Communication Techniques

Technique	Description
Active listening	Carefully noting what the client is saying and observing the client's nonverbal behavior
Broad openings	Encouraging the client to select topics for discussion
Clarifying	Providing a means for making the message clearer, to correct any misunderstandings, and to promote mutual understanding
Focusing	Directing the conversation on the topic being discussed
Informing	Giving information to the client
Offering self to help	Can include staying with the client or talking to the client
Open-ended questions	Encouraging conversation because these questions require more than one-word answers
Paraphrasing	Restating in different words what the client said
Reflecting	Directing the client's question or statement back to the client for consideration
Restating	Repeating what the client has said and directing the statement back to the client to provide the client the opportunity to agree or disagree or to clarify the message further
Silence	Allowing time for formulating thoughts
Summarizing	Stating briefly what was discussed during the conversation
Validating	Verifying that both the nurse and the client are interpreting the topic or message in the same way

What Are the Nontherapeutic Communication Techniques?

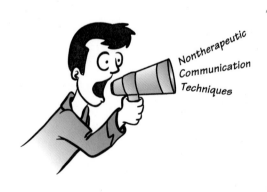

Nontherapeutic communication techniques are the techniques that impair or block the flow of a conversation. These techniques are also known as the barriers to an effective communication process. There are many nontherapeutic communication techniques. You are probably quite familiar with them and have learned that these techniques need to be avoided when communicating because of their ineffectiveness. The following section briefly reviews some of the nontherapeutic communication techniques.

Nontherapeutic Communication Techniques

Technique	Description
Approval	Implying that the client is thinking or doing the right thing and is not thinking or doing what is wrong; this may direct the client to focus on thinking or behavior that pleases the nurse
Asking excessive questions	Demanding information from the client without respect for the client's willingness or readiness to respond
Changing the subject	Avoiding addressing the client's thoughts, feelings, or concerns; implying that the client's statement is not important
Close-ended questions	Questions that ask for specific information such as a "yes" or "no" answer, and therefore inhibit communication
Disagreeing	Opposing the client's thinking or opinions, implying that the client is wrong
Disapproving	Indicating a negative value judgment about the client's behavior or thoughts
False reassurance	Statement implying that the client has no reason to be worried or concerned; belittling a client's concerns
Giving advice	Assuming that the client cannot think for himself or herself, which inhibits problem solving and fosters dependence
Minimizing the client's feelings	Statement implying that the client's feelings are not important
Parroting	Repeating the client's words before determining what the client has said
Placing the client's feelings on hold	Avoiding addressing the client's thoughts, feelings, or concerns; making a statement that places the responsibility of addressing the client's thoughts, feelings, or concerns elsewhere or on another person
Value judgments	Making a comment that addresses the client's morals; this can make the client feel angry or guilty, or as though he or she is not being supported
"Why?" questions	Questions that cause the client to feel defensive; these types of questions often imply criticism

▲ WHY ARE CULTURAL CONSIDERATIONS IMPORTANT?

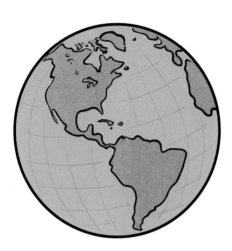

The nurse needs to be aware of certain cultural characteristics that relate to the communication process that may be different from his or her own cultural uniqueness. Questions on the NCLEX-RN examination may address the concept of communication with a client from a specific cultural group. If you note that a question contains information identifying a specific cultural group, you need to think about specific cultural characteristics to answer the question correctly.

With regard to communication, there are three cultural characteristics to consider. These include communication style, use of eye contact, and the meaning of touch. It is important to review the characteristics associated with a specific culture and to become familiar with them before taking the NCLEX-RN examination. Identified below are some of the characteristics of specific cultural groups that you need to consider. If you are unfamiliar with content related to the characteristics of various cultures, refer to the *Saunders Comprehensive Review for the NCLEX-RN Examination.* This product contains information about cultural characteristics and a specific chapter, entitled "Cultural Diversity," that describes many features related to cultural differences for various cultural groups.

> ### CULTURAL COMMUNICATION POINTS TO CONSIDER!
> Communication style
> Use of eye contact
> Meaning of touch

Communication Style

The following sections provide some background information to consider when developing your communication style with specific cultural groups.

African Americans

Personal questions asked on initial contact with the client may be viewed as intrusive.
Head nodding by the client does not necessarily mean agreement.

Asian Cultures

Asian cultures may believe that feelings and emotions are considered to be private, and an open expression of emotions is regarded as a weakness.
Silence is valued by the client.

Criticism or disagreement is not expressed verbally by the client.

Head nodding by the client does not necessarily mean agreement.

The client may interpret the word "no" as disrespect for others.

The client does not use hand gestures.

European (White) Americans

Silence can be used by the client to show respect or disrespect for another, depending on situation.

French and Italian Americans

The client may use expressive hand gestures and animated facial expressions during conversation.

German and British Americans

The client may show little facial emotion because these clients highly value the concept of self-control.

Hispanic Americans

The client may use dramatic body language such as gestures or facial expressions to express emotion or pain.

The client may tend to be verbally expressive, yet confidentiality is important.

Hispanic Americans may believe that direct confrontation is disrespectful, and the expression of negative feelings is impolite.

Native Americans

To Native Americans, silence indicates respect for the speaker.

Many of these clients speak in a low tone of voice and expect others to be attentive.

Body language is important.

Obtaining input from members of the extended family is important.

Use of Eye Contact

The following sections provide information regarding how the use of eye contact is viewed by clients of specific cultural groups.

African Americans

Direct eye contact may be interpreted as rude or aggressive behavior.

Asian Cultures

Eye contact is limited and may be considered inappropriate or disrespectful.

European (White) Americans

Eye contact may be viewed as indicating trustworthiness.

Native Americans

Eye contact may be viewed as a sign of disrespect.
The nurse needs to understand that the client may be attentive even when eye contact is absent.

Hispanic Americans

Some Hispanic Americans believe that avoiding eye contact with a person in authority indicates respect and attentiveness.

Meaning of Touch

The following sections discuss how touch is viewed in specific cultural groups.

African Americans

African Americans may be comfortable with close personal space when interacting with family and friends

Asian Cultures

These clients prefer a formal personal space except with family and close friends.
They usually do not touch others during conversation.
Touching is unacceptable with members of the opposite sex; if possible, a female client prefers a female health care provider.
The head is considered to be sacred; therefore, touching someone on the head may be considered disrespectful.
The nurse would avoid physical closeness and excessive touching and would only touch a client's head when necessary, informing the client before doing so.

European (White) Americans

European Americans tend to avoid close physical contact.
The nurse needs to respect the client's personal space.

Native Americans

Personal space is very important to Native Americans.

Native American clients may lightly touch another person's hand during greetings.

In this culture, massage is used for the newborn infant to promote bonding between the infant and mother.

Touching a dead body may be prohibited in some tribes.

Hispanic Americans

Hispanic Americans are comfortable with close proximity with family, friends, and acquaintances and value the physical presence of others.

The nurse needs to protect the client's privacy.

Hispanic Americans are very tactile and use embraces and handshakes.

The nurse needs to ask if it would be all right to touch a child before examining him or her.

SAMPLE COMMUNICATION QUESTIONS

Following are sample communication questions that illustrate the use of therapeutic and nontherapeutic communication techniques. Remember to use the following communication guidelines:

Use therapeutic communication techniques.

Avoid the use of nontherapeutic communication techniques.

Focus on the client's feelings, concerns, anxieties, or fears.

Consider cultural differences.

Sample Question

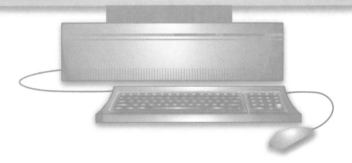

A mother says to the nurse in the physician's office, "I am afraid that my child might have another seizure." Which response by the nurse is therapeutic?
1. "Why worry about something that you cannot control?"
2. "Most children will never experience a second seizure."
3. "Tell me what frightens you the most about seizures."
4. "Phenytoin (Dilantin) can prevent another seizure from occurring."

Answer: 3

Test Taking Strategy:

Note the keyword *therapeutic*. Option 3 is the only option that addresses the client's fears. Option 1 is a nontherapeutic response because it states that the mother should not worry. Options 2 and 4 are incorrect because the nurse is giving false reassurance to the mother that a seizure will not reoccur or can be prevented in this child. Remember, use therapeutic communication techniques and focus on the client's feelings, concerns, anxieties, or fears!

Sample Question

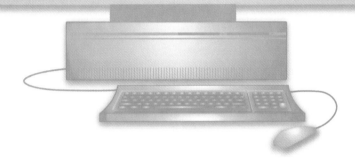

A client examined in the health care clinic has been diagnosed with hypertension and has been taking a prescribed antihypertensive medication. On a follow-up visit, the client says to the nurse, "I don't understand why I have to take this medication. It makes me feel awful." The appropriate nursing response is which of the following?

1. "You will need to ask your doctor about that."
2. "Everyone who takes that medication says the same thing."
3. "You have to take this medication if you want to prevent a stroke."
4. "Describe what you mean when you say that the medication makes you feel awful."

Answer: 4

Test-Taking Strategy:

Note the keyword *appropriate*. Option 1 avoids the client's concern and places the client's feelings on hold. Option 2 minimizes the client's feelings and implies that the client's complaint is not important. In option 3, the nurse gives advice and also provides false reassurance that the medication will prevent a stroke. In this option, the nurse also avoids the client's complaint and is threatening in a sense and may induce fear in the client. In option 4, the nurse uses the therapeutic communication technique of restating. In this technique, the nurse explores by repeating what the client has said and directing the statement back to the client to provide the client the opportunity to clarify the message further. Remember, use therapeutic communication techniques and focus on the client's feelings, concerns, anxieties, or fears!

Sample Question

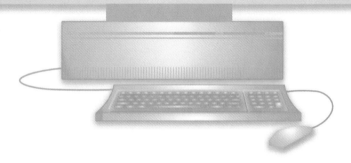

A client with a history of cardiac disease is brought to the emergency department because of experiencing an episode of chest pain while mowing the lawn. During the assessment, the client tells the nurse that he stopped taking his cardiac medication. The appropriate response by the nurse is which of the following?

1. "Tell me some of the reasons that led you to stop taking your medication."
2. "Why did you stop taking your medication?"
3. "Everything is going to be just fine. We'll get you started on those medications right away."
4. "You stopped the medication! Don't you know that you are never supposed to do that with cardiac medications?"

Answer: 1

Test-Taking Strategy:

Note the keyword *appropriate*. Option 1 is an open-ended and a broad opening question that will promote and encourage the client to communicate. The statement in option 2 uses the word *why*. Use of this word implies criticism and often makes the client feel defensive. In option 3, the nurse provides false reassurance by telling the client that everything is going to be fine. In addition, the nurse avoids exploring the reason(s) that led the client to stopping the medication. In option 4, the nurse demoralizes, belittles, and lectures the client, which is nontherapeutic. Remember, use therapeutic communication techniques and focus on the client's feelings, concerns, anxieties, or fears!

Sample Question

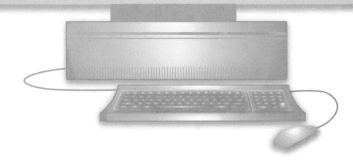

A client recently diagnosed with ovarian cancer says to the nurse, "I can't believe this has happened to me. I wish that I were dead!" Which nursing response is therapeutic?

1. "I know what you mean, but there are a lot of treatments available for ovarian cancer."
2. "Every client diagnosed with this type of cancer says the same thing."
3. "You must be feeling very upset. Are you thinking of hurting yourself?"
4. "Why are you talking that way? Your children wouldn't want to hear you say that, would they?"

Answer: 3

Test-Taking Strategy:
Note the keyword *therapeutic*. In option 3, the nurse focuses on the client's statement and addresses the client's feelings in the response. In options 1 and 2, the nurse minimizes the client's feelings. In addition, option 1 provides false reassurances. In option 4, the nurse uses the word *why*, which implies criticism and often makes the client feel defensive. In addition, option 4 focuses on the client's children and their feelings rather than on the client's feelings. Remember, use therapeutic communication techniques and focus on the client's feelings, concerns, anxieties, or fears!

Sample Question

Select all nursing responses that indicate the use of therapeutic communication techniques.

____ "I know how you feel."

____ "You're feeling anxious and it relates to your conversation that you had with your boss yesterday."

____ "You will do just fine, just wait and see."

____ "Let's talk more about why you are not following your diet."

____ "How come you still smoke when you know that you have cancer?"

Answer:

____ "I know how you feel."

__X__ "You're feeling anxious and it relates to your conversation that you had with your boss yesterday."

____ "You will do just fine, just wait and see."

__X__ "Let's talk more about why you are not following your diet."

____ "How come you still smoke when you know that you have cancer?"

Test-Taking Strategy:

Focus on the issue: therapeutic communication techniques. Review the following nursing responses:

"I know how you feel."—Nontherapeutic and minimizes the client's feelings.

"You're feeling anxious and it relates to your conversation that you had with your boss yesterday."—Therapeutic and indicates the use of reflection.

"You will do just fine, just wait and see."—Nontherapeutic and minimizes and avoids the client's feelings.

"Let's talk more about why you are not following your diet."—Therapeutic and uses the technique of focusing.

"How come you still smoke when you know that you have cancer?"—Nontherapeutic and demoralizes the client and also can make the client feel guilty, angry, anxious, or unsupported.

Remember, use therapeutic communication techniques and focus on the client's feelings, concerns, anxieties, or fears when answering communication questions!

Sample Question

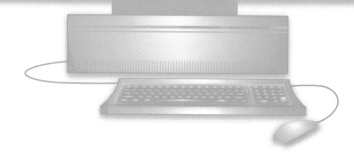

A nurse is providing instructions to an Asian client regarding obtaining a stool specimen for testing for occult blood.

As the nurse explains the instructions, the client continuously turns away from the nurse. Which nursing action is appropriate?

1. Continue with the instructions, verifying client understanding

2. Stress the importance of the instructions with the client

3. Walk around the client so that the nurse continuously faces the client

4. Give the client the list of instructions and return later to continue with the instructions

Answer: 1

Test-Taking Strategy:

In this question, you need to consider the characteristics of the Asian culture. Many Asian clients maintain a formal distance with others, which is a form of respect. Many Asian clients are uncomfortable with face-to-face communications, especially when there is direct eye contact. If the client turns away from the nurse during a conversation, the appropriate nursing action is to continue with the conversation. Walking around the client so that the nurse faces the client is in direct conflict with the cultural practice. Telling the client about the importance of the instructions may be viewed as degrading. The client may view returning later to continue with the explanation as a rude gesture. Remember, if the question identifies a specific cultural group, you need to consider the characteristics of the culture to answer the question!

Sample Question

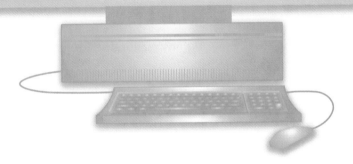

A nurse in an ambulatory care clinic is performing an admission assessment on an African-American client scheduled for a laparoscopic cholecystectomy. Which of the following questions would be inappropriate for the nurse to ask on initial assessment?

1. "Do you have any difficulty breathing?"
2. "Do you have a close family relationship?"
3. "Do you ever experience chest pain?"
4. "Do you frequently have episodes of abdominal pain?"

Answer: 2

Test-Taking Strategy:

In this question, you need to consider the characteristics of the African-American culture. Note the keywords *inappropriate* and *initial assessment*. In the African-American culture, it is considered to be intrusive to ask personal questions on the initial contact or meeting. African Americans are highly verbal and express feelings openly to family or friends, but what transpires within the family is viewed as private. Respiratory, cardiovascular, and gastrointestinal assessments include physiological assessments that are the priority assessments.

You can also use Maslow's Hierarchy of Needs theory to answer the question. Note that options 1, 3, and 4 address physiological needs. Option 2 addresses the psychosocial need. Remember, if the question identifies a specific cultural group, you need to consider the characteristics of the culture to answer the question!

REFERENCES

Harkreader H, Hogan MA: *Fundamentals of nursing: caring and clinical judgment,* ed 2, Philadelphia, 2004, WB Saunders.

Potter P, Perry A: *Fundamentals of nursing,* ed 6, St Louis, 2005, Mosby.

Stuart G, Laraia M: *Principles and practice of psychiatric nursing,* ed 7, St Louis, 2001, Mosby.

Varcarolis EM: *Foundations of psychiatric mental health nursing,* ed 4, Philadelphia, 2002, WB Saunders.

Chapter 12

Pharmacology Questions

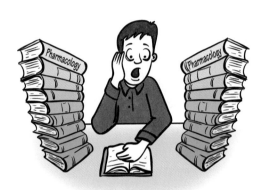

Pharmacology is one of the most difficult nursing content areas to master and feel comfortable with. One reason that it is so difficult is because of the enormous number of medications available. Another reason is that there is a vast amount of information to know about each medication. The National Council Licensure Examination for Registered Nurses (NCLEX-RN) Test Plan addresses pharmacological and parenteral therapies in the Physiological Integrity category and identifies 13% to 19% as the percentage of this type of test question that will possibly appear on your examination. What this means is, if you took a 100-question examination, 13 to 19 of the questions would be related to pharmacology and parenteral therapies. Therefore, it is important for you to spend ample time reviewing pharmacology in preparation for the NCLEX-RN, and it is best to do your review from a question and answer perspective.

> Questions related to pharmacological and parenteral therapies represent 13% to 19% of NCLEX-RN examination questions.

This chapter provides you with strategies for preparing to answer pharmacology questions and also guidelines and strategies to use when attempting to answer the questions correctly.

Remember to read the question carefully, noting the keywords and the issue of the question, and always use the process of elimination to select the correct option. As with any type of question, it is best to use your nursing knowledge to answer the question. However, a question may appear on your examination that contains a medication with which you are unfamiliar. When this occurs, the guidelines and the strategies to answer a pharmacology question correctly will be valuable. After you read this chapter, I recommend practicing as many pharmacology questions as you can. There are several resources available that contain hundreds of pharmacology practice questions. These resources include the *Saunders Comprehensive Review for the NCLEX-RN Examination, the Saunders Q & A Review for the NCLEX-RN Examination*, the *Saunders Computerized Review for the NCLEX-RN Examination*, the *Saunders Online Specialty Test for Pharmacology*, and the *Saunders Online Review Course for the NCLEX-RN Examination*. These products can be obtained at the Elsevier Health Web site (www.elsevierhealth.com).

> **GUIDELINES AND STRATEGIES**
> Read the question carefully.
> Note the keywords.
> Note the issue.
> Use the process of elimination.
> Use nursing knowledge.
> Use pharmacology guidelines.
> Use test-taking strategies.

PHARMACOLOGY GUIDELINES
How Will the Pharmacology Guidelines Be Helpful in Answering a Pharmacology Question, and What Are These Guidelines?

There are some specific guidelines to follow when you administer medication to a client. In addition to the five rights for medication administration, these guidelines include client assessment and assessment of other factors related to the medication, such as checking certain laboratory values or vital signs; checking for potential interactions or contraindications related to the medication; client teaching; monitoring for intended effects, side effects, adverse effects, or toxic effects; and evaluating the client's response to the medication therapy. When you are presented with a pharmacology question and are trying to select the correct option, using the guidelines will assist you in eliminating incorrect options. Some of these guidelines are listed below.

> **SIX MEDICATION RIGHTS**
>
> | Right client | Right time and frequency |
> |---|---|
> | Right medication | Right route |
> | Right dose | Right documentation |

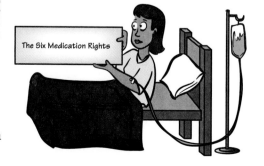

Pharmacology: Assessment Guidelines to Follow

Following is a list of assessment guidelines to follow when administering medication to a client:

Always assess for client allergies or hypersensitivity to a medication.

Always assess the client for existing medical disorders that are contraindicated with the administration of a prescribed medication.

Always assess for potential interactions related to the medication.

Always check pertinent laboratory results.

Always check the client's vital signs, particularly if medications such as antihypertensive or cardiac medications are being administered.

Always assess the client for intended effects, side effects, adverse effects, or toxic effects of the medication.

Always assess the client's response to the medication.

These guidelines will be particularly helpful if the question asks for the priority nursing action when administering a medication. Below is a sample pharmacology question illustrating how these guidelines may be helpful.

Sample Question: Pharmacology

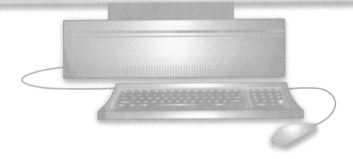

The nurse notes that a physician has prescribed co-trimoxazole (Bactrim) for a client with a urinary tract infection. Which priority action will the nurse take before administering this medication?

1. Call the pharmacy to order the medication
2. Ask the client about an allergy to sulfonamides
3. Check the medication supply room to find out whether the medication needs to be ordered
4. Inform the client about the need to increase fluid intake

Answer: 2

Test-Taking Strategy:

Remember to read the question carefully, noting the issue of the question and the keywords. In this question, the keyword is *priority*, and the issue is the action that the nurse will take. Using the pharmacology guidelines will direct you to option 2. Also, use of the steps of the nursing process will direct you to the correct option, because option 2 is the only option that addresses client assessment.

What Other Guidelines Will Be Helpful?

There are some general guidelines to keep in mind as you are trying to select the correct option.

Pharmacology: General Guidelines to Follow

Following is a list of general guidelines to follow when answering a question regarding medication administration:

Medication absorption, distribution, metabolism, and excretion are affected by age and physiological processes; the older client and the neonate and infant are at greater risk for toxicity than an adult.

Many medications are contraindicated in pregnancy and during breast-feeding.

Antacids are not usually administered with medication, because the antacid will affect the absorption of the medication.

Grapefruit juice is not usually administered with medication because it contains a substance that will interact with the absorption of the medication.

Enteric-coated and sustained-release tablets should not be crushed; also, capsules should not be opened.

Nursing interventions always include monitoring for intended effects, side effects, adverse effects, or toxic effects of the medication.

Nursing interventions always include client education.

The nurse or client should never adjust or change a medication dose, abruptly stop taking a medication, or discontinue a medication.

The nurse may withhold a medication if he or she suspects that the client is experiencing an adverse or toxic effect of a medication; the nurse must immediately contact the physician if either of these effects occurs.

The client needs to avoid taking any over-the-counter medications or any other medications, such as herbal preparations, unless they are approved for use by the health care provider.

The client needs to know how to correctly administer the medication.

The client needs to be aware of the side effects of medications and how to check his or her own temperature, pulse, and blood pressure.

The client needs to take the prescribed dose for the prescribed length of therapy and understand the necessity of compliance.

The client needs to avoid consuming alcohol and to avoid smoking.

The client should wear a Medic Alert bracelet if he or she is taking medications, such as but not limited to anticoagulants, oral hypoglycemics or insulin, certain cardiac medications, corticosteroids and glucocorticoids, antimyasthenic medications, anticonvulsants, and monoamine oxidase inhibitors.

The client needs to follow up with a health care provider as prescribed.

Below is a sample pharmacology question that illustrates how these general pharmacology guidelines may be helpful.

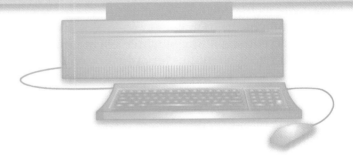

Sample Question: General Pharmacology Guidelines

A client taking amitriptyline hydrochloride (Elavil) calls the nurse at the physician's office and reports that he has an upset stomach whenever he takes the medication. The nurse most appropriately tells the client to:

1. Take the medication with an antacid
2. Stop the medication for 2 days, and then resume the prescribed medication schedule
3. Take the medication on an empty stomach
4. Take the medication with food

Answer: 4

Test-Taking Strategy:

Remember to read the question carefully, noting the issue of the question and the keywords. In this question, the keywords are *most appropriately*, and the issue is the client's complaint of an upset stomach. Recalling that antacids are not usually administered with medication and that the nurse would not tell a client to discontinue a medication will assist in eliminating options 1 and 2. From the remaining options, focusing on the issue will assist in eliminating option 3.

MEDICATION EFFECTS

What are the differences between an intended effect, a side effect, an adverse effect, and a toxic effect of a medication?

It is important to understand these differences; understanding them will assist in eliminating the incorrect options in a pharmacology question that asks about one of these effects. When you are presented with a question on the examination that asks about an effect of a medication, note the specific issue: is the issue of the question an intended effect, a side effect, an adverse effect, or a toxic effect? The differences are described in the following sections, and each section has a sample question related to the specific effect discussed in that section.

Intended Effect

An intended effect is the desired and expected effect of a medication. For example, the intended effect of morphine sulfate is pain relief. On the following page is a sample of a question that asks about an intended effect.

INTENDED EFFECT
A desirable effect

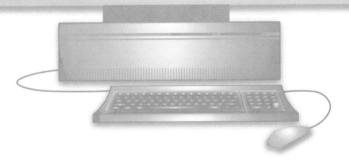

Sample Question: Intended Effect

Ibuproten (Motrin) is prescribed for a client with rheumatoid arthritis. On a follow-up visit to the physician's office, the nurse asks the client whether the medication has provided relief from which of the following symptoms?
1. Joint pain
2. Dyspepsia
3. Diarrhea
4. Flatulence

Answer: 1

Test-Taking Strategy:

Read the question carefully, noting the issue of the question and the keywords. In this question, the keywords are *provided relief from,* and the issue is an intended effect of the medication. Note that the question provides the client's diagnosis. Recalling the pathophysiology related to rheumatoid arthritis will assist in directing you to option 1. Also note that options 2, 3, and 4 are similar in that they all address gastrointestinal symptoms. When options are similar, it is best to eliminate those options because they are unlikely to be correct. In addition, options 2, 3, and 4 are side effects of ibuprofen, not intended effects.

Side Effect

A side effect is a physiological effect of a medication that is unrelated to the desired medication effects. For example, a side effect of an antihistamine medication is drowsiness. A side effect of a medication is not usually life-threatening, and normally there are measures that will either eliminate the side effect or alleviate the discomfort associated with it. On the following page is a sample of a question that asks about a side effect.

> **SIDE EFFECT**
> Not a desired effect
> Not usually life-threatening
> Can usually be alleviated with specific measures

Sample Question: Side Effect

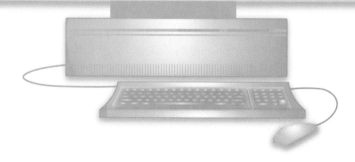

Erythromycin (E-Mycin) has been prescribed for a client with a respiratory infection. The nurse tells the client that which frequent side effect can occur from this medication?
1. Yellow discoloration to the white part of the eye
2. Abdominal cramping
3. Severe diarrhea
4. Yellow-colored skin

Answer: 2

Test-Taking Strategy:
Remember to read the question carefully, noting the issue of the question and the keywords. In this question, the keywords and the issue are a side effect of the medication. Eliminate options 1 and 4 first because they are similar and both indicate the presence of hepatitis, an adverse effect of the medication. From the remaining options, eliminate option 3 because of the word *severe*. Remember, the question asks about a side effect, not an adverse effect.

Adverse Effect

An adverse effect is more severe than a side effect and is always an undesirable effect. For example, an adverse effect of a sulfonamide is hypersensitivity that may be evidenced by a rash, fever, and shortness of breath. An adverse effect can range from a mild effect to a severe effect such as anaphylaxis. Adverse effects are always reported to the health care provider. Below is a sample question that asks about an adverse effect.

ADVERSE EFFECT
More severe than a side effect
Always an undesirable effect
Always reported to the health care provider

Sample Question: Adverse Effect

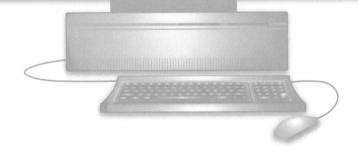

A client with congestive heart failure is receiving furosemide (Lasix). The nurse monitors the client for which adverse effect of the medication?
1. Nausea
2. Increase in urinary output
3. Gastric upset
4. Muscle weakness

Answer: 4

Test-Taking Strategy:

Read the question carefully, noting the issue of the question and the keywords. In this question, the keywords and the issue are an adverse effect of the medication. Eliminate options 1 and 3 first because they are similar and both relate to the gastrointestinal system. From the remaining options, eliminate option 2 because it is an intended effect of the medication. Also, recall that furosemide is a diuretic and can cause electrolyte imbalances, and that muscle weakness is an indication of hypokalemia. Remember, the question asks about an adverse effect.

Toxic Effect

A toxic effect (toxicity) of a medication occurs when the medication level in the body exceeds the therapeutic level either from overdosing or medication accumulation. Toxic effects are always reported to the health care provider. Toxic effects are most often identified by monitoring the plasma (serum) therapeutic range of the medication. For example, the therapeutic blood level of digoxin (Lanoxin) is 0.5 to 2 ng/mL; if the blood level is greater than 2 ng/mL, the client experiences toxicity. The client will normally exhibit certain signs and symptoms (depending on the medication) that indicate toxicity, and the nurse needs to monitor for these signs and symptoms. For example, in digoxin toxicity, the client may experience gastrointestinal disturbances, such as anorexia, nausea, and vomiting, or ocular disturbances, such as photophobia, light flashes, or halos around bright objects. Below is a list of medications commonly used in the clinical setting and their therapeutic blood level; a sample question that asks about a toxic effect also follows.

> **TOXIC EFFECT**
> Medication level in the body exceeds the therapeutic level

Therapeutic Blood Medication Levels

Medication	Therapeutic Range
Acetaminophen (Tylenol)	10–20 mcg/mL
Carbamazepine (Tegretol)	5–12 mcg/mL
Digoxin (Lanoxin)	0.5–2 ng/mL
Gentamicin (Garamycin)	5–10 mcg/mL
Lithium (Lithobid)	0.5–1.3 mEq/L
Magnesium sulfate	4–7 mg/dL
Phenytoin (Dilantin)	10–20 mcg/mL
Salicylate	100–250 mcg/mL
Theophylline/Aminophylline (Theo-Dur)	10–20 mcg/mL

Sample Question: Toxic Effect

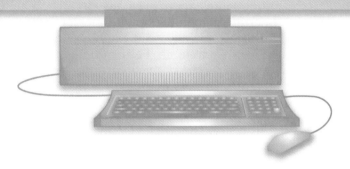

The nurse reviews the results of a therapeutic blood level that was drawn from a client taking theophylline (Theo-Dur) and notes that the level is 21 mcg/mL. The nurse would most appropriately:

1. Administer the next scheduled dose of theophylline
2. Place the results of the blood test in the client's medical record
3. Report the result to the health care provider
4. Ask the laboratory to draw another blood specimen to verify the result

Answer: 3

Test-Taking Strategy:

Remember to read the question carefully, noting the issue of the question and the keywords. In this question, the keywords are *most appropriately* and the issue is a toxic effect of the medication. Recalling that the therapeutic blood level of theophylline is 10 to 20 mcg/mL will assist in determining that the client is experiencing toxicity. Remember, toxic effects are always reported to the health care provider.

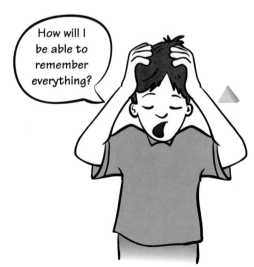

How will I be able to remember everything?

▲ MEDICATION NAMES

Do You Need to Memorize Both the Generic Name and the Trade Name of a Medication?

No memorizing is necessary! When a pharmacology question appears on the computer screen, both the generic name and the trade name will appear. This will be helpful to assist you in answering the question correctly. One medication name, perhaps the generic name, may be unfamiliar to you, but you may recognize the trade name. For example, a question may ask about a medication named furosemide (Lasix). You may not be familiar with the medication name furosemide, but it is very likely that you will be familiar with the medication name Lasix because it is a commonly administered medication.

How Will Medical Terminology Skills Help to Answer a Pharmacology Question?

If a pharmacology question appears on your examination that contains the name of a medication with which you are unfamiliar, try to break the generic or trade name of the medication into parts and use medical terminology to assist in determining the medication action. Following is a pharmacology question that illustrates how this strategy works.

Sample Question: Medical Terminology Skills

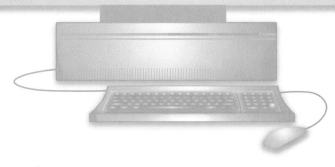

Metoprolol (Lopressor) has been prescribed for a client. The nurse performs which most important assessment before administering the medication to the client?
1. Checks the client's lung sounds
2. Checks the client for peripheral edema
3. Takes the client's blood pressure
4. Takes the client's temperature

BREAK THE WORD DOWN!

Answer: 3

Test-Taking Strategy:
Remember to read the question carefully, noting the issue of the question and the keywords. In this question, the keywords are *most important* and the issue is an assessment. Focus on the name of the medication; if you are unfamiliar with the medication, try to break the name of the medication into parts and use medical terminology to assist in determining the medication action. For example, Lopressor lowers (lo) the blood pressure (pressor).

MEDICATION CLASSIFICATIONS

How Will It Help to Identify a Medication by the Classification to Which It Belongs?

Medications that belong to a particular classification have similar medication actions and usually have commonalities in their side effects and nursing interventions related to administration. It is nearly impossible to learn every feature about every individual medication. Learning medications by a "classification system method" groups several medications with similar properties together and makes the amount of information that needs to be learned condensed and manageable.

With regard to side effects and nursing interventions, do not try to memorize every side effect and every nursing intervention for every medication. It is best if you associate side effects with nursing interventions. Learn to recognize the common side effects associated with each medication classification, and then relate the appropriate nursing interventions to each side effect. For example, if a side effect is hypertension, then the associated nursing intervention would be to monitor blood pressure; if a side effect is hypokalemia, then the associated nursing interventions are to monitor the client for signs of hypokalemia and to monitor the client's potassium blood level. Again, this makes the vast amount of information that you need to remember manageable.

> Relate nursing interventions to the side effects of a medication!

How Can You Determine the Medication Classification if You Are Unfamiliar with the Medication?

If you are presented with a pharmacology question that contains the name of a medication with which you are unfamiliar, some of the strategies to use include the following:

1. Note whether the question identifies the client's diagnosis. For example, if the question states: "Cyclophosphamide (Cytoxan) has been prescribed for a client with metastatic breast cancer," focusing on the client's diagnosis will help you to determine that cyclophosphamide is an antineoplastic medication.
2. Break down the name of the medication (either the generic or trade name) into parts. For example, if the question states: "Terbutaline sulfate (Brethine) has been prescribed for a client." Think about "breath" when you look at the medication name Brethine to help you determine that it is a respiratory medication.
3. Note the letters in the medication name and look for those letters that identify a particular medication classification. Several examples of commonalities in

medication names that belong to a particular classification are listed below. These examples are followed by sample questions.

COMMONALITIES IN MEDICATION NAMES

Following is a list of commonalities in medication names:

Androgens: Most medication names end with -*terone* such as testosterone (Androderm, Testoderm).

Angiotensin-converting enzyme (ACE) inhibitors: Most medication names end with -*pril* such as enalapril (Vasotec).

Antidiuretic hormones: Most medication names end with -*pressin* such as desmopressin (DDAVP).

Antilipemic medications: Most medication names end with -*statin* such as atorvastatin (Lipitor).

Antiviral medications: Most antiviral medications contain *vir* in their names such as ritonavir (Norvir).

Benzodiazepines: Benzodiazepines include alprazolam (Xanax), chlordiazepoxide (Librium), clorazepate (Tranxene), estazolam (ProSom), and triazolam (Halcion); most other benzodiazepines names end with -*pam* such as diazepam (Valium).

Beta-adrenergic blockers: Most medication names end with -*lol* such as atenolol (Tenormin).

Calcium channel blockers: Most medication names end with -*pine* such as amlodipine (Norvasc); some exceptions include diltiazem (Cardizem, Cardizem SR) and verapamil (Calan, Isoptin).

Carbonic anhydrase inhibitors: Most medication names end with -*mide* such as acetazolamide (Diamox).

Estrogens: Most estrogen medications contain -*est* in their names such as conjugated estrogen (Premarin).

Glucocorticoids and corticosteroids: Most medication names end with -*sone* such as prednisone (Deltasone).

Histamine H_2 receptor antagonists: Most medication names end with -*dine* such as cimetidine (Tagamet).

Nitrates: Most medications contain *nitr* in their names such as nitroglycerin (Nitrostat).

Pancreatic enzyme replacements: Most medications contain *pancre* in their names such as pancrelipase (Pancrease).

Phenothiazines: Most phenothiazine medication names end with -*zine* such as chlorpromazine (Thorazine).

Proton pump inhibitors: Most medication names end with -*zole* such as lansoprazole (Prevacid).

Sulfonamides: Most medications include *sulf* in their names such as sulfasalazine (Azulfidine).

Sulfonylureas: Most medication names end with -*mide* such as chlorpropamide (Diabinese).

Thiazide diuretics: Most medication names end with -*zide* such as hydrochlorothiazide (HydroDIURIL).

Thrombolytic medications: Most medication names end in -*ase* such as alteplase (Activase).

Thyroid hormones: Most medications contain *thy* in their names such as levothyroxine (Synthroid).

Xanthine bronchodilators: Most medication names end with *-line* such as aminophylline.

Sample Question: Commonalities in Medication Names

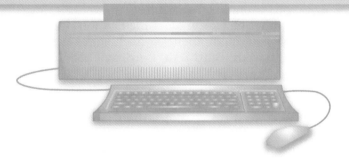

A home care nurse is performing an assessment on a client who is taking pantoprazole (Protonix). The nurse determines that the medication is effective if the client states relief of which of the following symptoms?

1. A nighttime cough

2. Heartburn

3. Constipation

4. Migraine headaches

Answer: 2

Test-Taking Strategy:

Remember to read the question carefully, noting the issue of the question and the keywords. In this question, the keywords are *is effective* and *relief of*, and the issue is an intended effect. Remembering that most gastric acid pump inhibitor medication names end with the suffix *-zole* will direct you to option 2.

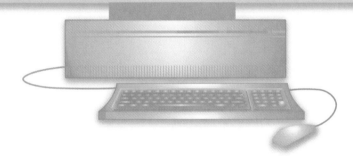

> A clinic nurse is taking a health history on a client seen at the health care clinic for the first time. When the nurse asks the client about current prescribed medications, the client tells the nurse that indinavir (Crixivan) is taken twice daily. Based on this finding, the nurse suspects the presence of which condition?
>
> **1.** Peptic ulcer disease
> **2.** Inflammatory bowel disease
> **3.** Human immunodeficiency virus (HIV)
> **4.** Diverticulitis

Answer: 3

Test-Taking Strategy:

Remember to read the question carefully, noting the issue of the question and the keywords. In this question, the keywords are *suspects the presence* and the issue is the nurse's finding. Remembering that many antiviral medication names contain the letters *vir* will direct you to option 3. Also note the similarity in options 1, 2, and 4. These options all relate to a gastrointestinal disorder.

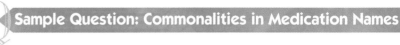

Sample Question: Commonalities in Medication Names

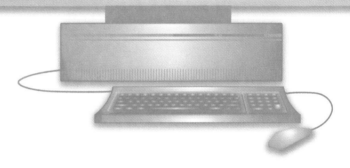

The nurse is preparing to administer atenolol (Tenormin) to a client. The nurse checks which of the following before administering the medication?
1. Potassium level
2. Blood glucose level
3. Blood pressure
4. Temperature

Answer: 3

Test-Taking Strategy:

Remember to read the question carefully, noting the issue of the question and the keywords. In this question, the keywords are *before administering* and the issue is an assessment. Note the name of the medication "atenolol." Recalling that most beta-blocker medication names end with -*lol* and that these medications are used to control blood pressure will direct you to option 3.

REFERENCES

Hodgson B, Kizior R: *Saunders nursing drug handbook 2005,* Philadelphia, 2005, WB Saunders.

Kee J, Hayes E: *Pharmacology: a nursing process approach,* ed 4, Philadelphia, 2003, WB Saunders.

Lehne R: *Pharmacology for nursing care,* ed 5, Philadelphia, 2004, WB Saunders.

Chapter 13

Additional Pyramid Strategies

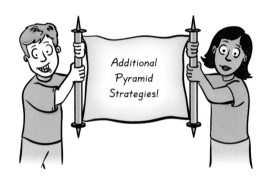

Additional Pyramid Strategies!

In addition to all of the test-taking strategies that you have reviewed so far in this book, there are other helpful strategies that you can use to assist in the process of elimination and answering questions correctly. This chapter reviews these helpful strategies and provides sample questions to illustrate how these strategies are used. Also included in this chapter are strategies that are useful for answering questions that relate to medication and intravenous (IV) calculations, questions that relate to laboratory values, and questions that relate to client positioning. The additional pyramid strategies include the following:

Eliminating options that contain absolute words and selecting options that contain not-so-absolute words

Eliminating options that contain medical rather than nursing interventions

Eliminating similar options

Ensuring that all components of an option are correct

Selecting the umbrella option

Visualizing the information in the case situation and in the options

Looking for similar concepts in the question and in one of the options

ELIMINATING OPTIONS THAT CONTAIN ABSOLUTE WORDS AND SELECTING OPTIONS THAT CONTAIN NOT-SO-ABSOLUTE WORDS: HOW WILL THIS HELP?

In most situations, if an option contains an absolute word, it is incorrect. As you read each option, if you note a word that is absolute, eliminate that option. Conversely, as you read an option and note a not-so-absolute word, then that may be the correct option. Below is a list of absolute and not-so-absolute words:

Absolute Words
  All
  Always
  Can't
  Every
  Must
  Never
  None
  Not
  Only
  Won't
Not-So-Absolute Words
  Generally
  May
  Possibly
  Usually

> Absolute words may indicate an incorrect option!
> Not-so-absolute words may indicate a correct option!

Following are sample questions that illustrate the strategy of absolute versus not-so-absolute words.

Sample Question: Eliminating Options That Contain Absolute Words

A nurse is providing dietary instructions to a client about a low-fat diet. The nurse tells the client to:
1. Never use butter for cooking
2. Read the labels on food items to determine the fat content
3. Eat only foods that have less than 1% fat content
4. Drink fluids only if they are fat-free

Answer: 2

Test-Taking Strategy:
Read every word in each option carefully. Note the absolute words *never* in option 1 and *only* in options 3 and 4. These options should be eliminated because they are incorrect. Remember, the use of an absolute word in an option will most likely make the option incorrect!

Sample Question: Selecting Options That Contain Not-So-Absolute Words

A client scheduled for a computerized tomography (CT) scan of the abdomen asks the nurse when the results of the test will be available. The nurse makes which most appropriate response to the client?

1. "The results won't be available for at least one week."
2. "You must ask the CT technician for that information."
3. "Your physician may have the results in about three days."
4. "Every scan is read by a radiologist and this process always takes one week."

Answer: 3

Test-Taking Strategy:

Read every word in each option carefully and note the keywords *most appropriate*. If you were unable to answer this question using nursing knowledge, note the use of the not-so-absolute word *may* in option 3. Also, note the absolute words *won't* in option 1, *must* in option 2, and *every* and *always* in option 4. These options should be eliminated because they are incorrect. Remember, the use of an absolute word in an option will most likely make the option incorrect, and the use of a not-so-absolute word in an option tends to make the option correct.

ELIMINATING OPTIONS THAT CONTAIN MEDICAL RATHER THAN NURSING INTERVENTIONS: HOW WILL THIS HELP?

An important point to remember is that the National Council Licensure Examination for Registered Nurses (NCLEX-RN) is a nursing examination, not a medical one. Therefore, focus on nursing and select the option that relates to a nursing intervention rather than a medical one. The only situation in which you may need to select a medical intervention is if the question indicates to do so. For example, if the question stem states, "Which intervention does the nurse anticipate the physician to prescribe?" then you may need to select the option that contains a medical action or prescription. Following is a review with sample questions that illustrate this strategy.

> Focus on nursing rather than medical interventions!

Sample Question: Eliminating Options That Contain Medical Rather Than Nursing Interventions

A nurse is caring for a client with a diagnosis of congestive heart failure who suddenly experiences severe dyspnea; the nurse suspects that pulmonary edema has developed. The nurse immediately:

1. Obtains a vial of furosemide (Lasix) and a syringe
2. Places the client in high-Fowler's position
3. Obtains a dose of morphine sulfate from the narcotic medication drawer
4. Inserts a Foley catheter

Answer: 2

Test-Taking Strategy:

Note the keyword *immediately* and note the issue of the question: a nursing action. Although options 1, 3, and 4 are interventions that would be done in this situation, they all require a medical order from the physician. Option 2 is a nursing action that does not require a medical order. Remember, this is a nursing examination, not a medical examination!

Sample Question: Selecting an Option That Indicates a Medical Intervention

A nurse is admitting an infant to the pediatric unit with a diagnosis of respiratory syncytial virus (RSV). The nurse anticipates that the physician will prescribe which of the following?

1. Ribavirin (Virazole)
2. Contact precautions
3. A private room
4. Strict hand washing procedures

Answer: 1

Test-Taking Strategy:

Note the issue of the question: the intervention that the physician will prescribe. Although the physician may document options 2, 3, and 4 on the medical order sheet, these are interventions that the nurse can implement for an infant with RSV. That is, a physician's order is not required for these interventions. In contrast, option 1 requires a physician's order. Remember, this is a nursing examination, not a medical examination, and the only situation in which you may need to select a medical intervention is if the question indicates to do so!

ELIMINATING SIMILAR OPTIONS: HOW WILL THIS HELP?

An important point for you to remember is that in multiple choice questions, there is only one correct option. As you read the options, if you note options that are similar with regard to their context, eliminate these options. The correct answer to the question will be the option that is different. Following is a sample question that illustrates this strategy of eliminating similar options.

Eliminate similar options!

Sample Question: Eliminating Similar Options

A nurse is preparing a plan of care for an older client with a history of heart failure who will be receiving a blood transfusion. The nurse writes in the plan which intervention that relates to monitoring for a transfusion reaction?

  1. Monitor the client's intake and output during the transfusion
  2. Weigh the client before and after the transfusion
  3. Monitor the client's temperature during the transfusion
  4. Check the client's lung sounds hourly for cackles

Answer: 3

Test-Taking Strategy:

Note the issue of the question: a transfusion reaction. If you know the signs of a transfusion reaction, you can answer this question easily. If you do not know these signs, read the options carefully. Note that options 1, 2, and 4 are similar in that they all relate to the complication of fluid overload. Because they are all similar, they are incorrect and need to be eliminated. Remember, the correct answer to the question will be the option that is different!

ENSURING THAT ALL PARTS OF AN OPTION ARE CORRECT: HOW WILL THIS HELP?

There may be some questions that contain options that include two parts, and each part of the option is separated by the word *and*. Read the question carefully, note the keywords, and focus on the issue. As you read the options, read both parts of the option. If you note that one part of the option is incorrect, then the entire option is incorrect; therefore, eliminate that option. In these types of questions, it is important to ensure that both parts of the option are correct. Following is a sample question that illustrates this strategy of ensuring that all parts of an option are correct.

Is everything correct?

> Ensure that all parts of an option are correct!

Sample Question: Ensuring That All Parts of an Option Are Correct

A nurse is performing an assessment on a client diagnosed with a cataract of the right eye. The nurse would expect to obtain which data on assessment?

1. Reports of blurred vision and excessive tearing of the eye
2. A cloudy white pupil and reports of eye pain
3. Reports of a gradual loss of vision and photophobia
4. Reports of a frontal headache and photophobia

Answer: 3

Test-Taking Strategy:
The options in this question contain two parts, and each part of the option is separated by the word *and*. Read the question carefully, note the keywords, and focus on the issue. The keywords are *expect to obtain*, and the issue of the question is assessment data noted in a client with a cataract. In this question, knowledge regarding the differences between the signs and symptoms of a cataract versus glaucoma will assist in answering the question correctly. Although a cloudy white pupil and photophobia occur in a client with a cataract, eye pain and frontal headaches do not. Therefore, these options are not entirely correct and need to be eliminated. Eye pain and frontal headaches occur in the client with glaucoma. From the remaining two options, recalling that excessive tearing occurs in the client with glaucoma, not the client with a cataract, will assist in eliminating option 1. Remember, all parts of the option need to be correct for the option to be correct!

SELECTING THE UMBRELLA OPTION: HOW WILL THIS HELP?

The umbrella option is the option that is a general statement and may incorporate the content of the other options within it. The umbrella option may also be termed as a global option or a comprehensive option. When you are answering a question and note that more than one option appears to be correct, look for the umbrella option. The umbrella option will be the correct answer. Following is a sample question that illustrates this strategy.

Look for the umbrella option!

Sample Question: Selecting the Umbrella Option

A nurse in the emergency department receives a telephone call from emergency medical services and is told that several victims who survived a plane crash and are suffering from cold exposure will be transported to the hospital. The initial nursing action of the emergency department nurse is which of the following?

1. Supply the trauma rooms with bottles of sterile water and normal saline
2. Call the laundry department and ask the department to send as many warm blankets as possible to the emergency room

3. Call the nursing supervisor to activate the agency disaster plan
4. Call the intensive care unit to request that nurses be sent to the emergency room

Answer: 3

Test-Taking Strategy:

Note the keyword *initial* and focus on the issue: the nursing action in the event of a disaster. As you read each option, you will note that all of the options are correct. In this type of question, look for the umbrella option. Option 3 is the umbrella option. Activating the agency disaster plan will ensure that the interventions in options 1, 2, and 4 will occur. Remember, the umbrella option incorporates the ideas of the other options within it.

VISUALIZING THE INFORMATION IN THE CASE SITUATION AND IN THE OPTIONS: HOW WILL THIS HELP?

As you read the question, it is helpful to visualize the case situation. Forming a mental image of the situation places you as the nurse into the scenario. This may be useful because as you create the mental image, you may recall a similar situation that you experienced in the actual clinical area and recall what the nurse did in the situation. In addition, visualize each option as you read it. This process will assist in determining the correct option. Visualizing and relating the case situation to a similar clinical experience can be a valuable strategy as you attempt to eliminate incorrect options. Following is a sample question that illustrates this strategy of visualizing the information.

> Visualize the information!

Sample Question: Visualizing the Information in the Case Situation and in the Options

A nurse prepares to perform a sterile dressing change on an abdominal incision. The nurse explains the procedure to the client, washes her hands, and sets up the sterile field. The nurse takes which action next?
1. Dons sterile gloves
2. Dons clean gloves and removes the old dressing
3. Cleans the wound with Betadine solution as prescribed
4. Assesses the integrity of the abdominal incision

Answer: 2

Test-Taking Strategy:

Note the keyword *next*. Form a mental image of this procedure and visualize the steps that you would take in this procedure.

You cannot clean the wound or assess the wound unless you remove the old dressing; therefore, eliminate options 3 and 4. From the remaining options, recall that sterile gloves are necessary for cleaning and dressing the incision once the old dressing is removed. This will direct you to option 2. Remember, visualizing and relating the case situation to a similar clinical experience can be a valuable strategy as you attempt to eliminate incorrect options!

LOOKING FOR SIMILAR CONCEPTS IN THE QUESTION AND IN ONE OF THE OPTIONS: HOW WILL THIS HELP?

Read the question carefully, noting the keywords and the issue of the question. As you read each option, look for the option that contains similar concepts or has a relationship to those identified in the question. This strategy may be helpful as you are eliminating the incorrect options. Following is a sample question that illustrates this strategy of looking for similar concepts.

> Look for similar concepts in the question and in one of the options!

Sample Question: Looking for Similar Concepts in the Question and in One of the Options

A client is admitted to the hospital with a diagnosis of pericarditis. The nurse assesses the client for which manifestation that differentiates pericarditis from other cardiopulmonary problems?
1. Chest pain that worsens on inspiration
2. Pericardial friction rub
3. Anterior chest pain
4. Weakness and irritability

Answer: 2

Test-Taking Strategy:
Note the keyword *differentiates* and focus on the issue: a manifestation that differentiates pericarditis from other cardiopulmonary problems. This tells you that the correct option will be one that is unique to this health problem. Note the relationship between the word *pericarditis* in the question and the word *pericardial* in the correct option. Also, recall that a pericardial friction rub is heard when there is inflammation of the pericardial sac, during the inflammatory phase of pericarditis. Remember, look for the option that contains a similar concept or has a relationship to the information in the question!

WHAT STRATEGIES WILL BE HELPFUL WHEN ANSWERING MEDICATION AND INTRAVENOUS (IV) CALCULATION QUESTIONS?

When a medication or IV calculation question is presented, you should always use the appropriate formula to solve the problem. Shortcuts should not be used in making these calculations. The problem and the answer should be expressed in the correct units of measure. Always be careful with decimal points. It is important to place the decimal points in the correct places, or the answer will be incorrect. When solving a medication calculation problem, always determine whether the answer is within reason and makes sense.

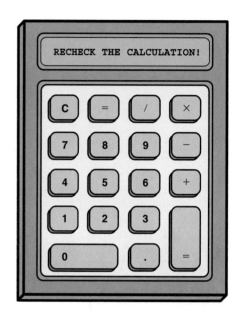

On the NCLEX-RN examination, medication and IV calculation questions will most likely be in a multiple choice or a fill in the blank format. You will be provided with an on-screen calculator for these medication and IV problems. Even if you use the calculator to calculate dosages and flow rates, it is important to recheck the calculation before selecting an option or typing the answer. Follow the formula, place the decimal points in the correct places, and check the accuracy of the calculation. Following are two sample questions that relate to medication and IV calculations.

MEDICATION AND INTRAVENOUS CALCULATIONS

Use the on-screen calculator!

Convert the unit of measure if necessary!

Follow the formula!

Place the decimal points in the correct places!

Recheck the accuracy of the calculation!

Sample Question: Medication Calculation

A physician's order reads phenytoin (Dilantin) 0.2 g orally twice daily. The medication label states 100-mg capsules. A nurse prepares how many capsule(s) to administer one dose?
1. 1 capsule
2. 2 capsules
3. 3 capsules
4. 4 capsules

Answer: 2

Test-Taking Strategy:

In this medication calculation problem, it is necessary to first convert grams to milligrams. Once you have done the conversion and reread the medication calculation problem, you will know that two capsules is the correct answer. Follow the formula for the calculation of the correct dose. Use the on-screen calculator, and then recheck your work, making sure that the answer makes sense.

In the metric system, to convert larger to smaller multiply by 1000 or move the decimal three places to the right; therefore, 0.2 g = 200 mg. The formula and the calculation using the formula are provided below. Remember, follow the formula, recheck your answer, and make sure that the answer makes sense before selecting an option or typing the answer!

Formula:

$$\frac{Desired}{Available} \times Capsules = Capsules \ per \ dose$$

Calculation:

$$\frac{200 \ mg}{100 \ mg} \times 1 \ Capsule = 2 \ Capsules$$

Sample Question: Intravenous Calculation

A physician orders 1000 mL one-half normal saline to infuse over 8 hours. The drop factor is 15 drops/mL. The nurse sets the flow rate at how many drops per minute? (Round the answer to the nearest whole number)

Answer: 31

Test-Taking Strategy:

This question is in the fill in the blank format. Use the formula for calculating IV flow rates when answering the question. Use the on-screen calculator, and then recheck your work, making sure that the answer makes sense. Be careful with the multiplication and division. The formula and the calculation using the formula are provided below. Remember, follow the formula, recheck your answer, and make sure that the answer makes sense before typing it!

Formula:

$$\frac{Total \ volume \times gtt \ factor}{Time \ in \ minutes} = gtt \ per \ min$$

$$\frac{1000 \ mL \times 15 \ gtt}{480 \ minutes} = \frac{15,000}{480} = 31.2, \ or \ 31 \ drops \ per \ minute$$

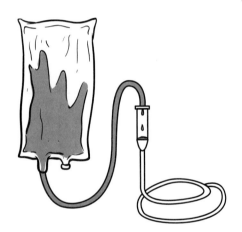

WHAT STRATEGIES WILL BE HELPFUL WHEN ANSWERING QUESTIONS THAT RELATE TO LABORATORY VALUES?

The questions on the NCLEX-RN related to laboratory values will require you to identify whether the laboratory value is normal or abnormal, and then you will be required to think critically about the effects of the laboratory value in terms of the client. If you are familiar with the normal values, you will be able to determine whether an abnormality exists when a laboratory value is

LEARN NORMAL LABORATORY VALUES!

presented in a question. Pyramid points to review are the normal values for the most common laboratory tests, therapeutic serum medication levels of commonly prescribed medications, and determination of the need to implement specific actions based on the findings. Remember that most blood specimens should not be drawn during hemodialysis.

When a question is presented on the NCLEX-RN regarding a specific laboratory value, note the disorder presented in the question and the associated body organ that is affected as a result of the disorder. This process will assist you in determining the correct option. For example, if the question is asking you about the immune status of a client receiving chemotherapy, assessment of laboratory values will focus on the white blood cell count and the neutrophils. You will need to analyze these results as possibly being low and determine the specific client need, which in this case would be the risk for infection. In the client receiving chemotherapy who has a low white blood cell count, your plan should center on the immune system, specifically protecting that client from infection. Interventions focus on preventive interventions related to infection, perhaps even protective isolation measures. Evaluation may focus on maintenance of a normal temperature in the client. Following is a review of a sample question that relates to a laboratory test.

LABORATORY VALUES

Identify whether the laboratory value is normal or abnormal!

Note the disorder presented in the question!

Identify the associated body organ that is affected as a result of the disorder!

Sample Question: Laboratory Values

A client with a diagnosis of sepsis is receiving antibiotics by the intravenous route. The nurse assesses for nephrotoxicity by monitoring which laboratory value most closely?

1. Blood urea nitrogen
2. White blood cell count
3. Platelet count
4. Lipase level

Answer: 1

Test-Taking Strategy:

Note the keywords *most closely*. Focus on the information in the question and note that the issue is nephrotoxicity. Read each option carefully and note that option 1 is the only option that relates to kidney function. Option 2 relates to the immune system. Option 3 relates to the hematological system. Option 4 relates to pancreatic function. Remember, note the disorder or issue presented in the question and the associated body organ that is affected as a result!

WHAT STRATEGIES WILL BE HELPFUL WHEN ANSWERING QUESTIONS THAT RELATE TO CLIENT POSITIONING?

Nursing responsibility includes positioning clients in a safe and appropriate manner to provide safety and comfort. Knowledge regarding the client position required for a certain procedure or condition is expected. It is the nurse's responsibility to reduce the likelihood and prevent the development of complications related to an existing condition, prescribed treatment, or medical or surgical procedure. It is imperative that the nurse review the physician's orders after treatments or procedures and take note of instructions regarding positioning and mobility.

When you are presented with a question that relates to positioning a client, focus on the information in the question, the client's diagnosis, the anatomic location of the client's diagnosis, and consider the pathophysiology of the disorder and the goals of care. That is, think about what complications you want to prevent. There are also some guidelines to remember when answering questions that relate to positioning. These guidelines are listed below.

CLIENT POSITIONING

Always review physician's orders!

Focus on the client's diagnosis!

Identify the anatomic location of the client's diagnosis!

Consider the pathophysiology of the disorder and the goals of care!

Think about what complications that you want to prevent!

 Guidelines Related to Positioning

Following is a list of guidelines related to positioning:

Elevation of an affected body part reduces edema.

Clients who have had neck or head surgery are placed in a semi-Fowler's or Fowler's position.

After a liver biopsy, the client is placed in a right lateral (side-lying) position to provide pressure to the site and prevent bleeding.

Clients receiving irrigations or feeding through a nasogastric, gastrostomy, or jejunostomy tube are placed in a semi-Fowler's or Fowler's position to prevent aspiration.

The left Sims' position is used to administer a rectal enema or irrigation to allow the solution to flow by gravity in the natural direction of the colon.

Clients with a respiratory disorder or cardiovascular disorder are placed in a semi-Fowler's or Fowler's position.

Clients with peripheral arterial disease may be advised to elevate their feet and legs at rest, because swelling can prevent arterial blood flow, but they should not raise their legs above the level of the heart because extreme elevation slows arterial blood flow; some clients may be advised to maintain a slightly dependent position to promote perfusion.

Clients with peripheral venous disease are usually advised to elevate their feet and legs.

Clients with a head injury are placed in a semi-Fowler's or Fowler's position.

If a client develops autonomic dysreflexia, the head of the bed is elevated.

In clients with hemorrhagic strokes, the head of the bed is usually elevated to 30 degrees to reduce intracranial pressure and to facilitate venous drainage.

For clients with ischemic strokes, the head of the bed is usually kept flat.

After craniotomy, the client should NOT be positioned on the site that was operated on, especially if the bone flap has been removed, because the brain has no bony covering on the affected site; a semi-Fowler's to Fowler's position is maintained with the head in a midline, neutral position to facilitate venous drainage from the head, and extreme hip and neck flexion is avoided.

With increased intracranial pressure, the client is placed in a semi-Fowler's to Fowler's position; the head is maintained in a midline, neutral position to facilitate venous drainage from the head, and extreme hip and neck flexion is avoided.

In a spinal cord injury, the client is immobilized on a spinal backboard, with the head in a neutral position, to prevent incomplete injury from becoming complete; head flexion, rotation, or extension is avoided and the client is log rolled.

In the client who underwent a total hip replacement, positioning will depend on the surgical techniques used, the method of implantation, the prosthesis, and the physician's preference; extreme internal and external rotation and adduction is avoided, and side-lying on the operative side is not allowed (unless specifically prescribed by the physician).

The following question relates to positioning a client.

Sample Question: Client Positioning

A nurse assists a physician in performing a liver biopsy. After the biopsy, the nurse plans to place the client in which of the following positions?

1. Supine
2. Prone
3. A left side-lying position with a small pillow or folded towel under the puncture site
4. A right side-lying position with a small pillow or folded towel under the puncture site

Answer: 4

Test-Taking Strategy:

Focus on the information in the question and the anatomic location of the procedure, and think about what complication that you want to prevent. In this situation, you want to prevent bleeding. Remember that the liver is on the right side of the body, and that the application of pressure on the right side will minimize the escape of blood or bile through the puncture site because this position compresses the liver against the chest wall at the biopsy site. Remember to focus on the information in the question, the client's diagnosis, and the anatomic location of the client's diagnosis, and consider the pathophysiology of the disorder and the goals of care!

REFERENCES

Chernecky C, Berger B: *Laboratory tests and diagnostic procedures,* ed 4, Philadelphia, 2004, WB Saunders, p 158.

Kee J, Marshall S: *Clinical calculations: with applications to general and specialty areas,* ed 5, Philadelphia, 2004, WB Saunders.

Lewis S, Heitkemper M, Dirksen S: *Medical-surgical nursing: assessment and management of clinical problems,* ed 6, St Louis, 2004, Mosby.

Peckenpaugh N: *Nutrition essentials and diet therapy,* ed 9, Philadelphia, 2003, WB Saunders.

Perry A, Potter P: *Clinical nursing skills and techniques,* ed 5, St Louis, 2002, Mosby.

Wong D, Perry S, Hockenberry M: *Maternal child nursing care,* ed 2, St Louis, 2002, Mosby.

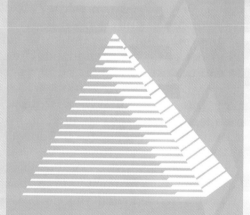

"*Answer questions every day! At least half an hour to an hour. I did Linda Silvestri's CD questions and I also purchased a strategies book and read over that. Also, when you answer the questions make sure you read over the strategies for why an answer was right or wrong. Often you learn a lot just from the responses. Don't study, just answer questions!! It really helps and it's important to use the critical thinking strategies that Linda talks about her books. It helped me to succeed and I highly recommend all of the products in Saunders Pyramid to Success for the NCLEX Examination.*"
—Mindy, Salve Regina University, Newport, Rhode Island

"*To prepare for the NCLEX exam, I used Saunders Computerized Review for the NCLEX-RN Examination. I found that taking the practice tests on my computer helped me understand the format of the NCLEX exam better. I also found that using the computerized review enabled me to move faster through material than reading the book alone. I practiced my test taking skills and increased my knowledge by using the review for one to two hours a day. This helped me balance my study time with work and personal time. I felt well prepared on the test day and passed my exam. Schedule the NCLEX exam for the afternoon so you can sleep in, relax for the morning, and miss rush-hour traffic! Most of all, believe in yourself!*"
—Melissa, Arizona State University, Tempe, Arizona

Part III

Additional Tips for Test-Takers

Chapter 14

Tips for Repeat Test-Takers

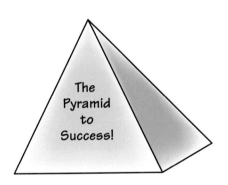

The Pyramid to Success!

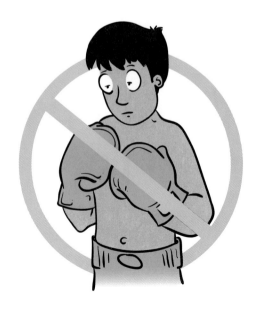

If you need to read this chapter because you have to retake the National Council Licensure Examination for Registered Nurses (NCLEX-RN) examination, do not be discouraged or lose hope. You will be successful when you retake the examination. If you believe in yourself and believe that you can be successful, you will pass this examination. Do not beat yourself up about the fact that you were initially unsuccessful!

You did the very best that you could! Never think that you are a failure because you did not pass this examination. Yes, you were unsuccessful, but you are not a failure. And never feel as if you are all alone. There are other nursing graduates who were unsuccessful when taking this examination the first time.

Part of the preparation for retaking the examination involves maintaining a positive attitude and confidence in yourself that you can be successful. Think about all of the achievements that you have made and all of your life goals that you have met. You have been successful in receiving your diploma from the nursing program that you have attended, and that is one major achievement.

Everyone faces obstacles during his or her lifetime that need to be overcome. Now you are faced with an obstacle. Can you overcome it? Yes, of course you can! You need to remember that success is like climbing a mountain. You will have challenging obstacles to deal with as you climb, but the only way to reach the top of the mountain is to face these challenges in a positive way.

Let's be realistic! Receiving the large envelope in the mail that contained retake information was a devastating experience, and you probably experienced a number of different feelings about the fact that you were unsuccessful. You probably needed to inform your family and perhaps children, friends, and your employer that you need to retake the examination. Sharing the news can be distressing and embarrassing. That you need to retake this examination may also have created a financial burden because you are unable to start your career as a registered nurse as you planned. So now what do you do? Stand tall, think about all of the accomplishments that you have achieved, stay positive, maintain your self-confidence, face those challenging obstacles, retake the examination, and think success!

This chapter provides you with tips and strategies that will help you to prepare to retake this examination. Specific tips and strategies address the procedure for self-assessment, development of a remediation plan, the steps in a remediation plan, and plans for a retake date.

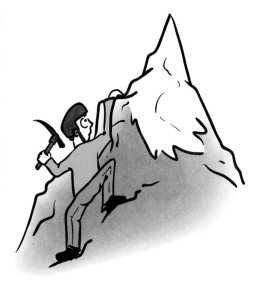

> Stand tall!
> Think about your accomplishments!
> Stay positive!
> Maintain your self-confidence!
> Face the challenges!
> Retake the examination!
> Think success!

POSITIVES: ARE THERE ANY?

There are many positive points that you can think about and focus on to help you remain optimistic. Think about it, you have been through the entire experience and know what the examination process is all about. Let's review some of these positives.

The Positives

You have seen the test and know what the test is all about.
You are familiar with the computer.
You are familiar with the test center.
You are familiar with the testing procedures.
You have reviewed nursing content once previously.
You know what content areas need some fine-tuning.

WHEN DO YOU SCHEDULE A DATE TO RETAKE THE EXAMINATION?

Retake policies vary from state to state; therefore, it is important to carefully review the materials that were sent to you for registering to retake the examination. Depending on your state's board of nursing, you will need to wait a minimum of 45 to 91 days before you can retake the examination. Readiness to retake this examination is highly individual, and your readiness may be very different from someone else's readiness. What you need to do is to develop your remediation plan and determine how much time it will take you to implement your plan. It is best to retake this examination as soon as you can, as long as you have prepared by following your remediation plan. The longer you wait, the greater the risk for forgetting critical nursing content that was learned in nursing school. So do not delay. Develop your remediation plan, get started with your review, and stick to your plan!

WHERE DO YOU START TO PREPARE FOR THE RETAKE EXAMINATION?

The first task that you have is to perform a self-assessment. Think about your testing experience and identify the factors or obstacles that you believe contributed to being unsuccessful. Write these factors down on a piece of paper, so that you can be sure to pay attention to them as you prepare. Some self-assessment questions that you may want to consider are detailed below.

> Your first task is self-assessment!

 ## Self-assessment Questions

Following is a list of self-assessment questions:
Did you adequately prepare?
Did you stick to your plan for review?
Did you review nursing content and practice test questions?
Do you understand how to use test-taking strategies?
Did you prepare for this examination holistically? That is, did you include exercise, fun, and relaxation, and did you eat a balanced diet?
Did you eat properly on the day of the examination? That is, did you eliminate caffeine and high-fat foods from your diet?
Did you have test anxiety on the day of the examination?
Were you able to control your test anxiety?
Did you face any obstacles on the way to the testing center that caused a delay, such as traffic or road construction?
Did you encounter any distractions as you were taking the examination? If so, what were they?
Were you able to focus and concentrate during the examination?
Were your expectations for yourself too high?
Did you expect the test to end after 75 questions? When it did not end, did you begin to lose your stamina, ability to concentrate, and self-confidence?

WHAT IS THE NCLEX-RN CANDIDATE PERFORMANCE REPORT, AND HOW WILL IT HELP WITH DEVELOPING A REMEDIATION PLAN?

The NCLEX-RN Candidate Performance Report is prepared by the National Council of State Boards of Nursing and is provided only to the nursing graduate who needs to retake the examination. This report provides extremely valuable information about your areas of strength and also areas of weakness that need particular focus as you prepare to retake the examination.

The NCLEX-RN Candidate Performance Report provides you with information about the number of questions that you answered and about your performance on specific content areas of the examination.

Specific Content Areas

Following is a list of specific content areas:
Growth and Development through the Life Span
Prevention and Early Detection of Disease
Coping and Adaptation
Pharmacological and Parenteral Therapies
Physiological Adaptation
Psychosocial Integrity
Reduction of Risk Potential
Safety and Infection Control
Health Promotion and Maintenance
Management of Care
Basic Care and Comfort

In addition to the specific content area, the report provides you with the percentage of test questions in the content area, a description of the content area and a list of subject matter related to it, and a report of your performance. The report of your performance is stated as either Above the Passing Standard, Near the Passing Standard, or Below the Passing Standard. This report is your guide in developing a remediation plan, because it identifies your specific strengths and areas that need improvement.

> Use the NCLEX-RN Candidate Performance Report as a guide in developing a remediation plan!

HOW DO YOU DEVELOP AN ACADEMIC REMEDIATION PLAN?

It is important to use the NCLEX-RN Candidate Performance Report as your guide in developing a remediation plan. There are some steps to follow in developing the plan. Let us review the Pyramid to Success 10-step remediation plan and how these steps can be implemented.

Steps of a Remediation Plan

1. Include nonacademic preparation strategies in the remediation plan.
2. Review the performance report.
3. Prioritize the content areas.
4. Start the review with content areas Below the Passing Standard with the greatest percentage of test questions.
5. Review nursing content using review resources.
6. Practice test questions.

7. Take an assessment test or online specialty test.
8. Take a practice Computerized Adaptive Test (CAT).
9. Review any content areas that still need some fine-tuning.
10. Retake the NCLEX-RN.

Step 1: Include Nonacademic Preparation Strategies in the Remediation Plan

Nonacademic preparation strategies are an important component of preparing for this examination. Review your self-assessment and identify the areas related to nonacademic preparation that were obstacles in your path to success. It is critical that you address these obstacles as part of your remediation plan because you do not want to have to face these barriers to success again when you retake the examination. Chapter 6 describes the ways to prepare yourself for this examination from a nonacademic perspective, and it identifies the methods that can be used to deal with any obstacles that you faced the first time you took the examination.

Step 2: Review the Performance Report

Start by reviewing your performance report sent to you by the National Council of State Boards of Nursing and identify the content areas that were most difficult for you. It is important to read the description of the subject matter tested in each reported content area because this provides you with information regarding what you need to review.

Step 3: Prioritize the Content Areas

Prioritize the content areas noted on your performance report that require review and write these content areas in order of priority in your remediation plan. Remember that all content areas of the test need to be reviewed, even those that were reported as Above the Passing Standard. But you need to prioritize the content areas, with those areas Below the Passing Standard as the priority, followed by those content areas Near the Passing Standard, and finally those areas Above the Passing Standard.

Step 4: Start the Review with Content Areas Below the Passing Standard with the Greatest Percentage of Test Questions

You need to start your review with the content areas that were most difficult for you. These content areas are those that were identified as Below the Passing Standard. If you have more than one content area Below the Passing Standard, look at the percentage of test questions in those areas and begin your review with the area that identifies the greatest percentage of test questions. Once you have completed your review in the content areas identified as Below the Passing Standard, proceed to review content areas identified as Near the Passing Standard, followed by content areas identified as Above the Passing Standard.

Step 5: Review Nursing Content Using NCLEX-RN Review Resources

In the Pyramid to Success, there are several NCLEX-RN review resources available to help you prepare for retaking this examination. It is extremely beneficial to use NCLEX-RN review resources because the content and practice test questions that they contain focus on the subject matter identified in the NCLEX-RN Test Plan. Do not attempt to prepare to retake this examination by studying all of the class notes that you have from nursing school because they are much too detailed and you will become overwhelmed. Also, do not prepare to retake this examination by planning to read all of your nursing textbooks. You have already read them, and now you need to focus specifically on the subject matter that will be tested on the NCLEX-RN. Several of the resources available to you are identified in the various steps of your remediation plan, and a description of how the resource(s) will be beneficial is provided. Any of these resources can be obtained online at the Elsevier Health Web site (www.elsevierhealth.com).

> Use NCLEX-RN review resources to prepare!

As you prepare for this examination, it is important to review nursing content areas, particularly the subject matter identified as an area requiring improvement on your performance report. Therefore, you need to use NCLEX-RN review resources. The resources available in the Pyramid to Success that contain nursing content are the *Saunders Comprehensive Review for the NCLEX-RN Examination* and the *Saunders Online Review Course for the NCLEX-RN Examination*. The choice is yours, and the resource that you select may depend on your own individual needs. Below is a description of each resource. The descriptions will help you make a decision regarding which resource will work best for you.

The *Saunders Comprehensive Review for the NCLEX-RN Examination* has the following features:
- The book contains both nursing content of all areas of nursing, including pharmacology, and practice questions.
- Nursing content areas include all of the areas identified in the NCLEX-RN Test Plan.
- The CD-ROM contains 4000 practice questions, and therefore provides you with practice questions on a computer.
- All practice questions are presented in multiple choice format and in the alternate test questions format that is used in the NCLEX-RN.

- All practice questions provide a rationale for the correct and incorrect answer(s), a test-taking strategy, question codes based on the NCLEX-RN Test Plan categories and nursing content areas, content area to review if you answered the question incorrectly, and a reference source and page number.

The *Saunders Online Review Course for the NCLEX-RN Examination* has the following features:

- It is available as a 4-, 8-, or 16-week course.
- It contains a 75-question pretest that provides feedback regarding your strengths and areas in need of improvement.
- It generates an individualized study schedule in a calendar format; if you need assistance with developing a remediation plan, this program will do it for you.
- It provides nursing content review and includes all of the areas identified in the NCLEX-RN Test Plan.
- This course contains a total of 10 modules and 47 lessons.
- Every lesson contains content for review, illustrations, practice questions, and a case study followed by questions related to the case study.
- Each module is followed by a 100-question examination that contains questions representative of the content in the module lessons.
- It includes a 265-question comprehensive (cumulative) examination.
- It includes a CAT examination.
- All practice questions are presented in multiple choice format and in the alternate test questions format that is used in the NCLEX-RN.
- All lesson and case study questions, module examination questions, and questions in the comprehensive examination provide a rationale for the correct and incorrect answer(s), a test-taking strategy, question codes based on the NCLEX-RN Test Plan categories and nursing content areas, content area to review if the question was answered incorrectly, and a reference source and page number.

Step 6: Practice Test Questions

Practicing answering test questions is a must! Practicing answering test questions yields a two-fold reward: (1) you will strengthen your knowledge base of nursing content, and (2) you will become skillful in the use of test-taking strategies. The more you practice, the more prepared you will be for this examination.

Both the *Saunders Comprehensive Review for the NCLEX-RN Examination* and the *Saunders Online Review Course for the NCLEX-RN Examination* contain a wealth of practice test questions and can be used in this step of your remediation plan.

Practicing answering test questions is a must!

One other extremely helpful resource for repeat test-takers is the *Saunders Q & A Review for the NCLEX-RN Examination*, which includes a CD-ROM containing 3500 practice questions that are different from those in other resources. The reason that this resource is so helpful is that the book is uniquely designed to contain chapters with practice questions specific to each Client Needs area identified in the NCLEX-RN Test Plan. Therefore, if you are having difficulty with a specific Client Needs category of the Test Plan, you can refer to that specific Client Needs area in the book or on the CD-ROM and obtain practice questions that relate specifically to the area in which improvement is needed.

Because strengthening your nursing knowledge base and improving your test-taking skills are your goals, it is important that you use the NCLEX-RN Review resources in the most effective manner. If you are using the CD-ROM accompanying either the *Saunders Comprehensive Review for the NCLEX-RN Examination* or the *Saunders Q & A Review for the NCLEX-RN Examination*, it is best to access the Study Mode because you are given important information immediately after answering the question. This information includes a rationale for the correct and incorrect answer(s), a test-taking strategy, question codes based on the NCLEX-RN Test Plan categories and nursing content areas, content area to review if you answered the question incorrectly, and a reference source and page number. Therefore, your study efforts will be most productive in achieving your goals of strengthening your nursing knowledge base and improving your test-taking skills because you will gain knowledge and become skilled as you move along through your review.

Step 7: Take an Assessment Test or Online Specialty Test

After you have reviewed nursing content and practiced answering test questions, it is time to determine your readiness to take the NCLEX-RN a second time. It is important to feel comfortable and reassured that you are ready, because this will help you to maintain self-confidence in your ability to be successful and to sustain your positive attitude. A special resource designed to determine your readiness for the NCLEX-RN is the *Saunders Computerized Review for the NCLEX-RN Examination*. This resource contains 2000 analysis and application types of questions on a CD-ROM and provides you with specific feedback regarding your performance. Once you receive this feedback, you will be able to identify any remaining content areas that need that fine-tuning. If you note any remaining content areas that need fine-tuning, you may want to return to *Saunders Comprehensive Review for the NCLEX-RN Examination* and review these areas.

If you feel that you need to strengthen your knowledge base in a specific nursing content area, you may want to use one of the *Saunders Online Specialty Tests*. Online specialty tests are available for adult health, maternal-newborn, pediatrics, mental health, and pharmacology. Each test provides you with 100 practice test questions. Each question provides the correct and incorrect answer(s), a test-taking strategy, question codes based on the NCLEX-RN Test Plan categories and nursing content areas, content area to review if you answered the question incorrectly, and a reference source and page number. You will also receive specific feedback regarding your performance on the test.

SAUNDERS ONLINE SPECIALTY TESTS
Adult health
Maternal-newborn
Pediatrics
Mental health
Pharmacology

Step 8: Take a Practice Computerized Adaptive Test

Taking a practice CAT examination is the last step in your remediation process before you retake the examination. It is important to feel comfortable and reassured that you are ready to retake this examination, because this will help you to maintain confidence in your ability to be successful and to sustain your positive attitude. A practice CAT examination simulates the actual NCLEX experience, and after taking the CAT examination, you will know whether you are ready to retake the NCLEX-RN because you will be given feedback indicating whether you have passed or failed the examination. The *Saunders Online Review Course for the NCLEX-RN Examination* contains a CAT examination.

Take a practice CAT exam!

Step 9: Review Any Content Areas That Still Need Some Fine-tuning

If you received passing results on the practice CAT examination, it is time to retake the examination. If you received failing results, you need to do additional content review and practice questions before retaking the examination. If you received failing results, review your performance report again and the practice test results that you printed out from all of the tests that you took from the CD-ROMs in the review resources. Again, identify the content areas in need of improvement and focus on these areas before retaking the NCLEX-RN. Any of the NCLEX-RN resources can be used to help you fine-tune those areas in need of improvement.

Step 10: Retake the NCLEX-RN

It is time! Are you ready? Of course you are! As long as you followed your remediation plan and strengthened those content areas that needed improvement, you are ready! Now, what do you do?

Think positive!
Groom yourself for success on the day of the examination!
Maintain confidence and belief in yourself!
Meet the challenges of the day!
Retake the examination!
Become a Registered Nurse!
And, of course, don't forget to smile!

REFERENCES

National Council of State Boards of Nursing: Test Plan for the National Council Licensure Examination for Registered Nurses (effective date: April 2004), Chicago, 2003, National Council of State Boards of Nursing.

National Council of State Boards of Nursing: Examination Candidate Bulletin, Chicago, 2005, National Council of State Boards of Nursing.

National Council of State Boards of Nursing online: Available at www.ncsbn.org

Chapter 15

Tips for International Nurses

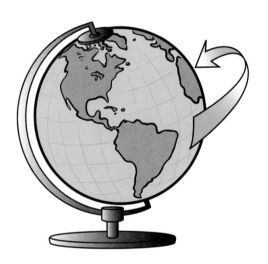

For an international or foreign-educated nurse, preparation to take the National Council Licensure Examination for Registered Nurses (NCLEX-RN) involves basically four processes. These processes include meeting the requirements defined by the U.S. immigration laws, meeting the eligibility requirements defined by the National Council of State Board of Nursing (NCSBN) and the specific state board of nursing for the state in which you intend to obtain licensure, registering to take the NCLEX-RN, and academic preparation for the examination.

This chapter provides information regarding the processes that you will have to pursue to become a registered nurse in the United States. An important factor to keep in mind is that some of the requirements may vary from state to state. Therefore, an important first step for you may be to contact the board of nursing for the state in which you are planning to obtain licensure. State board of nursing contact information can be obtained through the NCSBN Web site (http://www.ncsbn.org). Once you have accessed the NCSBN Web site, select the link titled "Boards of Nursing." In addition, you can write to, call, or fax the NCSBN regarding the NCLEX-RN (NCSBN, 111 E. Wacker Drive, Suite 2900, Chicago, IL 60601; [312] 525-3600 voice; [312] 279-1032 fax).

EXAMINATION PREPARATION

Meeting the requirements defined by U.S. immigration laws

Meeting the eligibility requirements defined by the NCSBN and your state's board of nursing

Registering to take the NCLEX-RN

Academic preparation for the NCLEX-RN

WHAT DO YOU NEED TO DO TO MEET THE REQUIREMENTS DEFINED BY UNITED STATES IMMIGRATION LAWS?

To meet the requirements defined by U.S. immigration laws, you are required to obtain a VisaScreen™ Certificate. The VisaScreen components include an educational analysis, license verification, assessment of proficiency in the English language, and an examination that tests nursing knowledge. All documents that verify eligibility must be submitted by the school or nursing program, licensure agency, or testing agency.

VISASCREEN COMPONENTS
Educational analysis
License verification
Assessment of proficiency in the English language
An examination that tests nursing knowledge

The VisaScreen

U.S. immigration law requires certain health care professionals to successfully complete a screening program before receiving an occupational visa (Section 343 of the Illegal Immigration Reform and Immigration Responsibility Act of 1996). Therefore, you are required to obtain a VisaScreen Certificate.

The Commission on Graduates of Foreign Nursing Schools (CGFNS) is the organization that offers this federal screening program. The International Commission on Health Care Professions (ICHP), a division of CGFNS, administers the VisaScreen. Once each of the VisaScreen components has been successfully achieved, you will be presented with a VisaScreen Certificate. Information related to the VisaScreen can be obtained through the CGFNS Web site (http://www.cgfns.org).

Educational Analysis

The educational analysis component of the VisaScreen requires the following documentation:
- Proof of completion of senior secondary school education, separate from any professional certification.
- Proof of completion from a government-approved professional health care program of at least 2 years in length.
- Proof of completion of a minimum number of clock and/or credit hours in specific theoretical and clinical areas while attending nursing school.

Licensure Verification

You must present all current and past licensure for review.

Proficiency in the English Language

You must submit proof of a passing score on an approved U.S. Department of Education and Health and Human Services English language proficiency examination. Acceptable English language proficiency examinations include the following:
- Test of English as a Foreign Language (TOEFL)
- Test of Written English (TWE) and Test of Spoken English (TSE)
- The Test of English for International Communication (TOEIC)

The testing organizations that administer the English language proficiency examinations include:

1. The Educational Testing Service (ETS; P.O. Box 6151, Princeton, NJ 08541-6151; [609] 771-7100; e-mail: toefl@ets.org) and
2. The International English Language Testing System (IELTS Administrator, Cambridge Examinations and IELTS International, 100 East Corson Street, Suite 200, Pasadena, CA 91103; [626] 564-2954; e-mail: ielts@ceii.org; Web site: http://www.ielts.org).

Examination to Test Nursing Knowledge

An examination to test nursing knowledge includes the following components:

1. The one-day Qualifying Exam that is administered as part of the process for obtaining a CGFNS Certificate tests nursing knowledge; therefore, a CGFNS Certificate provides proof of adequate nursing knowledge. This Qualifying Exam is described later in the section "What Are the Components of the Commission on Graduates of Foreign Nursing Schools Certification Program?"
2. A foreign-educated nurse who is licensed and practicing nursing in the United States also is required to obtain a VisaScreen; if the nurse does not have a CGFNS Certificate, the nurse may be granted eligibility to take the NCLEX-RN to provide proof of nursing knowledge.

WHAT ARE THE NATIONAL COUNCIL OF STATE BOARD OF NURSING AND SPECIFIC STATE BOARD OF NURSING REQUIREMENTS?

State requirements are developed based on the guidelines and requirements set by the NCSBN. Most states in the United States require that you receive certification from the CGFNS before you can be eligible to take the NCLEX-RN. If the state in which you intend to obtain licensure does not require CGFNS certification, it may require submission of some of the same documents that CGFNS required. Therefore, in addition to what CGFNS requires, a state may require the following:

- Proof of citizenship or lawful alien status
- Official transcripts of educational credentials sent directly to the board of nursing from your school of nursing
- Validation of theoretical instruction and clinical practice in a variety of nursing areas including medical nursing, surgical nursing, pediatric nursing, maternity and newborn nursing, and mental health nursing
- Copy of nursing license, diploma, or both
- Proof of proficiency in the English language
- Photographs of yourself
- Application fees

> Find out what the NCSBN and the specific state board of nursing require!

WHAT DOES THE COMMISSION ON GRADUATES OF FOREIGN NURSING SCHOOLS PROVIDE?

The CGFNS provides a certification program for nurses educated and licensed outside of the United States.

The Certificate Program offered by the CGFNS is a requirement of most state boards of nursing, and the certificate may be required before you can take the NCLEX-RN. The Certificate Program ensures that you are eligible and qualified to meet licensure and other practice requirement in the United States, and it predicts your success on the NCLEX-RN. This program also assists you in obtaining your VisaScreen Certificate. Additional information relating to CGFNS and its Certification Program can be obtained through the CGFNS Web site (http://www.cgfns.org).

> CGFNS provides a certification program for nurses educated and licensed outside of the United States!

WHAT ARE THE ELIGIBILITY REQUIREMENTS FOR THE COMMISSION ON GRADUATES OF FOREIGN NURSING SCHOOLS CERTIFICATION PROGRAM?

The CGFNS Certification Program is designed for nurses educated outside of the United States who hold both an initial and current registration/licensure as a first-level general registered nurse. According to the CGFNS, a first-level nurse is called a registered nurse or professional nurse in most countries. As a general nurse, the foreign-educated nurse must have obtained theoretical instruction and clinical practice in a variety of nursing areas. These nursing areas include medical nursing, surgical nursing, pediatric nursing, maternity and newborn nursing, and mental health nursing. If the nurse educated outside of the United States does not meet these requirements, he or she is not eligible for the Certification Program.

WHAT ARE THE COMPONENTS OF THE COMMISSION ON GRADUATES OF FOREIGN NURSING SCHOOLS CERTIFICATION PROGRAM?

The CGFNS Certification Program contains three parts, and all parts must be successfully completed to be awarded a CGFNS Certificate. The three parts include a credentials review, a 1-day qualifying examination that tests nursing knowledge, and an English language proficiency examination. The qualifying examination and the English language proficiency examination can be taken at various locations throughout the world. This provides you with the opportunity to obtain the CGFNS Certificate before coming to the United States to take the NCLEX-RN. These three parts of the Certificate Program are described in detail below.

COMPONENTS OF THE CGFNS CERTIFICATION PROGRAM

Credentials review

One-day qualifying examination that tests nursing knowledge

English language proficiency examination

Credentials Review

CGFNS requires validation of your education and your licensing history to ensure that you have the appropriate credentials to seek certification. CGFNS must receive transcripts and validation documents directly from your nursing program and the licensing agency. Transcripts and validation documents will not be accepted from the applicant. The specific credentialing requirements are similar to those needed for the VisaScreen Certificate and include the following:

- Completed senior secondary school education
- Graduated from a government approved nursing program of at least 2 years in length

- Obtained theoretical instruction and clinical practice in the areas of medical nursing, surgical nursing, pediatric nursing, maternity and newborn nursing, and mental health nursing
- Hold a full and unrestricted license or registration to practice as a first-level general nurse in the country where you completed your general nursing education
- Hold a current license or registration as a first-level general nurse

Qualifying Examination

The Qualifying Examination tests your knowledge in nursing in the areas of adult health, pediatrics, maternity and newborn, mental health, and community health. The examination is designed to ensure that you have the knowledge to provide nursing care to various client groups at the same level as recent U.S. nursing graduates.

English Language Proficiency Examination

You must take and pass an English language proficiency examination; the examination can be taken before or after the Qualifying Examination. This examination needs to be taken from a testing organization that is approved by CGFNS, and you must apply directly with the testing organization to take the examination. The examination scores must be sent directly to CGFNS from the testing organization. CGFNS will not accept test scores from the applicant. The types of English proficiency examinations, approved testing organizations, and their contact information were listed previously in the section "Proficiency in the English Language."

CGFNS identifies certain applicants as exempt from the English language proficiency requirement. For an applicant to be exempt, he or she must meet all of the following criteria: native language is English; country of nursing education is Australia, Canada (except Quebec), Ireland, New Zealand, or the United Kingdom; and language of instruction and textbooks was English.

Once you have successfully met each of the three required components of the CGFNS Certification Program, CGFNS will issue a certificate of completion. Unless the state in which you intend to obtain licensure indicates additional requirements, and if you have received your VisaScreen Certificate, you are eligible to take the NCLEX-RN.

HOW DO YOU REGISTER TO TAKE THE NATIONAL COUNCIL LICENSURE EXAMINATION FOR REGISTERED NURSES?

If you are planning to take the NCLEX-RN in the United States, the initial step in the registration process is to submit an application to the state board of nursing in the state in which you intend to obtain licensure. You need to obtain information from your state's board of nursing regarding the specific registration process because the process may vary from state to state. In most states, you may register for the examination through the Internet (the NCLEX-RN candidate Web site is http://www.vue.com/nclex), by mail, or by telephone. It is important that you follow the registration instructions and complete the registration forms precisely and accurately. Registration forms not properly completed, or not accompanied by the proper fees in the required method of payment, will be returned to you and will delay testing. There is a fee for taking the examination, and you may also have to pay additional fees to the board of nursing in the state in which you are applying. You will be sent confirmation indicating that your registration was received. If you do not receive a confirmation within 4 weeks of submitting your registration, you should contact the candidate services. Contact information can be obtained at the NCLEX-RN candidate Web site (http://www.vue.com/nclex).

> **REGISTERING FOR THE EXAMINATION**
> You may register for the examination through the Internet (http://www.vue.com/nclex), by mail, or by telephone.

Once your eligibility to take the NCLEX-RN has been verified by the board of nursing in the state in which licensure is requested, your registration form is processed and an Authorization to Test form will be sent to you. You cannot make an appointment until the board of nursing declares your eligibility and you receive an Authorization to Test form. The examination will take place at Pearson Professional Centers. An appointment can be made through the Internet or by telephone; and you can schedule an appointment at any Pearson Professional Center. You do not have to take the examination in the same state in which you are seeking licensure. A confirmation of your appointment will be sent to you. (See Chapters 1 and 2 for additional information regarding the NCLEX-RN and testing procedures.)

IS THE NATIONAL COUNCIL LICENSURE EXAMINATION FOR REGISTERED NURSES ADMINISTERED IN ANY LOCATIONS OUTSIDE OF THE UNITED STATES?

According to the NCSBN, as of January 2005, NCLEX-RN testing abroad is available. The places that provide this testing service are Seoul, South Korea; London, United Kingdom; and Hong Kong. Testing services abroad provide the nurse who is interested in becoming a licensed nurse in the United States an opportunity to pass the NCLEX-RN before traveling to the United States.

HOW DO YOU PREPARE ACADEMICALLY TO TAKE THE NATIONAL COUNCIL LICENSURE EXAMINATION FOR REGISTERED NURSES?

The challenge that is presented to you is one that requires patience and endurance. The positive result of your endeavor will certainly reward you professionally and give you the personal satisfaction of knowing you have become part of a family of highly skilled professionals, the Registered Nurse. After you have successfully completed the requirements to become eligible to take the NCLEX-RN, you will have one other important goal to achieve: passing the NCLEX-RN.

Adequate preparation for the NCLEX-RN is critical. Not only is this examination difficult, but it also tests you on your competence to practice as a registered nurse in the United States. What does this mean in terms of what you need to do to prepare academically? Some of these critical points are listed as follows:

> Know what you need to know!

You need to be knowledgeable with regard to nursing content in all areas of nursing as practiced in the United States. There may be some variations in the methods of delivering care from country to country, but you need to be familiar with the U.S. way of nursing care, so to speak.

You need to know the roles and responsibilities of the registered nurse practicing in the United States.

You need to understand the purpose and use of a Nurse Practice Act.

You need to understand words and acceptable abbreviations used in nursing in the United States.

You need to be knowledgeable about the communication process used in the United States and be able to use therapeutic communication techniques effectively.

You need to be knowledgeable about the medications that are used to treat health conditions in the United States and how to administer medications.

You need to understand each step of the Nursing Process.

You need to understand the NCLEX-RN Test Plan and the testing procedures.

You need to be familiar with the types of questions that are used in the NCLEX-RN.

You need to be skillful in the use of test-taking strategies to answer questions.

You need to know how to develop a study plan.

You need to know how to prepare yourself from a nonacademic perspective.

You need to know when you are adequately prepared to take the NCLEX-RN.

These are some of the critical points that you need to address as you prepare to take this examination. The task of preparing may seem overwhelming, but do not despair. An important step that you have already taken in preparing is that you are using this book and, as a result, are becoming familiar with the NCLEX-RN Test Plan, the examination process, the types of questions on the examination, nonacademic preparation strategies, and test-taking strategies. There are also additional resources available to you that will help you to address all of the critical points related to this examination. It is vital that you use review resources to prepare, because they will focus your review on essential content areas. Several of these review resources are described below, together with suggestions regarding their use. As you decide on a review resource for preparation, think about your needs and determine which resource or resources will meet your needs. These review resources can be obtained online at the Elsevier Health Web site (www.elsevierhealth.com).

> Review resources can be obtained online at:
> http://www.elsevierhealth.com

Saunders Comprehensive Review for the NCLEX-RN Examination

The *Saunders Comprehensive Review for the NCLEX-RN Examination* is a valuable tool that contains both content and practice questions. Its accompanying CD-ROM contains 4000 practice questions; therefore, the format provides you with questions on a computer. The questions are presented in multiple choice format and in the alternate test questions format that is used in the NCLEX-RN. When using this CD-ROM, it is best to access the Study Mode because you are given important information immediately after answering the question. This information includes the correct answer, rationale for the correct and incorrect options, the test-taking strategy for answering the question correctly, content area to review if you answered the question incorrectly, and the reference source and page number. Therefore, you learn as you move along through your review. As you are studying, if you have difficulty with a specific topic, make a note of it and be sure to review the topic.

> *Saunders Comprehensive Review for the NCLEX-RN Examination* contains nursing content and 4000 practice questions!

Saunders Online Review Course for the NCLEX-RN Examination

The *Saunders Online Review Course for the NCLEX-RN Examination* is an online course that is available as a 4-, 8-, or 16-week course. It contains a 75-question pretest that provides feedback regarding your strengths and areas in need of improvement. Based on the pretest, the program generates an individualized study schedule in a calendar format; therefore, if you need assistance with developing a study plan, this program will do it for you. The program provides nursing content review and includes all of the areas identified in the NCLEX-RN Test Plan. It contains a total of 10 modules and 47 lessons. Every lesson contains content for review, illustrations, practice questions, and a case study followed by questions related to the case study, and each module is followed by a 100-question examination that contains questions representative of the content in the module lessons. The program also includes a 265-question comprehensive (cumulative) examination and a Computerized Adaptive Testing (CAT) examination that simulates the NCLEX-RN testing experience.

All of the practice questions are presented in multiple choice format and in the alternate test questions format that is used in the NCLEX-RN. All lesson and case study questions, module examination questions, and comprehensive examination questions provide a rationale for the correct and incorrect answer(s), a test-taking strategy, question codes based on the NCLEX-RN Test Plan categories and nursing content areas, content area to review if you answered the question incorrectly, and a reference source and page number.

> *Saunders Online Review Course for the NCLEX-RN Examination* contains a CAT examination!

Saunders Q & A Review for the NCLEX-RN Examination

Another extremely helpful resource is the *Saunders Q & A Review for the NCLEX-RN Examination,* which includes a CD-ROM containing 5000 practice questions that are different from those in the other resources. The reason that this resource is so helpful is that the book is uniquely designed to contain chapters with practice questions specific to each Client Needs area identified in the NCLEX-RN Test Plan. Therefore, as you are reviewing, if you are having difficulty with a specific Client Needs category of the Test Plan, you can refer to that specific Client Needs area in the book or on the CD-ROM and obtain practice questions that relate specifically to the area in which improvement is needed.

As with the *Saunders Comprehensive Review for the NCLEX-RN Examination*, when using this CD-ROM, it is best to access the Study Mode because you are given important information immediately after answering the question. This information includes the correct answer, rationale for the correct and incorrect options, the test-taking strategy for answering the question correctly, content area to review if you answered the question incorrectly, and the reference source and page number. Therefore, you learn as you move along through your review.

> *Saunders Q & A Review for the NCLEX-RN Examination* is uniquely designed to contain chapters with practice questions specific to each Client Needs area identified in the NCLEX-RN Test Plan.

Saunders Computerized Review for the NCLEX-RN Examination

A special resource designed to determine your readiness for the NCLEX-RN is the *Saunders Computerized Review for the NCLEX-RN Examination*. This resource contains 2000 analysis and application types of questions on a CD-ROM and provides you with specific feedback regarding your performance. Once you receive this feedback, you will be able to identify any remaining content areas that need further review. Using this resource will help to determine your readiness. If you determine that there are any remaining content areas that need review, you will need to return to *Saunders Comprehensive Review for the NCLEX-RN Examination* and review these areas.

> *Saunders Computerized Review for the NCLEX-RN Examination* determines your readiness to take the examination!

Saunders Online Specialty Tests

If you believe that you need to strengthen your knowledge base in a specific nursing content area, you may want to use one of the *Saunders Online Specialty Tests*. Online specialty tests are available for adult health, maternal-newborn, pediatrics, mental health, and pharmacology. Each test provides you with 100 practice test questions. Each question provides the correct and incorrect answer(s), a test-taking strategy, question codes based on the NCLEX-RN Test Plan categories and nursing content areas, content area to review if you answered the question incorrectly, and a reference source and page number. You also will receive specific feedback regarding your performance on the test.

> **SAUNDERS ONLINE SPECIALTY TESTS**
> Adult health
> Maternal-newborn
> Pediatrics
> Mental health
> Pharmacology

WISHING YOU SUCCESS!

Never lose sight of the goals that you want to achieve. Patience and dedication will contribute significantly to achieving the status of Registered Nurse. Remember, success is climbing a mountain, facing the challenge of obstacles, and reaching the top of the mountain. I wish you the best success in your career as a registered nurse in the United States of America!

REFERENCES

Commission on Graduates of Foreign Nursing Schools online: Available at http://www.cgfns.org

Educational Testing Service online: Available at http://www.ets. org/toefl

International English Testing System online: Available at http://www. ielts.org

National Council of State Boards of Nursing online: Available at http://www.ncsbn.org

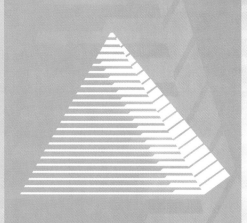

"A study method that I used to help me pass NCLEX exam involved three easy steps. First, I did several practice questions from my review books and CD-ROMS and made a list of every disease process or drug with which I was not familiar. Next, I took the list and made flash cards with all of the pertinent details of the content area in which I was unfamiliar. I then studied each flash card and attempted to learn the 'hows' and 'whys' of the material instead of just memorizing it. In the third and final step, I decided to 'teach' the information to another person – either a nursing school buddy, family member, or my roommate. I found that teaching the material to another person dramatically helped to reinforce my own understanding of each concept. I hope that this method helps someone else – good luck to everyone studying for the NCLEX exam!"
—Robert, Clayton College and State University, Morrow, Georgia

"STUDY, STUDY, STUDY! & PRACTICE, PRACTICE, PRACTICE! As part of our last semester we were required to complete no less than 10 practice NCLEX exams with a score of at least 85% correct. In accomplishing this, the average number of practice exams completed per student was at least 25 to 30. Each exam had to be at least 50 questions with the recommended number being 100 questions each. I personally used four review products including the complete NCLEX review series from Saunders by Linda Silvestri. I also attended a review course to prepare for the exam. I know that this sounds like a lot (and it was!) but when it came time to take the test for real, I had no anxiety and knew that I had done everything I could to prepare for a successful outcome. Considering that I spent 45 minutes and only had 75 questions on the exam and passed on the first attempt, I would say that all of the effort paid off. I wish each of you much success in your preparation for the exam and know that each of you possess the required knowledge to pass the exam. You just need to know how to take the test and this is where the prep courses and practice exams will truly prove invaluable."
—Tom, Wallace Community College, Dothan, Alabama

Part IV

Practice Test

1. A client receiving therapy at a mental health clinic says to the nurse, "When I have a stressful day at work and when my boss 'is on my case all day,' I go home and take my frustrations out on my children." The most appropriate response to this client is which of the following?

   1   "Why do you do this? Can you think of another way to take out your frustrations?"

   2   "The only way to take out your frustrations is to join a health care center that provides equipment for weight-lifting and boxing."

   3   "Is there someplace that you can go after work to relieve your frustrations before going home?"

   4   "Let's talk about some other ways that you can handle your frustrations."

Answer: 4

Rationale: The nursing response in option 4 provides the client the opportunity to problem solve. Option 1 uses the word *why*, and this word can make the client feel defensive and often implies criticism. Option 2 is incorrect because physical activity is not the only way to relieve frustrations. In addition, this suggestion may not be appropriate for this client. Option 3 avoids the fact that the client needs to deal with the issue: taking her frustrations out on her children.

Test-Taking Strategy: Note the keywords *most appropriate* and use therapeutic communication techniques. Eliminate option 1 because of the word *why*. Next, eliminate option 2 because of the absolute word *only*. From the remaining options, note that option 3 is similar to option 2 (options that are similar are incorrect), and that option 4 provides the client the opportunity to problem solve. Review therapeutic communication techniques and the test-taking strategies for answering communication questions if you had difficulty with this question.

Level of Cognitive Ability: Application
Client Needs: Psychosocial Integrity
Integrated Process: Communication and Documentation
Content Area: Mental Health

Reference
Stuart G, Laraia M: *Principles and practice of psychiatric nursing*, ed 7, St Louis, 2001, Mosby, p 29.

---

2. A physician orders 3000 mL 0.9% normal saline solution to be administered intravenously (IV) over a 24-hour period. The nurse sets the flow rate to infuse how many milliliters per hour?
   Answer: _____

Answer: 125

Rationale: Use the IV formula to determine milliliters per hour.

Formula:

$$\frac{\text{Total volume (mL)}}{\text{Number of hours}} = \text{mL/hr}$$

$$\frac{3000 \text{ mL}}{24 \text{ hours}} = 125 \text{ mL/hr}$$

Test-Taking Strategy: Use the formula for calculating IV infusion rates. Remember, use a calculator, follow the formula, recheck your answer, and make sure that the answer makes sense before documenting the answer. Review the test-taking strategies for answering IV calculation questions if you had difficulty with this question.

Level of Cognitive Ability: Application
Client Needs: Physiological Integrity

Integrated Process: Nursing Process/Implementation
Content Area: Fundamental Skills

Reference
Kee J, Marshall S: *Clinical calculations: with applications to general and specialty areas,* ed 5, Philadelphia, 2004, WB Saunders, pp 204–205.

---

3. A female client admitted to the mental health unit for treatment of depression says to a female nurse, "Women always get put down. It's as if we are useless members of society." The most appropriate nursing response is which of the following?
   1   "Tell me how you feel as a woman."
   2   "Yes, that does happen to women, but it doesn't mean that women have to stand for that kind of treatment."
   3   "I never let anyone make me feel as though I am useless!"
   4   "Think about it. That's no longer true in today's society."

Answer: 1
Rationale: In option 1, the nurse uses the therapeutic technique of focusing and encourages the client to verbalize and expand on her feelings. In option 2, the nurse agrees with the client, and then takes a forceful stance with regard to how the client should deal with these feelings. In option 3, the nurse provides an opinion; in addition, this option uses the absolute word *never.* In option 4, the nurse disagrees with the client.

Test-Taking Strategy: Note the keywords *most appropriate* and use therapeutic communication techniques. Eliminate option 3 first because of the absolute word *never;* in addition, in this option, the nurse provides an opinion, which is nontherapeutic. Next, eliminate options 2 and 4. In option 2, the nurse agrees with the client; in option 4, the nurse disagrees with the client. Review therapeutic communication techniques and the test-taking strategies for answering communication questions if you had difficulty with this question.

Level of Cognitive Ability: Application
Client Needs: Psychosocial Integrity
Integrated Process: Communication and Documentation
Content Area: Mental Health

Reference
Stuart G, Laraia M: *Principles and practice of psychiatric nursing,* ed 7, St Louis, 2001, Mosby, p 31.

---

4. Erythromycin has been prescribed for a client with otitis media. To ensure optimal absorption, the nurse tells the client to take the medication
   1   On an empty stomach
   2   Immediately after a meal
   3   Just before eating
   4   With a snack such as peanut butter and crackers

Answer: 1
Rationale: Erythromycin is an antibiotic. It may be taken without regard to meals, but optimal absorption occurs when taken on an empty stomach.

Test-Taking Strategy: If you are unfamiliar with the medication identified in the question (erythromycin), noting that it is prescribed to treat otitis media provides the clue that it is an antibiotic. Focus on the issue: ensuring optimal absorption. Note that options 2, 3, and 4 are similar in that they all indicate taking the medication with food. Review this medication and the test-taking strategies for answering pharmacology questions if you had difficulty with this question.

Level of Cognitive Ability: Application
Client Needs: Physiological Integrity

Integrated Process: Nursing Process/Implementation
Content Area: Pharmacology

Reference

Hodgson B, Kizior R: *Saunders nursing drug handbook 2004,* Philadelphia, 2004, WB Saunders, p 373.

---

5. A nurse employed in a mental health unit is meeting with a client for the first time. Which nursing statement would be most appropriate to initiate the conversation?
   1 "Have psychiatric medications ever been prescribed for you?"
   2 "What would you like to discuss?"
   3 "Are you feeling sad?"
   4 "Have you ever been admitted to a mental health facility?"

Answer: 2

Rationale: The nursing statement in option 2 is an open-ended question and encourages conversation because it requires more than a one-word answer. In options 1, 3, and 4, the nurse attempts to obtain information from the client; however, these statements are close-ended in that the client can respond by a "yes" or "no" response. These statements do not encourage discussion.

Test-Taking Strategy: Note the keywords *most appropriate* and use therapeutic communication techniques. Eliminate options 1, 3, and 4 because they are similar and all are close-ended questions. Review therapeutic communication techniques and the test-taking strategies for answering communication questions if you had difficulty with this question.

Level of Cognitive Ability: Application
Client Needs: Psychosocial Integrity
Integrated Process: Communication and Documentation
Content Area: Mental Health

Reference

Varcarolis EM: *Foundations of psychiatric mental health nursing,* ed 4, Philadelphia, 2002, WB Saunders, p 254.

---

6. Metoprolol tartrate (Toprol XL) has been prescribed for a client to treat hypertension. To enhance absorption, the nurse tells the client to take the medication
   1 Crushed in apple sauce
   2 With a meal
   3 With 8 oz grapefruit juice
   4 With 1 oz aluminum hydroxide (Amphojel)

Answer: 2

Rationale: Metoprolol tartrate is a beta-adrenergic blocker that is used to treat hypertension. To enhance absorption, it is administered with or immediately after meals.

Test-Taking Strategy: If you are unfamiliar with the medication identified in the question (metoprolol tartrate), noting that its name ends with *-lol* provides the clue that it is a beta-adrenergic blocker. Noting the letters *XL* after the medication name provides the clue that the medication is extended release. Focus on the issue: enhancing optimal absorption. Also use pharmacology guidelines to answer the question. Remember, sustained (extended)-release tablets should not be crushed, and grapefruit juice and antacids are not administered with medication because these items affect absorption. Review this medication and the test-taking strategies for answering pharmacology questions if you had difficulty with this question.

Level of Cognitive Ability: Application
Client Needs: Physiological Integrity

Integrated Process: Nursing Process/Implementation
Content Area: Pharmacology

Reference
Hodgson B, Kizior R: *Saunders nursing drug handbook 2004,* Philadelphia, 2004, WB Saunders, p 664.

---

7. A nurse is having a conversation with a client admitted to a mental health unit. The client says to the nurse, "I work in a factory doing piece work, and I am very competitive with the people that I work with." Which of the following is the most appropriate nursing response?
   1   "In other words, you seem to be saying that you try to do better than your fellow employees."
   2   "When you are being paid by piece work, you need to be competitive."
   3   "Why are you competitive? After all, you get paid based on the amount of work that you do, not your fellow employees."
   4   "Do you find that your fellow employees are competitive also?"

Answer: 1
Rationale: Option 1 uses the therapeutic technique of paraphrasing. In paraphrasing, the nurse restates in different words what the client has stated to confirm an understanding of what the client has said. In option 2, the nurse agrees with the client. In option 3, the nurse uses the word *why,* and this word can make the client feel defensive and often implies criticism. Option 4 focuses on fellow employees, not the client.

Test-Taking Strategy: Note the keywords *most appropriate* and use therapeutic communication techniques. Eliminate option 4 first because it does not focus on the client. Next, eliminate option 3 because the nurse uses the word *why.* From the remaining options, eliminate option 2 because the nurse agrees with the client. In addition, option 1 uses the therapeutic technique of paraphrasing. Review therapeutic communication techniques and the test-taking strategies for answering communication questions if you had difficulty with this question.

Level of Cognitive Ability: Application
Client Needs: Psychosocial Integrity
Integrated Process: Communication and Documentation
Content Area: Mental Health

Reference
Varcarolis EM: *Foundations of psychiatric mental health nursing,* ed 4, Philadelphia, 2002, WB Saunders, p 254.

---

8. A physician's order reads, "morphine sulfate, gr 1/8 intramuscularly stat." The medication ampule reads, "morphine sulfate, 10 mg/mL." A nurse prepares how many milliliters to administer the correct dose?
   Answer: _____

Answer: 0.75
Rationale: It is necessary to convert gr 1/8 to milligrams. After converting grains to milligrams, use the formula to calculate the correct dose.

Conversion:

$$60 \text{ mg} : \text{gr } 1 :: \text{x mg} : \text{gr } 1/8$$

$$1x = 1/8 \times 60/1$$

$$x = 60/8 = 7.5 \text{ mg}$$

Formula:

$$\frac{\text{Desired}}{\text{Available}} \times \text{X mL} = \text{milliliters per dose}$$

$$\frac{7.5 \text{ mg}}{10 \text{ mg}} \times 1 \text{ mL} = 0.75 \text{ mL}$$

Test-Taking Strategy: In this medication calculation problem, it is necessary to first convert grains to milligrams. Next, use a calculator and follow the formula for the calculation of the correct dose. Label each figure, including the answer. Recheck your work, making sure that the answer makes sense. Review the test-taking strategies for answering medication calculation questions if you had difficulty with this question.

Level of Cognitive Ability: Application
Client Needs: Physiological Integrity
Integrated Process: Nursing Process/Implementation
Content Area: Fundamental Skills

Reference
Kee J, Marshall S: *Clinical calculations: with applications to general and specialty areas,* ed 5, Philadelphia, 2004, WB Saunders, p 80.

---

9. A client says to the nurse, "Ever since my wife passed on, my life is empty and has no meaning." Which of the following is the most appropriate nursing response?
   1. "What would your children think if they knew how you felt?"
   2. "Most people who lose a loved one feel empty."
   3. "Your life has no meaning?"
   4. "Let's talk about the positive things that you have in your life."

Answer: 3
Rationale: In option 3, the nurse uses the therapeutic technique of restating. In this technique, the nurse explores more thoroughly topics that are significant to the client. Option 1 does not focus on the client's feelings; rather, it focuses on the client's children. Option 2 generalizes and does not focus on the client. Option 4 avoids the client's feelings.

Test-Taking Strategy: Note the keywords *most appropriate* and use therapeutic communication techniques. Eliminate options 1 and 4 first because they are similar and do not focus on the client's feelings. Next, eliminate option 2 because it is a generalized statement and stereotypes the client. Option 3 uses the therapeutic technique of restating. Review therapeutic communication techniques and the test-taking strategies for answering communication questions if you had difficulty with this question.

Level of Cognitive Ability: Application
Client Needs: Psychosocial Integrity
Integrated Process: Communication and Documentation
Content Area: Mental Health

Reference
Varcarolis EM: *Foundations of psychiatric mental health nursing,* ed 4, Philadelphia, 2002, WB Saunders, p 255.

---

10. Flurbiprofen (Ocufen) is prescribed for a client with osteoarthritis. On a follow-up visit to the physician's office, the nurse asks the client whether the medication has provided relief from which of the following?
    1. Indigestion
    2. Diarrhea
    3. Abdominal cramps
    4. Pain

Answer: 4
Rationale: Flurbiprofen is a nonsteroidal antiinflammatory medication that reduces inflammatory response and the intensity of pain stimulus that reaches sensory nerve endings. In the client with osteoarthritis, the intended effect is pain relief. Indigestion, diarrhea, and abdominal cramps are occasional side effects of the medication.

Test-Taking Strategy: Note the keywords *provided relief from.* Also note that the question provides the client's diagnosis. Recalling the pathophysiology related to osteoarthritis will assist in directing you to option 4. In addition, options 1, 2, and 3 are similar in that they all address gastrointestinal symptoms. Review this medication and the test-taking strategies for answering pharmacology questions if you had difficulty with this question.

Level of Cognitive Ability: Analysis
Client Needs: Physiological Integrity
Integrated Process: Nursing Process/Evaluation
Content Area: Pharmacology

Reference
Hodgson B, Kizior R: *Saunders nursing drug handbook 2004,* Philadelphia, 2004, WB Saunders, p 432.

---

11. Select all nursing statements that indicate the use of a therapeutic communication technique.

___ "You will do just fine. You'll see."
___ "What would you like to discuss?"
___ "I wouldn't worry about that."
___ "Can you describe your feelings?"
___ "Can you tell me what the voices are saying?"

Answer:

___ "You will do just fine. You'll see."
_X_ "What would you like to discuss?"
___ "I wouldn't worry about that."
_X_ "Can you describe your feelings?"
_X_ "Can you tell me what the voices are saying?"

Rationale: The nursing statement "What would you like to discuss?" is therapeutic and is an open-ended question that invites the client to share personal feelings. The nursing statements "Can you describe your feelings?" and "Can you tell me what the voices are saying?" are therapeutic and are focused statements that are exploratory. The nursing statements "I wouldn't worry about that," and "You will do just fine. You'll see," are nontherapeutic and provide false reassurance.

Test-Taking Strategy: Read each nursing statement and focus on the issue: use of therapeutic communication techniques. Recalling the therapeutic and nontherapeutic techniques will assist in answering the question. Review therapeutic communication techniques and the test-taking strategies for answering communication questions if you had difficulty with this question.

Level of Cognitive Ability: Application
Client Needs: Psychosocial Integrity
Integrated Process: Communication and Documentation
Content Area: Mental Health

Reference
Varcarolis EM: *Foundations of psychiatric mental health nursing,* ed 4, Philadelphia, 2002, WB Saunders, pp 255, 258.

---

12. Adalimumab (Humira) is added to the medication regimen for a client with severe rheumatoid arthritis. The nurse provides instructions to

Answer: 2

Rationale: Adalimumab is a disease-modifying antirheumatic drug and a monoclonal antibody that binds to, and thereby neutralizes, tumor necrosis factor. It reduces the client about the medication and tells the client that

1   The medication is used to slow the progression of joint damage but cannot be coadministered with an analgesic
2   The medication is used to slow the progression of joint damage and can be coadministered with an analgesic
3   The medication is available in an oral liquid form only
4   The medication never needs to be refrigerated

symptoms and slows the progression of joint damage. This medication can be used alone or in combination with methotrexate or other antirheumatic medicines. It is administered by subcutaneous injection. It should be stored in a cold environment at 2 to 8°C (36 to 46°F) and protected from light.

Test-Taking Strategy: Eliminate option 3 because of the absolute word *only* and eliminate option 4 because of the absolute word *never*. Also note that options 1 and 2 indicate opposite statements; this may indicate that one of these options is correct. Note that the client has severe rheumatoid arthritis and that adalimumab is *added to the medication regimen*. This will direct you to option 2. Review this medication and the test-taking strategies for answering pharmacology questions if you had difficulty with this question.

Level of Cognitive Ability: Application
Client Needs: Physiological Integrity
Integrated Process: Teaching/Learning
Content Area: Pharmacology

Reference
Lehne R: *Pharmacology for nursing care,* ed 5, Philadelphia, 2004, WB Saunders, pp 770t, 772.

---

13. A psychiatrist prescribes aripiprazole (Abilify) for a client with a diagnosis of schizophrenia. Which of the following nursing interventions would be most therapeutic?

1   Administer the medication only after meals.
2   Instruct the client that the medication may cause sedation and should be taken at bedtime.
3   Advise the client to increase his usual exercise pattern threefold to help with medication absorption.
4   Advise the client to limit his alcohol intake to one drink each day.

Answer: 2

Rationale: Aripiprazole is an antipsychotic agent that may be referred to as a dopamine system stabilizer. Because antipsychotic agents cause sedation, bedtime dosing helps promote sleep and decreases daytime drowsiness. It may be administered with or without food and is well absorbed in the presence or absence of food. It is not necessary for the client to increase his or her usual exercise pattern to assist in absorption of the medication. Alcohol is avoided, not limited.

Test-Taking Strategy: Noting that the client has schizophrenia will assist in determining that the medication is an antipsychotic. Eliminate option 1 because of the absolute word *only*. Eliminate option 4 recalling that alcohol intake is avoided, not limited. From the remaining options, eliminate option 3 because of the words *increase his usual exercise pattern threefold*. Also note that option 2 is the more global (umbrella) option. Review the characteristics of this medication and the test-taking strategies for answering pharmacology questions if you had difficulty with this question.

Level of Cognitive Ability: Application
Client Needs: Physiological Integrity
Integrated Process: Teaching/Learning
Content Area: Pharmacology

Reference
Lehne R: *Pharmacology for nursing care,* ed 5, Philadelphia, 2004, WB Saunders, pp 284t, 293–294.

14. A nurse is having a conversation with a client and responds to the client's statement by saying, "You say that your mother left you when you were six years old." What therapeutic communication technique is the nurse using?

1 Sharing observations
2 Restating
3 Summarizing
4 Focusing

Answer: 2

Rationale: In restating, the nurse repeats the main thought that the client expressed. The nurse shares observations by commenting on how the client looks, sounds, or acts. Summarizing is a concise review of key aspects of a conversation. Focusing centers on key elements of a message.

Test-Taking Strategy: Focus on the nursing statement. Also, noting the keywords *You say that* in the nursing statement will assist in identifying the technique that the nurse is using. Review therapeutic communication techniques and the test-taking strategies for answering communication questions if you had difficulty with this question.

Level of Cognitive Ability: Application
Client Needs: Psychosocial Integrity
Integrated Process: Communication and Documentation
Content Area: Mental Health

Reference
Stuart G, Laraia M: *Principles and practice of psychiatric nursing,* ed 7, St Louis, 2001, Mosby, p 34.

---

15. A client says to the nurse, "My doctor ordered adefovir (Hespera) for me, so I guess I'll soon be cured." Which nursing response would be most therapeutic?

1 "Yes. Although it's relatively new and its results remain tentative, it does seem so."
2 "Yes, it will cure the disease, but you will want to monitor for side effects and stop the medication immediately if any occur."
3 "Although this medication cannot cure your disease, it will control it."
4 "Yes, but just be certain to divide the dosage as the doctor has indicated in his instructions."

Answer: 3

Rationale: Adefovir is an antiviral medication that is used to treat clients with chronic hepatitis B who exhibit active viral replication and persistent increases of liver function blood levels. It controls the disease but does not cure it. Its mechanism is similar to acyclovir (Zovirax), and it is used with caution in older adults and people who may have untreated human immunodeficiency virus infection. Nephrotoxicity is the primary concern with use of this medication. Administration of this medication should not be stopped suddenly. It is usually administered once daily without regard to food.

Test-Taking Strategy: If you are unfamiliar with this medication, note the letters *vir* in its name. These letters indicate that the medication is an antiviral. Note that options 1, 2, and 4 are similar in that they all indicate that the client will be cured of the disease. Option 3 is the option that is different. Review the characteristics of this medication and the test-taking strategies for answering pharmacology questions if you had difficulty with this question.

Level of Cognitive Ability: Application
Client Needs: Physiological Integrity
Integrated Process: Teaching/Learning
Content Area: Pharmacology

Reference
Lehne R: *Pharmacology for nursing care,* ed 5, Philadelphia, 2004, WB Saunders, pp 975–976.

16. A clinic nurse is performing a medication assessment on a client being seen in that clinic for the first time. The nurse notes that the client takes terbutaline (Brethine) and asks the client about a history of which disorder that is treated with this medication?

  1   Ulcerative colitis
  2   Congestive heart failure
  3   Asthma
  4   Hypothyroidism

Answer: 3

Rationale: Terbutaline is an oral beta-adrenergic agonist bronchodilator that is used to treat asthma. It is not used to treat ulcerative colitis, congestive heart failure, or hypothyroidism.

Test-Taking Strategy: Focus on the name of the medication. Recalling that most xanthine bronchodilator medication names end with *-line* will direct you to option 3. Review the characteristics of this medication and the test-taking strategies for answering pharmacology questions if you had difficulty with this question.

Level of Cognitive Ability: Analysis
Client Needs: Physiological Integrity
Integrated Process: Nursing Process/Assessment
Content Area: Pharmacology

Reference
Lehne R: *Pharmacology for nursing care*, ed 5, Philadelphia, 2004, WB Saunders, p 798.

---

17. A nurse is preparing to administer medications to a client in the hospital and notes that the client takes levothyroxine (Synthroid) daily. The nurse suspects that the client has a history of

  1   Hypothyroidism
  2   Hyperthyroidism
  3   Hypotension
  4   Hypertension

Answer: 1

Rationale: Levothyroxine is a synthetic thyroid hormone used to treat hypothyroidism. It is not used to treat hyperthyroidism, hypotension, or hypertension.

Test-Taking Strategy: Focus on the name of the medication. Recalling that most thyroid medications contain the letters *thy* in their name will assist in eliminating options 3 and 4. From the remaining options, eliminate option 2 because it would be harmful to administer thyroid to a client who is in a hyperthyroid state. Review this medication and the test-taking strategies for answering pharmacology questions if you had difficulty with this question.

Level of Cognitive Ability: Analysis
Client Needs: Physiological Integrity
Integrated Process: Nursing Process/Analysis
Content Area: Pharmacology

Reference
Hodgson B, Kizior R: *Saunders nursing drug handbook 2004*, Philadelphia, 2004, WB Saunders, p 596.

---

18. Sucralfate (Carafate) is prescribed for a client with a gastric ulcer. The nurse tells the client to take the medication

  1   One hour before meals and at bedtime
  2   Just after meals
  3   With meals and at bedtime
  4   With a snack at bedtime

Answer: 1

Rationale: Sucralfate is an antiulcer medication and should be scheduled for administration 1 hour before meals and at bedtime. Administration at these times allows it to form a protective coating over the ulcer before food intake stimulates gastric acid production and mechanical irritation. The bedtime dose protects the stomach lining during sleep.

Test-Taking Strategy: Note the similarities in options 2, 3, and 4, and then eliminate these options. Each of these options indicates taking the medication with a food item. Review the characteristics of this medication and the test-taking strategies for answering pharmacology questions if you had difficulty with this question.

Level of Cognitive Ability: Application
Client Needs: Health Promotion and Maintenance
Integrated Process: Teaching/Learning
Content Area: Pharmacology

Reference
Hodgson B, Kizior R: *Saunders nursing drug handbook 2004,* Philadelphia, 2004, WB Saunders, p 940.

---

19. Sulfasalazine (Azulfidine) is prescribed for a client with ulcerative colitis. The nurse determines that the medication is achieving the intended effect if the client reports which of the following?
1 Increased urinary output
2 Formed stools
3 Absence of nausea
4 Relief of headaches

Answer: 2

Rationale: Sulfasalazine is a sulfonamide that is used to treat acute ulcerative colitis and to prevent recurrences. It acts by inhibiting prostaglandin synthesis, thus reducing inflammation. The intended effect that occurs as a result of reducing bowel inflammation is the relief of diarrhea and production of formed stools. Options 1, 3, and 4 are not intended effects of this medication.

Test-Taking Strategy: Focus on the issue: an intended effect of the medication. Noting that the client has ulcerative colitis will assist in directing you to option 2. Also, remember that medication names that include the letters *sulf* are sulfonamides; this will also assist in answering the question correctly. Review the characteristics of this medication and the test-taking strategies for answering pharmacology questions if you had difficulty with this question.

Level of Cognitive Ability: Analysis
Client Needs: Physiological Integrity
Integrated Process: Nursing Process/Evaluation
Content Area: Pharmacology

Reference
Ignatavicius D, Workman M: *Medical-surgical nursing: critical thinking for collaborative care,* ed 4, Philadelphia, 2002, WB Saunders, p 1285.

---

20. A nurse is reviewing the plan of care for a child with juvenile rheumatoid arthritis (JRA). The nurse determines that which of the following is a priority nursing diagnosis?
1 Disturbed Body Image
2 Risk for Bathing/Hygiene Self-care Deficit
3 Risk for Injury
4 Acute Pain

Answer: 4

Rationale: All of the nursing diagnoses are appropriate for the child with JRA. The priority nursing diagnosis relates to pain. Acute pain needs to be managed before other problems can be addressed.

Test-Taking Strategy: Note the keyword *priority.* Using Maslow's Hierarchy of Needs theory, remember that physiological needs (option 4) receive greatest priority. Option 3 addresses safety and security needs. Option 1 addresses self-esteem needs. Option 2 identifies an at-risk (potential), not an actual, problem. Review care to the child with JRA and the test-taking strategies for answering prioritizing questions if you had difficulty with this question.

Level of Cognitive Ability: Analysis
Client Needs: Physiological Integrity
Integrated Process: Nursing Process/Planning
Content Area: Delegating/Prioritizing

Reference
Wong D, Hockenberry M: *Wong's nursing care of infants and children,* ed 7, St Louis, 2003, Mosby, p 1823.

---

21. The nurse is assessing for the presence of cyanosis in a dark-skinned client. The nurse checks which best site for the presence of cyanosis?
    1 Soles of the feet
    2 Back of the hands
    3 Conjunctiva of the eye
    4 Ear lobes

Answer: 3

Rationale: In a dark-skinned client, the presence of cyanosis can be best seen in the areas where the epidermis is thin and pigmentation is lighter. These areas include the conjunctiva of the eye, mucous membranes, and nail beds. In a light-skinned client, cyanosis can be most easily detected in nail beds, ear lobes, lips, mucous membranes, and palms and soles of the feet.

Test-Taking Strategy: Focus on the issue: cyanosis. Also note the keyword *best* and that the client has dark skin. Eliminate options 1, 2, and 4 because these options are similar, and they identify body areas where the epidermis is thick. Review skin assessment techniques and the various test-taking strategies if you had difficulty with this question.

Level of Cognitive Ability: Application
Client Needs: Health Promotion and Maintenance
Integrated Process: Nursing Process/Assessment
Content Area: Adult Health/Cardiovascular

Reference
Lewis S, Heitkemper M, Dirksen S: *Medical-surgical nursing: assessment and management of clinical problems,* ed 6, St Louis, 2004, Mosby, p 483.

---

22. A nurse is assessing the risk factors for acquiring pneumonia during hospitalization for a group of clients. The nurse determines that which of the following clients is at lowest risk?
    1 An older client with diabetes mellitus
    2 A client with human immunodeficiency virus (HIV)
    3 A client with a spinal cord injury who is immobile
    4 A postoperative client who is ambulating

Answer: 4

Rationale: The postoperative client who is ambulating is at lowest risk. This client has had no direct insult to the respiratory tract. Clients with HIV, an upper respiratory infection, or a chronic disease (e.g., heart, lung, or kidney disease; diabetes mellitus; or cancer) are at greater risk for development of pneumonia. Clients who are on bed rest and are immobilized also are at risk for development of pneumonia.

Test-Taking Strategy: This is a false response question. Note the keywords *lowest risk,* which tell you that the correct option will be the client who does not have a significant risk for development of pneumonia. Focusing on these keywords will direct you to option 4. Review the risk factors related to development of pneumonia and the test-taking strategies for answering false response questions if you had difficulty with this question.

Level of Cognitive Ability: Analysis
Client Needs: Health Promotion and Maintenance
Integrated Process: Nursing Process/Assessment
Content Area: Adult Health/Respiratory

Reference
Lewis S, Heitkemper M, Dirksen S: *Medical-surgical nursing: assessment and management of clinical problems,* ed 6, St Louis, 2004, Mosby, p 593.

---

23. A physician orders 500 mL normal saline to infuse intravenously (IV) over 5 hours. The drop factor is 10 drops/mL. A nurse sets the flow rate at how many drops per minute? (Round answer to the nearest whole number.)
Answer:_____

Answer: 17
Rationale: Use the IV flow rate formula.

Formula:

$$\frac{\text{Total volume} \times \text{gtt factor}}{\text{Time in minutes}} = \text{gtt per min}$$

$$\frac{500 \text{ mL} \times 10 \text{ gtt}}{300 \text{ minutes}} = \frac{5000}{300} = 16.6, \text{ or } 17 \text{ drops/min}$$

Test-Taking Strategy: Use the formula for calculating IV flow rates. Remember, use a calculator, follow the formula, recheck your answer, and make sure that the answer makes sense before documenting the answer. Review the test-taking strategies for answering IV calculation questions if you had difficulty with this question.

Level of Cognitive Ability: Application
Client Needs: Physiological Integrity
Integrated Process: Nursing Process/Implementation
Content Area: Fundamental Skills

Reference
Kee J, Marshall S: *Clinical calculations: with applications to general and specialty areas,* ed 5, Philadelphia, 2004, WB Saunders, pp 204–205.

---

24. A client with an iron deficiency anemia is taking an iron supplement and tells the nurse that she is going to stop the medication because it causes constipation. The nurse responds most appropriately by stating which of the following?
  1 "Constipation is bothersome, but it is much more important to take the medication."
  2 "Constipation is most intense during initial therapy and becomes less bothersome with continued use."

Answer: 2
Rationale: Constipation is a side effect of iron supplements, but this side effect becomes less bothersome with continued use. In addition, there are measures to take to alleviate this side effect. Option 2 addresses the client's concern. In options 1 and 3, the nurse disapproves of the client's feelings. In addition, the nurse lectures the client in these options. Option 4 places the client's issue on hold.

Test-Taking Strategy: Use therapeutic communication techniques. Eliminate option 3 because of the absolute word *never.* Next, eliminate option 4 because it places the client's issue on hold. From the remaining options, remembering to focus on the client's feelings and concerns will direct you to option 2. Review client teaching points for

3 "Never stop taking any medication without talking to the doctor first."

4 "In time you will get used to this side effect."

administering iron tablets and the test-taking strategies for answering communication questions if you had difficulty with this question.

Level of Cognitive Ability: Application
Client Needs: Psychosocial Integrity
Integrated Process: Communication and Documentation
Content Area: Fundamental Skills

Reference
Harkreader H, Hogan MA: *Fundamentals of nursing: caring and clinical judgment,* ed 2, Philadelphia, 2004, WB Saunders, pp 251, 255–257.

---

25. A client has been recently diagnosed with diabetes mellitus. The nurse does which of the following as the first step in teaching the client about the disorder?

1 Gathers all available resource materials

2 Plans for the evaluation of the session

3 Identifies the client's knowledge and needs

4 Decides on the teaching approach

Answer: 3

Rationale: Determining what to teach a client begins with an assessment of the client's own knowledge and learning needs. Once these factors have been determined, the nurse can effectively plan a teaching approach, the actual content, and resource materials that may be needed. The evaluation is done after teaching is completed.

Test-Taking Strategy: Note the keyword *first.* Use the steps of the nursing process. Remember that assessment is the first step. Review teaching and learning principles and the test-taking strategies for answering prioritizing questions if you had difficulty with this question.

Level of Cognitive Ability: Application
Client Needs: Health Promotion and Maintenance
Integrated Process: Teaching/Learning
Content Area: Delegating/Prioritizing

Reference
Harkreader H, Hogan MA: *Fundamentals of nursing: caring and clinical judgment,* ed 2, Philadelphia, 2004, WB Saunders, p 262.

---

26. A client with heart disease says to the nurse, "I guess I'll never be able to eat ice cream again." The nurse most appropriately responds with which of the following statements?

1 "There are lots of other foods you can eat."

2 "Ice cream has too much fat content, so why would you even want to eat it."

3 "You don't think you will be able to eat ice cream at all?"

4 "Why do you say that?"

Answer: 3

Rationale: The nurse most appropriately responds by rephrasing the client's statement. Option 3 is a therapeutic response and rephrases the client's statement. Options 1, 2, and 4 are examples of nontherapeutic communication techniques. Options 1 and 2 give advice. In addition, option 2 lectures to the client. Option 4 requests an explanation from the client.

Test-Taking Strategy: Use therapeutic communication techniques. Option 3 is the only therapeutic response and rephrases the client's statement. Review therapeutic communication techniques and the test-taking strategies for answering communication questions if you had difficulty with this question.

Level of Cognitive Ability: Application
Client Needs: Psychosocial Integrity

Integrated Process: Communication and Documentation
Content Area: Fundamental Skills

Reference
Harkreader H, Hogan MA: *Fundamentals of nursing: caring and clinical judgment,* ed 2, Philadelphia, 2004, WB Saunders, pp 251, 255–257.

---

27. A client scheduled for a coronary artery bypass graft states to the nurse, "I'm not sure if I should have this surgery." Which of the following responses by the nurse is most appropriate?
  1 "Don't worry. Everything will be fine."
  2 "It's your decision."
  3 "Why don't you want to have this surgery?"
  4 "Tell me what concerns you have about the surgery."

Answer: 4
Rationale: The nurse needs to gather more data and assist the client in exploring his or her feelings about the surgery. Options 1, 2, and 3 are nontherapeutic. Option 1 provides false reassurance. Option 2 is a blunt response and does not address the client's concern. Option 3 can make the client feel defensive.

Test-Taking Strategy: Use therapeutic communication techniques. Option 4 is the only option that addresses the client's concern. Review therapeutic communication techniques and the test-taking strategies for answering communication questions if you had difficulty with this question.

Level of Cognitive Ability: Application
Client Needs: Psychosocial Integrity
Integrated Process: Communication and Documentation
Content Area: Fundamental Skills

Reference
Harkreader H, Hogan MA: *Fundamentals of nursing: caring and clinical judgment,* ed 2, Philadelphia, 2004, WB Saunders, pp 251, 255–257.

---

28. A client states, "It will be so hard to wait for the results of this biopsy. I don't know what I will do if the results are positive." What is the most appropriate response by the nurse?
  1 "It's not good for you to worry."
  2 "Most biopsies end up being negative, so don't worry about it."
  3 "You sound concerned about the results of this test."
  4 "You are in good hands; even if it is positive, your doctor is the best."

Answer: 3
Rationale: The nurse needs to gather more data and assist the client in exploring his or her feelings about the results of the biopsy. The nurse should not disregard the client's feelings. Options 1, 2, and 4 are incorrect. These statements provide false reassurances and do not focus on the client's feelings.

Test-Taking Strategy: Use therapeutic communication techniques. Options 1, 2, and 4 are nontherapeutic, provide false reassurances, and do not focus on the client's feelings. Option 3 addresses the client's concern. Review therapeutic communication techniques and the test-taking strategies for answering communication questions if you had difficulty with this question.

Level of Cognitive Ability: Application
Client Needs: Psychosocial Integrity
Integrated Process: Communication and Documentation
Content Area: Fundamental Skills

Reference
Harkreader H, Hogan MA: *Fundamentals of nursing: caring and clinical judgment,* ed 2, Philadelphia, 2004, WB Saunders, pp 251, 255–257.

29. A client will be receiving long-term continuous total parenteral nutrition (TPN) at home. The nurse formulates which priority nursing diagnosis for the client?
  1   Ineffective Coping
  2   Hopelessness
  3   Social Isolation
  4   Risk for Situational Low Self-esteem

Answer: 3

Rationale: The client will be receiving TPN long term and continuously at home. Therefore, the client will be socially isolated from stimuli outside the home. There are no data in the question to support options 1, 2, or 4.

Test-Taking Strategy: Focus on the data provided in the question and note the keywords *long-term*, *continuous*, and *at home*. Eliminate options 1, 2, and 4 because there are no data in the question to support these options. Review care to the client receiving TPN and the various test-taking strategies if you had difficulty with this question.

Level of Cognitive Ability: Analysis
Client Needs: Psychosocial Integrity
Integrated Process: Nursing Process/Planning
Content Area: Fundamental Skills

Reference
Lewis S, Heitkemper M, Dirksen S: *Medical-surgical nursing: assessment and management of clinical problems,* ed 6, St Louis, 2004, Mosby, p 991.

---

30. A physician orders 1000 mL normal saline to infuse intravenously at a rate of 125 mL/hr. A nurse determines that it will take how many hours for 1 L to infuse?
  Answer: _____

Answer: 8

Rationale: It is necessary to determine that 1 L = 1000 mL. Next, use the formula for determining infusion time in hours.

Formula:

$$\frac{\text{Total volume to infuse}}{\text{Milliliters per hour being infused}} = \text{Infusion time}$$

$$\frac{1000 \text{ mL}}{125 \text{ mL}} = 8 \text{ hours}$$

Test-Taking Strategy: Read the question carefully and note that the question is asking about infusion time in hours. First, recall that 1 L = 1000 mL. Next, use a calculator and use the formula for determining infusion time in hours. Review the test-taking strategies for answering intravenous calculation questions if you had difficulty with this question.

Level of Cognitive Ability: Analysis
Client Needs: Physiological Integrity
Integrated Process: Nursing Process/Analysis
Content Area: Fundamental Skills

Reference
Kee J, Marshall S: *Clinical calculations: with applications to general and specialty areas,* ed 5, Philadelphia, 2004, WB Saunders, p 202.

31. A client has been taking fosinopril (Monopril). The nurse determines that the medication is having the intended effect if the nurse notes which of the following?
1. Relief of diarrhea
2. Decreased pulse rate
3. Relief of headaches
4. Decreased blood pressure

Answer: 4

Rationale: Monopril is an angiotensin-converting enzyme (ACE) inhibitor that decreases blood pressure. It can cause tachycardia as a side effect of therapy. Other side effects of the medication are neutropenia and agranulocytopenia. Options 1, 2, and 3 are not intended effects of the medication.

Test-Taking Strategy: Note the keywords *intended effect.* Recalling that most ACE inhibitors end with *-pril* and that these medications are used to treat hypertension will direct you to option 4. Review this medication and the test-taking strategies for answering pharmacology questions if you had difficulty with this question.

Level of Cognitive Ability: Analysis
Client Needs: Physiological Integrity
Integrated Process: Nursing Process/Evaluation
Content Area: Pharmacology

Reference
Hodgson B, Kizior R: *Saunders nursing drug handbook 2004,* Philadelphia, 2004, WB Saunders, p 446.

---

32. A nurse is caring for a client who is receiving a potassium-sparing diuretic. The nurse monitors for which side effect of the medication?
1. Hypernatremia
2. Hyperkalemia
3. Constipation
4. Diaphoresis

Answer: 2

Rationale: A potassium-sparing diuretic spares potassium, which means that potassium is retained in the body. Side effects of potassium-sparing diuretics usually include hyperkalemia, dehydration, hyponatremia, and lethargy. Although hypokalemia is a concern with the administration of most diuretics, hyperkalemia is a concern with the administration of a potassium-sparing medication. Additional side effects of this type of medication include nausea, vomiting, cramping, diarrhea, headache, ataxia, drowsiness, confusion, and fever.

Test-Taking Strategy: Note the keywords *potassium-sparing* and focus on the issue: a side effect. Recalling that a potassium-sparing diuretic spares potassium will direct you to option 2. Review the characteristics of this medication and the test-taking strategies for answering pharmacology questions if you had difficulty with this question.

Level of Cognitive Ability: Analysis
Client Needs: Physiological Integrity
Integrated Process: Nursing Process/Assessment
Content Area: Pharmacology

Reference
Lehne R: *Pharmacology for nursing care,* ed 5, Philadelphia, 2004, WB Saunders, pp 406–407.

33. A client is scheduled for a diagnostic procedure requiring the injection of a radiopaque dye. The nurse checks which most critical information before the procedure?
1   Intake and output
2   Baseline vital signs
3   Height and weight
4   History of allergy to iodine or shellfish

Answer: 4

Rationale: Procedures that involve the injection of a radiopaque dye require an informed consent. The risk for allergic reaction exists if the client has an allergy to iodine or shellfish. The risk for allergic reaction and possible anaphylaxis must be determined before the procedure. Although options 1, 2, and 3 identify information obtained before the procedure, these are not the most critical items.

Test-Taking Strategy: Note the keywords *most critical.* Use the ABCs—airway, breathing, and circulation. The risk for an allergic reaction and anaphylaxis makes option 4 correct. Review the complications associated with injection of a radiopaque dye and the test-taking strategies for answering prioritizing questions if you had difficulty with this question.

Level of Cognitive Ability: Application
Client Needs: Physiological Integrity
Integrated Process: Nursing Process/Assessment
Content Area: Delegating/Prioritizing

Reference
Black J, Hawks J: *Medical-surgical nursing: clinical management for positive outcomes,* ed 7, Philadelphia, 2005, WB Saunders, p 103.

---

34. Cefuroxime axetil (Ceftin), 1 g in 50 mL normal saline, is to be administered over 30 minutes. The drop factor is 15 drops/mL. A nurse sets the flow rate at how many drops per minute?
Answer: _____

Answer: 25

Rationale: Use the intravenous (IV) flow rate formula.

Formula:

$$\frac{\text{Total volume} \times \text{gtt factor}}{\text{Time in minutes}} = \text{gtt per min}$$

$$\frac{50 \text{ mL} \times 15 \text{ gtt}}{30 \text{ minutes}} = \frac{750}{30} = 25 \text{ drops/min}$$

Test-Taking Strategy: Use the formula for calculating IV flow rates. Remember, use a calculator, follow the formula, recheck your answer, and make sure that the answer makes sense before documenting the answer. Review the test-taking strategies for answering IV calculation questions if you had difficulty with this question.

Level of Cognitive Ability: Application
Client Needs: Physiological Integrity
Integrated Process: Nursing Process/Implementation
Content Area: Fundamental Skills

Reference
Kee J, Marshall S: *Clinical calculations: with applications to general and specialty areas,* ed 5, Philadelphia, 2004, WB Saunders, pp 204–205.

35. A nurse is preparing to perform a venipuncture to initiate continuous intravenous (IV) therapy with 0.9% normal saline solution. The nurse gathers the needed supplies and does which of the following before performing the venipuncture?
1 Applies a tourniquet below the chosen venipuncture site
2 Inspects the 0.9% normal saline solution for particles or contamination
3 Places an armboard at the joint located above the venipuncture site
4 Places cool compresses over the vein to be used for the venipuncture

Answer: 2
Rationale: All IV solutions should be free of particles or precipitates. A tourniquet is applied above the chosen venipuncture site. Cool compresses cause vasoconstriction, making the vein less visible. Armboards are applied only if necessary and after the IV infusion is started.

Test-Taking Strategy: Visualize the procedure for preparing to initiate an IV infusion. This will assist in eliminating options 1 and 3. From the remaining options, use principles related to heat and cold to eliminate option 4. Review the procedure for performing a venipuncture and the various test-taking strategies if you had difficulty with this question.

Level of Cognitive Ability: Application
Client Needs: Physiological Integrity
Integrated Process: Nursing Process/Implementation
Content Area: Fundamental Skills

Reference
Harkreader H, Hogan MA: *Fundamentals of nursing: caring and clinical judgment*, ed 2, Philadelphia, 2004, WB Saunders, pp 594–598.

---

36. A nurse is caring for a client after an allogeneic liver transplant and is receiving tacrolimus (Prograf). The nurse monitors the client for which adverse effect of the medication?
1 Decrease in urine output
2 Hypotension
3 Profuse sweating
4 Photophobia

Answer: 1
Rationale: Tacrolimus is an immunosuppressant medication used in the prophylaxis of organ rejection in clients receiving allogeneic liver transplants. Frequent side effects include headache, tremor, insomnia, paresthesia, diarrhea, nausea, constipation, vomiting, abdominal pain, and hypertension. Adverse and toxic effects include nephrotoxicity, neurotoxicity, and pleural effusion. Nephrotoxicity is characterized by an increase in serum creatinine level and a decrease in urine output. Neurotoxicity, including tremor, headache, and mental status changes, can occur.

Test-Taking Strategy: Use medical terminology to identify the medication. Look at the medication name, Prograf (*pro* means "for," and *graf* means "graft"). This assists you in identifying the action of the medication (to prevent transplant rejection) and classifying it as an immunosuppressant (which may, in turn, assist you in remembering the side effects and adverse and toxic effects of the medication). Review this medication and the test-taking strategies for answering pharmacology questions if you had difficulty with this question.

Level of Cognitive Ability: Analysis
Client Needs: Physiological Integrity
Integrated Process: Nursing Process/Assessment
Content Area: Pharmacology

Reference
Hodgson B, Kizior R: *Saunders nursing drug handbook 2004*, Philadelphia, 2004, WB Saunders, p 948.

37. An antepartum client is diagnosed with bacterial vaginosis. The nurse expects to note which of the following on assessment of the client?
  1 Hematuria and hypertension
  2 Itching and vaginal discharge
  3 Proteinuria and hematuria
  4 Costovertebral angle pain

Answer: 2

Rationale: Clinical manifestations of bacterial vaginosis include pain, itching, and a thick, white vaginal discharge. Proteinuria, hematuria, hypertension, and costovertebral angle pain are clinical manifestations associated with urinary tract infections.

Test-Taking Strategy: Focus on the information in the question. Note the relation between the words *vaginosis* in the question and *vaginal* in option 2. Also, remember that when options contain two parts and each part is separated by the word *and*, all parts of the option must be correct. Review the clinical manifestations of bacterial vaginosis and the various test-taking strategies if you had difficulty with this question.

Level of Cognitive Ability: Analysis
Client Needs: Physiological Integrity
Integrated Process: Nursing Process/Assessment
Content Area: Maternity/Antepartum

Reference
Lowdermilk D, Perry A: *Maternity & women's health care*, ed 8, St Louis, 2004, Mosby, p 206.

38. A nurse is caring for a client who has pheochromocytoma. The nurse is monitoring for the major symptom of pheochromocytoma when the nurse
  1 Tests the client's urine for occult blood
  2 Takes the client's weight
  3 Palpates the client's skin for its temperature
  4 Takes the client's blood pressure

Answer: 4

Rationale: Hypertension is the major symptom associated with pheochromocytoma. The blood pressure status is monitored by taking the client's blood pressure. Glycosuria, weight loss, and diaphoresis are clinical manifestations as well; however, hypertension is the major symptom. Hematuria is not associated with this disorder.

Test-Taking Strategy: Note the keyword *major*. Use the ABCs—airway, breathing, and circulation. A method of monitoring circulation is to take the blood pressure. Review the clinical manifestations associated with this disorder and the various test-taking strategies if you had difficulty with this question.

Level of Cognitive Ability: Application
Client Needs: Physiological Integrity
Integrated Process: Nursing Process/Assessment
Content Area: Adult Health/Endocrine

Reference
Lewis S, Heitkemper M, Dirksen S: *Medical-surgical nursing: assessment and management of clinical problems*, ed 6, St Louis, 2004, Mosby, p 1335.

39. A nurse is assessing a client who was treated for an asthma attack. The nurse determines that the client's respiratory status has worsened if which of the following is noted?

Answer: 4

Rationale: Diminished breath sounds are an indication of obstruction and possible impending respiratory failure. Wheezing is not a reliable manifestation to determine the severity of an asthma attack. For wheezing to occur, the

1   Loud wheezing
2   Wheezing during inspiration and expiration
3   Wheezing on expiration only
4   Diminished breath sounds

client must be able to move sufficient air to produce breath sounds. The client with a severe asthma attack may have no audible wheezing because of the decrease of airflow. Clients may experience loud wheezes with minor attacks, whereas others may not wheeze with severe attacks. Wheezing usually occurs first on expiration. The client may wheeze during both inspiration and expiration as the asthma attack progresses.

Test-Taking Strategy: Eliminate option 3 because of the absolute word *only*. From the remaining options, focus on the keywords *respiratory status has worsened.* Use the ABCs—airway, breathing, and circulation. Remember that diminished breath sounds indicate obstruction and possibly respiratory failure. Review assessment of the client experiencing an asthma attack and the various test-taking strategies if you had difficulty with this question.

Level of Cognitive Ability: Analysis
Client Needs: Physiological Integrity
Integrated Process: Nursing Process/Analysis
Content Area: Adult Health/Respiratory

Reference
Lewis S, Heitkemper M, Dirksen S: *Medical-surgical nursing: assessment and management of clinical problems,* ed 6, St Louis, 2004, Mosby, p 640.

---

40. A physician's office nurse is assessing a client who recently had a renal transplant. The nurse monitors for which signs of acute graft rejection?
1   Hypotension, graft tenderness, and anemia
2   Hypertension, oliguria, thirst, and hypothermia
3   Fever, vomiting, hypotension, and copious amounts of dilute urine
4   Fever, hypertension, graft tenderness, and malaise

Answer: 4
Rationale: Acute rejection usually occurs within the first 3 months after transplantation, although it can occur for up to 2 years after transplantation. The client exhibits fever, hypertension, malaise, and graft tenderness. Options 1, 2, and 3 do not completely identify signs of acute rejection.

Test-Taking Strategy: Focus on the issue: acute graft rejection. Remember that when an option contains more than one part, all parts of the option need to be correct. Begin to answer this question by eliminating options 1 and 3, because hypotension is not part of the clinical picture with graft rejection. Select option 4 instead of option 2 because fever accompanies this complication, not hypothermia. Review the signs of acute graft rejection and the various test-taking strategies if you had difficulty with this question.

Level of Cognitive Ability: Analysis
Client Needs: Physiological Integrity
Integrated Process: Nursing Process/Assessment
Content Area: Adult Health/Renal

Reference
Lewis S, Heitkemper M, Dirksen S: *Medical-surgical nursing: assessment and management of clinical problems,* ed 6, St Louis, 2004, Mosby, p 1242.

41. A nurse is caring for a client who has a fungal infection and is receiving amphotericin B (Fungizone) intravenously. Which of the following indicates that the client is experiencing an adverse or toxic effect from the medication?
1 Lethargy
2 Decreased urinary output
3 Muscle weakness
4 Confusion

Answer: 2

Rationale: Amphotericin B is an antifungal agent. Adverse reactions include nephrotoxicity evidenced by decreased urinary output. Cardiovascular toxicity, as evidenced by hypotension and ventricular fibrillation, and anaphylactic reaction rarely occur. Vision and hearing alterations, seizures, hepatic failure, and coagulation defects also may occur. Options 1, 3, and 4 are not associated with an adverse effect.

Test-Taking Strategy: Focus on the information in the question. Noting that the client has a fungal infection will assist in determining that an antifungal medication is being administered. Remembering that this medication causes nephrotoxicity, cardiovascular toxicity, and vision and hearing alterations leads you to option 2. Review the characteristics of this medication and the test-taking strategies for answering pharmacology questions if you had difficulty with this question.

Level of Cognitive Ability: Analysis
Client Needs: Physiological Integrity
Integrated Process: Nursing Process/Assessment
Content Area: Pharmacology

Reference
Hodgson B, Kizior R: *Saunders nursing drug handbook 2004,* Philadelphia, 2004, WB Saunders, p 55.

42. Penicillin V potassium (Pen-Vee K) has been prescribed to treat a client in the hospital with a respiratory tract infection. Which priority action will the nurse take before administering the medication?
1 Call the pharmacy to order the medication
2 Ask the client about a history of allergies
3 Inform the client about the importance of deep-breathing exercises
4 Tell the client to report symptoms of a rash or itching immediately

Answer: 2

Rationale: Penicillin V potassium is an antibiotic. Before administering the medication, the nurse performs a baseline assessment and questions the client about a history of allergies to penicillin or to a cephalosporin. Although the nurse would need to order the medication and teach the client about the adverse effects of the medication, assessment for allergy is the priority (the medication would not be given to the client if an allergy exists). Although deep-breathing exercises are important for a client with a respiratory infection, this action is not directly related to administering penicillin V potassium.

Test-Taking Strategy: If you are unfamiliar with the medication identified in the question (penicillin V potassium), noting that it is prescribed for a respiratory infection provides the clue that it is an antibiotic. Note the keyword *priority* and the issue of the question: the action that the nurse will take. Using pharmacology guidelines will direct you to option 2. Also, using the steps of the nursing process will direct you to option 2 because it is the only option that addresses assessment. Options 1, 3, and 4 address implementation. Review the characteristics of this medication and the test-taking strategies for answering pharmacology questions if you had difficulty with this question.

Level of Cognitive Ability: Application
Client Needs: Physiological Integrity
Integrated Process: Nursing Process/Implementation
Content Area: Pharmacology

Reference

Hodgson B, Kizior R: *Saunders nursing drug handbook 2004*, Philadelphia, 2004, WB Saunders, p 791.

---

43. Gentamicin sulfate (Garamycin), 80 mg in 100 mL normal saline, is to be administered over 30 minutes. The drop factor is 10 drops/mL. A nurse sets the flow rate at how many drops per minute? (Round answer to the nearest whole number.)
Answer: _____

Answer: 33

Rationale: Use the intravenous (IV) flow rate formula.

Formula:

$$\frac{\text{Total volume} \times \text{gtt factor}}{\text{Time in minutes}} = \text{gtt per minute}$$

$$\frac{100 \text{ mL} \times 10 \text{ gtt}}{30 \text{ minutes}} = \frac{1000}{30} = 33.3, \text{ or } 33 \text{ drops/min}$$

Test-Taking Strategy: Use the formula for calculating IV flow rates. Remember, use a calculator, follow the formula, recheck your answer, and make sure that the answer makes sense before documenting the answer. Review the test-taking strategies for answering IV calculation questions if you had difficulty with this question.

Level of Cognitive Ability: Application
Client Needs: Physiological Integrity
Integrated Process: Nursing Process/Implementation
Content Area: Fundamental Skills

Reference

Kee J, Marshall S: *Clinical calculations: with applications to general and specialty areas*, ed 5, Philadelphia, 2004, WB Saunders, pp 204–205.

---

44. A physician's order reads 150 mcg levothyroxine (Synthroid) PO daily. The medication label reads 0.1 mg Synthroid per tablet. A nurse administers how many tablet(s) to the client?
Answer: _____

Answer: 1.5

Rationale: It is necessary to convert 150 mcg to milligrams. In the metric system, to convert smaller to larger, divide by 1000 or move the decimal three places to the left. Therefore, 150 mcg = 0.15 mg. Next, use the formula to calculate the correct dose.

Formula:

$$\frac{\text{Desired}}{\text{Available}} \times \text{tablet(s)} = \text{tablets per dose}$$

$$\frac{0.15 \text{ mg}}{0.1 \text{ mg}} \times 1 \text{ tablet} = 1.5 \text{ tablets}$$

Test-Taking Strategy: In this medication calculation problem, it is necessary first to convert micrograms to milligrams. Remember, use a calculator, follow the formula, recheck your answer, and make sure that the answer makes sense before documenting the answer. Review the test-taking strategies for answering medication calculation questions if you had difficulty with this question.

Level of Cognitive Ability: Application
Client Needs: Physiological Integrity
Integrated Process: Nursing Process/Implementation
Content Area: Fundamental Skills

Reference
Kee J, Marshall S: *Clinical calculations: with applications to general and specialty areas,* ed 5, Philadelphia, 2004, WB Saunders, p 80.

---

45. The nurse notes that a hospitalized client is receiving sotalol (Betapace). The nurse monitors the client for which side effect related to the medication?
1   Difficulty swallowing
2   Diaphoresis
3   Dry mouth
4   Bradycardia

Answer: 4

Rationale: Sotalol is a beta-adrenergic blocking agent. Side effects include bradycardia, palpitations, difficulty breathing, irregular heart beat, signs of congestive heart failure, and cold hands and feet. Gastrointestinal disturbances, anxiety and nervousness, and unusual tiredness and weakness also can occur. Options 1, 2, and 3 are not side effects.

Test-Taking Strategy: Focus on the issue: a side effect. Remember that medication names ending with *-lol* are beta-blockers, which are commonly used for cardiac disorders. The only option that is directly cardiac related is option 4. Review the characteristics of this medication and the test-taking strategies for answering pharmacology questions if you had difficulty with this question.

Level of Cognitive Ability: Analysis
Client Needs: Physiological Integrity
Integrated Process: Nursing Process/Assessment
Content Area: Pharmacology

Reference
Hodgson B, Kizior R: *Saunders nursing drug handbook 2004,* Philadelphia, 2004, WB Saunders, p 928.

---

46. A nurse is developing a plan of care for a client in Buck's extension traction. The nurse identifies which nursing diagnosis as the priority?
1   Deficient diversional activity
2   Risk for social isolation
3   Risk for impaired skin integrity
4   Risk for loneliness

Answer: 3

Rationale: Buck's skin traction is a type of traction in which weights are attached to the skin with the use of a boot. The priority nursing diagnosis for the client is impaired skin integrity. Risk for altered neurovascular status also is a concern. Options 1, 2, and 4 may also be appropriate for the client in Buck's skin traction, but risk for impaired skin integrity presents the greatest risk.

Test-Taking Strategy: Note the keyword *priority.* Use Maslow's Hierarchy of Needs theory. The only option that indicates a physiological need is option 3. Options 1, 2, and 4 indicate psychosocial needs. Review care to the client in Buck's extension traction and the test-taking strategies for answering prioritizing questions if you had difficulty with this question.

Level of Cognitive Ability: Analysis
Client Needs: Physiological Integrity
Integrated Process: Nursing Process/Planning
Content Area: Adult Health/Musculoskeletal

Reference
Lewis S, Heitkemper M, Dirksen S: *Medical-surgical nursing: assessment and management of clinical problems*, ed 6, St Louis, 2004, Mosby, pp 1660, 1664.

---

47. A client is being taught how to self-administer insulin. The client says to the nurse, "I'm not sure I will be able to do this." Which of the following statements by the nurse is the most appropriate?
1   "What are your concerns about giving yourself insulin?"
2   "Don't worry. Everyone is unsure at first."
3   "You'll be fine once you get used to giving your own shots."
4   "Maybe your wife or daughter can give you your shot."

Answer: 1
Rationale: Option 1 restates the client's concern and provides the client the opportunity to verbalize. Options 2 and 3 indicate false reassurances, which invalidate the client's concerns. Option 4 offers advice without knowing what the client's concerns really are.

Test-Taking Strategy: Use therapeutic communication techniques. Remembering to focus on the client's feelings will direct you to option 1. Review therapeutic communication techniques and the test-taking strategies for answering communication questions if you had difficulty with this question.

Level of Cognitive Ability: Application
Client Needs: Psychosocial Integrity
Integrated Process: Communication and Documentation
Content Area: Adult Health/Endocrine

Reference
Harkreader H, Hogan MA: *Fundamentals of nursing: caring and clinical judgment*, ed 2, Philadelphia, 2004, WB Saunders, pp 251, 255–257.

---

48. A physician orders 3000 mL normal saline to infuse intravenously (IV) over 24 hours. The drop factor is 15 drops/mL. The nurse prepares to set the flow rate at how many drops per minute? (Round answer to the nearest whole number.)
Answer: _____

Answer: 31
Rationale: Use the IV flow rate formula.

Formula:

$$\frac{\text{Total volume} \times \text{gtt factor}}{\text{Time in minutes}} = \text{gtt per minute}$$

$$\frac{3000 \text{ mL} \times 15 \text{ gtt}}{1440 \text{ minutes}} = \frac{45000}{1440} = 31.2, \text{ or } 31 \text{ drops/min}$$

Test-Taking Strategy: Use the formula for calculating IV flow rates. Remember, use a calculator, follow the formula, recheck your answer, and make sure that the answer makes sense before documenting the answer. Review the test-taking strategies for answering IV calculation questions if you had difficulty with this question.

Level of Cognitive Ability: Application
Client Needs: Physiological Integrity
Integrated Process: Nursing Process/Implementation
Content Area: Fundamental Skills

Reference
Kee J, Marshall S: *Clinical calculations: with applications to general and specialty areas,* ed 5, Philadelphia, 2004, WB Saunders, pp 204–205.

---

49. Nitroprusside sodium (Nipride) is being administered to a client. The nurse monitors for which intended effect of the medication?
1   Headache
2   Flushing of the skin
3   Hypotension
4   Relief of chest pain

Answer: 4

Rationale: Nitroprusside sodium is an antihypertensive and vasodilator. Its therapeutic or intended effect is to dilate coronary arteries, decrease oxygen consumption, and relieve chest pain. Flushing of the skin is an occasional side effect. Although the medication is used to reduce increased blood pressure, a too rapid rate of infusion of the medication reduces the blood pressure too rapidly, resulting in hypotension. Headache is an adverse effect of the medication.

Test-Taking Strategy: If you are unfamiliar with the medication identified in the question (nitroprusside sodium), noting that its name contains *nitr* provides the clue that it is a nitrate. Focus on the issue: an intended effect. Recalling that an intended effect is a desirable and expected effect and that nitrates vasodilate will direct you to option 4. Review the characteristics of this medication and the test-taking strategies for answering pharmacology questions if you had difficulty with this question.

Level of Cognitive Ability: Analysis
Client Needs: Physiological Integrity
Integrated Process: Nursing Process/Evaluation
Content Area: Pharmacology

Reference
Hodgson B, Kizior R: *Saunders nursing drug handbook 2004,* Philadelphia, 2004, WB Saunders, p 736.

---

50. A client seeks treatment for a fractured radius. There is an open wound on the arm through which jagged bone edges protrude. The nurse determines that the client has a
1   Greenstick fracture
2   Comminuted fracture
3   Open fracture
4   Simple fracture

Answer: 3

Rationale: An open fracture (compound fracture) is one in which the skin has been broken and the wound extends to the depth of the fractured bone. A greenstick fracture is an incomplete fracture, which occurs through part of the cross section of a bone; one side of the bone is fractured, and the other side is bent. A comminuted fracture is a complete fracture across the shaft of a bone, with splintering of the bone into fragments. A simple fracture is a fracture of the bone across its entire shaft, with some possible displacement but without breaking the skin.

Test-Taking Strategy: Note the keywords *open* and *bone edges protrude*. Note the relation between these words and option 3. Review types of fractures and the various test-taking strategies if you had difficulty with this question.

Level of Cognitive Ability: Analysis
Client Needs: Physiological Integrity
Integrated Process: Nursing Process/Assessment
Content Area: Adult Health/Musculoskeletal

Reference

Lewis S, Heitkemper M, Dirksen S: *Medical-surgical nursing: assessment and management of clinical problems*, ed 6, St Louis, 2004, Mosby, p 1657.

---

51. A 4-year-old child is admitted to the hospital for surgery. The nurse asks the parents which priority question to identify the adequacy of support for the child's psychosocial needs?
    1   "What signs and symptoms has your child been having?"
    2   "Will a family member be able to stay with the child most of the time?"
    3   "How much do you know about the surgery and its expected outcome?"
    4   "What are your child's favorite toys?"

Answer: 2

Rationale: Separation from family is the most stressful aspect of hospitalization in young children. A primary goal is to prevent separation from family in children younger than 5 years. Identifying support and the ability of family members to stay with the child takes priority over favorite toys or diversional activities. Options 1 and 3 relate to physiological needs.

Test-Taking Strategy: Focus on the issue: adequacy of support and the child's psychosocial needs. Eliminate options 1 and 3 because they relate to physiological needs. From the remaining options, use Maslow's Hierarchy of Needs theory to select the security issue rather than the diversional activity. Review psychosocial needs of a 4-year-old child and the test-taking strategies for answering prioritizing questions if you had difficulty with this question.

Level of Cognitive Ability: Application
Client Needs: Psychosocial Integrity
Integrated Process: Nursing Process/Assessment
Content Area: Child Health

Reference

Wong D, Hockenberry M: *Wong's nursing care of infants and children*, ed 7, St Louis, 2003, Mosby, pp 1032–1034.

---

52. A nurse is assessing a child who has just returned from surgery in a hip spica cast. Which of the following is the priority?
    1   The head of the bed is elevated
    2   The hips are abducted
    3   Circulation is adequate
    4   The child is on the right side

Answer: 3

Rationale: The priority concern during the first few hours after a cast is applied is swelling, which may cause the cast to act as a tourniquet and constrict circulation. Therefore, circulatory assessment is a high priority. Elevating the head of a bed for a child in a hip spica causes discomfort. Using pillows to abduct the hips is not necessary, because a hip spica cast immobilizes the hip and knee. Turning the child side to side at least every 2 hours is important because it allows the body cast to dry evenly and prevents complications related to immobility; however, it is not a greater priority than checking circulation.

Test-Taking Strategy: Note the keyword *priority*. Use the ABCs—airway, breathing, and circulation. Option 3 reflects circulation. Review care to the child in a hip spica cast and the test-taking strategies for answering prioritizing questions if you had difficulty with this question.

Level of Cognitive Ability: Application
Client Needs: Physiological Integrity
Integrated Process: Nursing Process/Implementation
Content Area: Child Health

Reference
Wong D, Hockenberry M: *Wong's nursing care of infants and children*, ed 7, St Louis, 2003, Mosby, pp 1785–1786.

---

53. A nurse is caring for a client with a brainstem injury. The nurse monitors which of the following as the priority?
1   Respiratory rate and rhythm
2   Electrolyte results
3   Peripheral vascular status
4   Radial pulse rate

Answer: 1
Rationale: The respiratory center is located in the brainstem. Monitoring the respiratory status is critical in a client with a brainstem injury, although the nurse may also monitor laboratory results, pulse rate, and peripheral vascular status.

Test-Taking Strategy: Use the ABCs—airway, breathing, and circulation. Option 1 relates to airway. Also, recalling the anatomic location of the respiratory center will direct you to the correct option. Review care to the client with a brainstem injury and the test-taking strategies for prioritizing questions if you had difficulty with this question.

Level of Cognitive Ability: Application
Client Needs: Physiological Integrity
Integrated Process: Nursing Process/Assessment
Content Area: Delegating/Prioritizing

Reference
Lewis S, Heitkemper M, Dirksen S: *Medical-surgical nursing: assessment and management of clinical problems*, ed 6, St Louis, 2004, Mosby, p 1470.

---

54. A nurse is caring for a client with a diagnosis of rheumatoid arthritis who is receiving 5 g aspirin (acetylsalicylic acid [ASA]) orally daily. The nurse recognizes which of the following as an adverse effect related to the medication?
1   Tinnitus
2   Urinary retention
3   Joint pain
4   Difficulty voiding

Answer: 1
Rationale: Aspirin is a nonsteroidal antiinflammatory drug. Adverse effects include gastrointestinal bleeding or gastric mucosal lesions, ringing in the ears (tinnitus), or generalized pruritus. Headache, dizziness, flushing, tachycardia, hyperventilation, sweating, and thirst are also adverse effects. Options 2, 3, and 4 are not adverse effects. In addition, aspirin is administered to the client with rheumatoid arthritis to relieve joint pain.

Test-Taking Strategy: Focus on the issue: an adverse effect. Eliminate options 2 and 4 first because they are similar. Next, eliminate option 3 because aspirin is administered to relieve joint pain. Finally, remembering that aspirin can cause gastrointestinal disturbances and ototoxicity will direct you to the correct option. Review this medication and the test-taking strategies for pharmacology questions if you had difficulty with this question.

Level of Cognitive Ability: Analysis
Client Needs: Physiological Integrity
Integrated Process: Nursing Process/Assessment
Content Area: Pharmacology

Reference
Hodgson B, Kizior R: *Saunders nursing drug handbook 2004,* Philadelphia, 2004, WB Saunders, p 75.

---

55. A child with hemophilia is brought into the emergency department after being hit on the neck with a baseball. The nurse should immediately check the child for
   1   Spontaneous hematuria
   2   Airway obstruction
   3   Headache
   4   Slurred speech

Answer: 2
Rationale: Trauma to the neck may cause bleeding into the tissues of the neck, which may compromise the airway. Hematuria is a symptom of hemophilia, but it is not associated with neck injury. Headache and slurred speech are associated with head trauma and are not the priority in this situation.

Test-Taking Strategy: Note the keyword *immediately.* Use the ABCs—airway, breathing, and circulation. Airway assessment is always a first priority. This directs you to option 2. Review care to the child with hemophilia and the test-taking strategies for answering prioritizing questions if you had difficulty with this question.

Level of Cognitive Ability: Application
Client Needs: Physiological Integrity
Integrated Process: Nursing Process/Assessment
Content Area: Child Health

Reference
Wong D, Hockenberry M: *Wong's nursing care of infants and children,* ed 7, St Louis, 2003, Mosby, p 1565.

---

56. A client received a thermal burn caused by the inhalation of steam. The client's mouth is edematous, and the nurse notes blisters in the client's mouth. Based on these data, the nurse monitors the client most closely for
   1   Difficulty swallowing
   2   Pain
   3   Fluid and electrolyte imbalances
   4   Wheezing

Answer: 4
Rationale: Thermal burns to the airway can occur with the inhalation of steam or explosive gases or with the aspiration of scalding liquids. Thermal burns to the upper airway are more common and result in edema in the mouth with mucosal blisters or ulcerations. The mucosal edema can lead to upper airway obstruction, manifested by wheezing, particularly during the first 24 to 48 hours after burn injury. The client should be maintained on NPO (nothing by mouth) status after a burn injury. Although options 2 and 3 are components of care, they are not the priority.

Test-Taking Strategy: Note the keywords *most closely.* Use the ABCs—airway, breathing, and circulation. Wheezing relates to airway. Review care to the client with a thermal burn to the airway and the test-taking strategies for answering prioritizing questions if you had difficulty with this question.

Level of Cognitive Ability: Application
Client Needs: Physiological Integrity
Integrated Process: Nursing Process/Implementation
Content Area: Adult Health/Integumentary

Reference
Lewis S, Heitkemper M, Dirksen S: *Medical-surgical nursing: assessment and management of clinical problems*, ed 6, St Louis, 2004, Mosby, p 517.

---

57. A nurse is caring for a client who is receiving aminophylline (Theophylline) intravenously. The nurse reviews the client's laboratory results and determines that the drug plasma level is therapeutic if which value is noted?
1   5 mcg/mL
2   8 mcg/mL
3   15 mcg/mL
4   25 mcg/mL

Answer: 3
Rationale: Aminophylline is a bronchodilator. The therapeutic serum level range is 10 to 20 mcg/mL. Options 1 and 2 identify low levels. Option 4 identifies an increased level requiring physician notification.

Test-Taking Strategy: Focus on the name of the medication and recall that most xanthine bronchodilator medication names end with *-line*. Remember that the therapeutic serum level range is 10 to 20 mcg/mL. This will direct you to option 3. Review this drug plasma level and the test-taking strategies for answering pharmacology questions if you had difficulty with this question.

Level of Cognitive Ability: Analysis
Client Needs: Physiological Integrity
Integrated Process: Nursing Process/Analysis
Content Area: Pharmacology

Reference
Lehne R: *Pharmacology for nursing care*, ed 5, Philadelphia, 2004, WB Saunders, p 803.

---

58. A client taking divalproex sodium (Depakote) for the management of seizure disorder reports to the laboratory for follow-up blood tests. The clinic nurse checks the results of which laboratory test to monitor for medication toxicity?
1   Liver function studies
2   Sedimentation rate
3   Glucose
4   Electrolytes

Answer: 1
Rationale: Divalproex sodium is an anticonvulsant that can cause potentially fatal hepatotoxicity. The nurse checks the results of liver function studies to monitor for toxicity. Options 2, 3, and 4 are not associated with monitoring for medication toxicity.

Test-Taking Strategy: Focus on the keyword *toxicity*. Recall that toxicity occurs when the medication level in the body exceeds the therapeutic level either from overdosing or medication accumulation. Think about the organs involved in the absorption and elimination of medications. The body systems most often affected are the liver and the kidneys, although some medications are ototoxic or neurotoxic. Keeping these guidelines in mind, look for the option that relates to one of these body systems. This will direct you to option 1. Review the characteristics of this medication and the test-taking strategies for answering pharmacology questions if you had difficulty with this question.

Level of Cognitive Ability: Analysis
Client Needs: Physiological Integrity
Integrated Process: Nursing Process/Assessment
Content Area: Pharmacology

Reference
Hodgson B, Kizior R: *Saunders nursing drug handbook 2004,* Philadelphia, 2004, WB Saunders, p 1036.

---

59. A nurse is caring for a client with a history of cardiac disease. The nurse monitors the client focusing on which priority assessment item?
1 Peripheral pulse rate
2 Apical heart rate
3 Body temperature
4 Bowel sounds

Answer: 2
Rationale: Monitoring the apical heart rate is a priority component of assessment in a client with cardiac disease. Monitoring the peripheral pulse rate also is important, but it is not as important as the apical heart rate. Bowel sounds and body temperature may be a component of an assessment but are unrelated to the information in the question.

Test-Taking Strategy: Use the ABCs—airway, breathing, and circulation. This will direct you to the correct option. Also note the relation of the words *cardiac disease* in the question and *heart* in the correct option. Review care to the client with a history of cardiac disease and the test-taking strategies for answering prioritizing questions if you had difficulty with this question.

Level of Cognitive Ability: Application
Client Needs: Physiological Integrity
Integrated Process: Nursing Process/Assessment
Content Area: Adult Health/Cardiovascular

Reference
Lewis S, Heitkemper M, Dirksen S: *Medical-surgical nursing: assessment and management of clinical problems,* ed 6, St Louis, 2004, Mosby, p 764.

---

60. A nurse is monitoring a client with a tracheostomy tube for complications related to the tube. The nurse suspects tracheoesophageal fistula if which of the following is noted?
1 Abdominal distention
2 Excess mucus production
3 Abnormal skin and mucous membrane color
4 Use of accessory muscles to assist with breathing

Answer: 1
Rationale: Necrosis of the tracheal wall can lead to an artificial opening between the posterior trachea and esophagus. This problem is called tracheoesophageal fistula. The fistula allows air to escape into the stomach, causing abdominal distention. It also causes aspiration of gastric contents. Options 2, 3, and 4 are not findings associated with this complication.

Test-Taking Strategy: Use medical terminology to assist you in answering this question. A fistula is an artificial opening. *Tracheoesophageal* indicates trachea to esophagus. Based on this medical terminology, review the options. Think of air from the trachea moving to the esophagus. If this occurs, you would note abdominal distention. Review care to the client with a tracheostomy tube and the various test-taking strategies if you had difficulty with this question.

Level of Cognitive Ability: Analysis
Client Needs: Physiological Integrity
Integrated Process: Nursing Process/Assessment
Content Area: Adult Health/Respiratory

Reference
Ignatavicius D, Workman M: *Medical-surgical nursing: critical thinking for collaborative care*, ed 4, Philadelphia, 2002, WB Saunders, p 499.

---

61. A nurse suctioning a client through an endotracheal tube monitors the client for complications associated with the procedure. Which of the following indicates a complication?
    1. A blood pressure of 138/88 mm Hg
    2. An irregular heart rate
    3. A reddish coloration in the client's face
    4. A pulse oximetry level of 95%

Answer: 2

Rationale: The client should be monitored closely for complications related to suctioning, including hypoxemia, cardiac irregularities resulting from vagal stimulation, mucosal trauma, and paroxysmal coughing. If complications occur during the procedure, especially cardiac irregularities, the procedure is stopped, and the client is reoxygenated.

Test-Taking Strategy: Eliminate options 1 and 4 first because they identify normal findings. From the remaining options, use the ABCs—airway, breathing, and circulation—to direct you to option 2. Review the complications of suctioning and the various test-taking strategies if you had difficulty with this question.

Level of Cognitive Ability: Analysis
Client Needs: Physiological Integrity
Integrated Process: Nursing Process/Assessment
Content Area: Adult Health/Respiratory

Reference
Harkreader H, Hogan MA: *Fundamentals of nursing: caring and clinical judgment*, ed 2, Philadelphia, 2004, WB Saunders, pp 866–868.

---

62. A clinic nurse is assessing the neurological status of a client. The nurse would assess for new memory by asking the client
    1. To state the city of birth
    2. What type of transportation was used to get to the clinic
    3. What the client ate for lunch yesterday
    4. To repeat three unrelated words spoken to the client immediately and 5 minutes later

Answer: 4

Rationale: Remote memory, or long-term memory, is tested by asking the client about something from the past (option 1). The nurse must be able to verify this information. Recent (recall) memory tests information within days, weeks, or months (options 2 and 3). New (immediate) memory is tested by asking the client to repeat three unrelated words that the examiner speaks. The client repeats them immediately so the nurse knows they have been heard correctly, and the nurse asks the client to repeat them again 5 minutes later.

Test-Taking Strategy: Note the keywords *new memory.* Each of the incorrect options can be eliminated by comparing which of the pieces of information would be *newest* to the client. This will direct you to option 4. Review neurological assessment and the various test-taking strategies if you had difficulty with this question.

Level of Cognitive Ability: Application
Client Needs: Health Promotion and Maintenance

Integrated Process: Nursing Process/Assessment
Content Area: Adult Health/Neurological

Reference
Ignatavicius D, Workman M: *Medical-surgical nursing: critical thinking for collaborative care*, ed 4, Philadelphia, 2002, WB Saunders, p 885.

---

63. A nurse is performing an assessment on a client with a disorder of the inner ear. Which question will the nurse ask the client to determine whether the client is experiencing the most common symptom of this type of ear disorder?
 1 "Do you have any hearing loss?"
 2 "Do you have any itching around your ear?"
 3 "Do you have any ringing in the ears?"
 4 "Do you have any pain in the ear?"

Answer: 3
Rationale: Tinnitus is the most common report of clients with otological disorders, especially disorders involving the inner ear. Symptoms of tinnitus range from mild ringing in the ear that can go unnoticed during the day to a loud roaring in the ear that can interfere with the client's thinking process and attention span. The client may experience some pain or hearing loss depending on the disorder, but these are not the most common symptoms. Itching around the ear may be associated with a disorder other than an inner ear disorder.

Test-Taking Strategy: Note the keywords *most common* and focus on the issue: a disorder of the inner ear. Recalling the anatomy and physiology of the inner ear will assist in directing you to option 3. Review the characteristics of inner ear infections and the various test-taking strategies if you had difficulty with this question.

Level of Cognitive Ability: Application
Client Needs: Physiological Integrity
Integrated Process: Nursing Process/Assessment
Content Area: Adult Health/Ear

Reference
Ignatavicius D, Workman M: *Medical-surgical nursing: critical thinking for collaborative care*, ed 4, Philadelphia, 2002, WB Saunders, p 1067.

---

64. A client arrives at the health care clinic after sustaining an eye injury in which paint thinner splashed into the eye. The nurse would initially ask the client which of the following questions?
 1 "Did you bring the container of paint thinner with you?"
 2 "What time did the injury occur?"
 3 "Did you flush the eye after the injury?"
 4 "What brand of paint thinner caused the injury?"

Answer: 3
Rationale: Emergency care after a chemical burn to the eye includes irrigating the eye immediately with tap water or sterile normal saline or ocular irrigating solution if available. The irrigation should be maintained for at least 10 minutes. After this emergency treatment, visual acuity is assessed. The initial assessment should focus on the type of treatment that took place immediately after the injury.

Test-Taking Strategy: Note the keyword *initially* and note the type of injury to the eye. Eliminate options 1 and 4 first because they are similar. From the remaining options, use Maslow's Hierarchy of Needs theory. The treatment of the injury is the priority. Review care to the client with an eye injury and the test-taking strategies for answering prioritizing questions if you had difficulty with this question.

Level of Cognitive Ability: Application
Client Needs: Physiological Integrity

Integrated Process: Nursing Process/Assessment
Content Area: Adult Health/Eye

Reference
Ignatavicius D, Workman M: *Medical-surgical nursing: critical thinking for collaborative care*, ed 4, Philadelphia, 2002, WB Saunders, p 1043.

---

65. A nurse is observing a client who is ambulating after a prolonged period of bed rest. The nurse determines that the client should immediately stop the activity if the client exhibits

1   An increase in pulse rate from 78 to 80 beats/min
2   An increase in respiratory rate from 16 to 18 breaths/min
3   Some arm and leg weakness
4   Shortness of breath and diaphoresis

Answer: 4

Rationale: Bed rest decreases the client's strength and endurance. Shortness of breath and diaphoresis are systemic signs of fatigue indicating that the client should rest. Options 1, 2, and 3 are normal findings.

Test-Taking Strategy: Note the keywords *immediately stop*. Use the ABCs—airway, breathing, and circulation. Option 4 indicates that the client is not tolerating the activity from a cardiopulmonary standpoint. Options 1, 2, and 3 are expected effects. Review the effects of mobility and the various test-taking strategies if you had difficulty with this question.

Level of Cognitive Ability: Analysis
Client Needs: Physiological Integrity
Integrated Process: Nursing Process/Evaluation
Content Area: Adult Health/Musculoskeletal

Reference
Ignatavicius D, Workman M: *Medical-surgical nursing: critical thinking for collaborative care*, ed 4, Philadelphia, 2002, WB Saunders, p 129.

---

66. A client who has been raped arrives at the emergency department. Which of these observations would be most important for the nurse to consider when planning the immediate care for the client?

1   The victim states she "feels like it didn't happen."
2   The victim states that she "feels numb."
3   The victim states the rapist knows where she lives and has stated: "He will kill me if I tell anyone about the rape."
4   The victim states she knows the rapist well; in fact, they had been dating for several weeks.

Answer: 3

Rationale: Providing safety is the primary concern for the nurse. The priority statement by the victim is that the rapist will kill her. The victim who states she "feels like it didn't happen" or that she "feels numb" is most likely in the denial stage, which can be a helpful defense mechanism for the victim. That the rapist and the victim know each other is a common phenomenon; in many situations of abuse, the victim does know the rapist.

Test-Taking Strategy: Note the keywords *most important* and *immediate*. Eliminate options 1 and 2 first because they are similar. From the remaining options, use Maslow's Hierarchy of Needs theory. Option 3 is concerned with safety. Review care to the rape victim and the test-taking strategies for answering prioritizing questions if you had difficulty with this question.

Level of Cognitive Ability: Application
Client Needs: Physiological Integrity
Integrated Process: Nursing Process/Planning
Content Area: Mental Health

Reference
Varcarolis E: *Foundations of psychiatric mental health nursing*, ed 4, Philadelphia, 2002, WB Saunders, p 727.

67. A nurse is monitoring a client with acute pulmonary emboli who is receiving streptokinase (Streptase) by intravenous infusion through an infusion pump. Which finding would indicate an adverse effect related to the medication and the need to notify the physician?
  1 Positive peripheral pulses
  2 A radial pulse rate of 58 beats/min
  3 A blood pressure of 140/90 mm Hg
  4 Client reports back pain

Answer: 4

Rationale: Streptokinase is a thrombolytic medication that acts directly on the fibrinolytic system to convert plasminogen to plasmin, an enzyme that degrades fibrin clots, fibrinogen, and other plasma proteins. The nurse should monitor the client for bleeding during administration of this medication, because severe internal hemorrhage can occur as an adverse effect. Signs of bleeding or internal hemorrhage include a decrease in blood pressure, an increase in pulse, or reports of abdominal or back pain. Positive peripheral pulses are a normal finding.

Test-Taking Strategy: Eliminate option 1 first because it is a normal finding. Focus on the name of the medication and recall that most thrombolytic medication names end with *-ase*. Recalling that bleeding is a concern with the use of this type of medication will assist in answering the question. Options 2 and 3 are not signs of bleeding or shock. If a client is bleeding internally, the client will report back or abdominal pain. Also, remember that the physician should be notified if a client is experiencing a life-threatening situation. Review the characteristics of this medication and the various test-taking strategies if you had difficulty with this question.

Level of Cognitive Ability: Analysis
Client Needs: Physiological Integrity
Integrated Process: Nursing Process/Assessment
Content Area: Pharmacology

Reference
Hodgson B, Kizior R: *Saunders nursing drug handbook 2004,* Philadelphia, 2004, WB Saunders, p 938.

---

68. A nurse is monitoring an infant diagnosed with congenital hypothyroidism. The nurse would expect to note which of the following assessment findings?
  1 Excessive sleepiness
  2 Hypertonic reflexes
  3 Hyperactivity
  4 Frequent, loose stools

Answer: 1

Rationale: Signs and symptoms of hypothyroidism may be nonspecific and may include feeding difficulty, prolonged jaundice, respiratory problems, hypotonia, constipation, large posterior fontanel, excessive sleepiness, large tongue, rare crying, dry and mottled skin, and slow, deep tendon reflexes.

Test-Taking Strategy: Focus on the diagnosis: hypothyroidism. Recall that the physiological action of thyroid hormone is to regulate metabolism. Use medical terminology and recall that a condition that is *hypo-* will demonstrate signs of depressed function. Also note that options 2, 3, and 4 indicate *hyper*activity of body systems. Review care to the infant with congenital hypothyroidism and the various test-taking strategies if you had difficulty with this question.

Level of Cognitive Ability: Analysis
Client Needs: Physiological Integrity

Integrated Process: Nursing Process/Assessment
Content Area: Maternity/Postpartum

Reference
Wong D, Hockenberry M: *Wong's nursing care of infants and children*, ed 7, St Louis, 2003, Mosby, p 320.

---

69. A nurse is caring for a client with a diagnosis of acute lymphocytic leukemia who is receiving chemotherapy intravenously. The nurse reviews the client's laboratory results and determines that the client is experiencing an adverse effect of the medication if which of the following is noted?

1 White blood cell (WBC) count: 5000/μL

2 Blood urea nitrogen (BUN) level: 15 mg/dL

3 Platelet count: 200,000 cells/μL

4 Alkaline phosphatase: 25 units/dL

Answer: 4

Rationale: Adverse effects can occur from chemotherapy and can include effects such as hematological reactions, hepatotoxicity, neurotoxicity, and nephrotoxicity. The normal WBC count is 5000 to 10,000/μL. The normal platelet count is 150,000 to 450,000 cells/μL. The normal BUN level is 5 to 20 mg/dL. The normal alkaline phosphatase is 4.5 to 13 units/dL.

Test-Taking Strategy: Focus on the issue: an adverse effect. Review the laboratory values presented in the options and note that the only abnormal laboratory result is the alkaline phosphatase. Review these normal laboratory values and the various test-taking strategies if you had difficulty with this question.

Level of Cognitive Ability: Analysis
Client Needs: Physiological Integrity
Integrated Process: Nursing Process/Analysis
Content Area: Pharmacology

Reference
Ignatavicius D, Workman M: *Medical-surgical nursing: critical thinking for collaborative care*, ed 4, Philadelphia, 2002, WB Saunders, pp 562–563.

---

70. A nurse is caring for a client with a tracheostomy tube and is monitoring the client for subcutaneous emphysema. The nurse identifies this complication by noting which of the following?

1 Crackling sounds heard in the upper lobes bilaterally

2 A puffy and crackling sensation on palpation of the tissues surrounding the tracheostomy site

3 Signs of respiratory distress

4 Dyspnea

Answer: 2

Rationale: Subcutaneous emphysema occurs when air escapes from the tracheostomy incision into the tissues, dissects fascial planes under the skin, and accumulates around the face, neck, and upper chest. These areas appear puffy, and slight finger pressure produces a crackling sound and sensation. Generally, this is not a serious condition, because the air eventually will be absorbed. Options 1, 3, and 4 are not signs of subcutaneous emphysema, but they could be signs of other complications.

Test-Taking Strategy: Eliminate options 3 and 4 first because they are similar. Next, note the word *subcutaneous* in the question and the relation of this word to the description in option 2. Review the characteristics of subcutaneous emphysema and the various test-taking strategies if you had difficulty with this question.

Level of Cognitive Ability: Analysis
Client Needs: Physiological Integrity
Integrated Process: Nursing Process/Assessment
Content Area: Adult Health/Respiratory

Reference
Ignatavicius D, Workman M: *Medical-surgical nursing: critical thinking for collaborative care*, ed 4, Philadelphia, 2002, WB Saunders, p 498.

---

71. A nurse is caring for a client with chronic stable angina who is receiving amlodipine (Norvasc). Which of the following would indicate to the nurse that the client is experiencing an adverse effect of the medication?
    1 Bradycardia
    2 Hypotension
    3 Constipation
    4 Abdominal cramping

Answer: 2

Rationale: Amlodipine is a calcium channel blocker. Adverse or toxic effects may produce excessive peripheral vasodilation and marked hypotension with reflex tachycardia. Frequent side effects include peripheral edema, headache, and flushing.

Test-Taking Strategy: Focus on the issue: an adverse effect. Note the name of the medication, recall that most calcium channel blocker medication names end with *-pine*, and recall that these medications are used to treat hypertension. This will direct you to option 2. Review the characteristics of this medication and the various test-taking strategies if you had difficulty with this question.

Level of Cognitive Ability: Analysis
Client Needs: Physiological Integrity
Integrated Process: Nursing Process/Evaluation
Content Area: Pharmacology

Reference
Hodgson B, Kizior R: *Saunders nursing drug handbook 2004*, Philadelphia, 2004, WB Saunders, p 51.

---

72. A mother tells the clinic nurse that she doesn't want her child to receive any immunizations because she has heard that they cause serious illnesses. The nurse makes which most appropriate statement to the mother?
    1 "Why are you afraid? Children are immunized everyday without a problem."
    2 "There will be a slight discomfort at the time of the injection, but that is all that will happen."
    3 "I can see you are very concerned about your child. What do you think might happen after an immunization is given?"
    4 "Are you afraid the child is going to die from the injection?"

Answer: 3

Rationale: Option 3 acknowledges the mother's concern and provides an opportunity for the mother to respond to the nurse's open-ended question. Options 1, 2, and 4 are nontherapeutic. Option 1 can make the mother feel defensive, devalues the mother's feelings, and requires an explanation from the mother. Option 2 provides false reassurance. Option 4 is an attempt to verify an assumption not supported in the question.

Test-Taking Strategy: Use therapeutic communication techniques. The correct option demonstrates empathy and helps the mother focus on specific fears, so that the nurse can clarify information. Remember, focus on the client's feelings. Review therapeutic communication techniques and the test-taking strategies for answering communication questions if you had difficulty with this question.

Level of Cognitive Ability: Application
Client Needs: Psychosocial Integrity
Integrated Process: Communication and Documentation
Content Area: Child Health

Reference
Harkreader H, Hogan MA: *Fundamentals of nursing: caring and clinical judgment*, ed 2, Philadelphia, 2004, WB Saunders, pp 251, 255–257.

73. A nurse is reviewing the laboratory results of a client with cancer and notes that the calcium level is 14 mg/dL. The nurse determines that this calcium level is consistent with which oncological emergency?
  1 Syndrome of inappropriate antidiuretic hormone (SIADH)
  2 Spinal cord compression
  3 Superior vena cava syndrome
  4 Hypercalcemia

Answer: 4

Rationale: One potentially life-threatening complication of cancer is hypercalcemia, which is characterized by calcium levels greater than 11 mg/dL. Although spinal cord compression and superior vena cava syndrome also are oncological emergencies, they are not characterized by high calcium levels. SIADH also is an oncological emergency, but it is characterized by hyponatremia.

Test-Taking Strategy: Note the similarity of the calcium level in the question and the word *hypercalcemia* in the correct option. Review the significance of an increased calcium level and the various test-taking strategies if you had difficulty with this question.

Level of Cognitive Ability: Analysis
Client Needs: Physiological Integrity
Integrated Process: Nursing Process/Analysis
Content Area: Adult Health/Oncology

Reference
Ignatavicius D, Workman M: *Medical-surgical nursing: critical thinking for collaborative care,* ed 4, Philadelphia, 2002, WB Saunders, p 441.

---

74. A nurse is caring for a client admitted to the hospital with a musculoskeletal injury. The nurse monitors for the major symptom associated with neurovascular compromise by
  1 Counting the client's apical pulse for one full minute
  2 Observing for drainage on the dressing of the affected extremity
  3 Taking the client's blood pressure on the unaffected side
  4 Determining whether pain is experienced with passive motion of the affected extremity

Answer: 4

Rationale: Neurovascular compromise in a client with a musculoskeletal injury is created by increased pressure within a compartment. The pressure occurs because fascia is unable to expand when muscle swelling occurs. The only option that addresses neurovascular compromise is option 4.

Test-Taking Strategy: Focus on the keywords *major symptom* and *neurovascular compromise.* The only option that addresses neurovascular compromise is option 4. Review the signs of neurovascular compromise and the various test-taking strategies if you had difficulty with this question.

Level of Cognitive Ability: Application
Client Needs: Physiological Integrity
Integrated Process: Nursing Process/Implementation
Content Area: Adult Health/Musculoskeletal

Reference
Lewis S, Heitkemper M, Dirksen S: *Medical-surgical nursing: assessment and management of clinical problems,* ed 6, St Louis, 2004, Mosby, p 1672.

---

75. A postpartum mother reports severe pain and an intense feeling of swelling and pressure in the vaginal area. The nurse immediately checks the client's

Answer: 3

Rationale: Hematoma is suspected when pain or pressure in the vaginal area is reported by the client. Massive hemorrhage can occur into the tissues resulting in hypovolemia and shock. Options 1, 2, and 4 are not associated with the client's complaint.

1 Episiotomy site for drainage
2 Rectum for hemorrhoids
3 Vulva for a hematoma
4 Vagina for lacerations

Test-Taking Strategy: Note the keyword *immediately* and focus on the client's descriptions. Note that option 3 indicates a bleeding disorder, which is a priority. Review postpartum assessment and the various test-taking strategies if you had difficulty with this question.

Level of Cognitive Ability: Application
Client Needs: Physiological Integrity
Integrated Process: Nursing Process/Assessment
Content Area: Maternity/Postpartum

Reference
Lowdermilk D, Perry A: *Maternity & women's health care,* ed 8, St Louis, 2004, Mosby, p 1037.

---

76. A nurse is caring for a client receiving hemodialysis who has an internal arteriovenous fistula. The nurse expects to note which finding if the fistula is patent?

1 White fibrin specks noted in the fistula
2 Palpation of a thrill over the site of the fistula
3 Lack of a bruit at the site of the fistula
4 Warmth and redness at the site of the fistula

Answer: 2

Rationale: An internal arteriovenous fistula is created through a surgical procedure in which an artery in the arm is anastomosed to a vein. The fistula is internal. To determine patency, the nurse palpates over the fistula for a thrill and auscultates for a bruit. The nurse would not note white fibrin specks in the fistula, because the fistula is internal. Warmth and redness may indicate a potential inflammatory process.

Test-Taking Strategy: Focus on the issue: a patent fistula. Option 1 can be eliminated first; the nurse would not note white fibrin specks in the fistula, because the fistula is internal. Next, eliminate option 4 because warmth and redness may indicate a potential inflammatory process. From the remaining options, recall that the presence of a bruit or a thrill indicates a patent fistula. Review care to the client with an internal arteriovenous fistula and the various test-taking strategies if you had difficulty with this question.

Level of Cognitive Ability: Analysis
Client Needs: Physiological Integrity
Integrated Process: Nursing Process/Assessment
Content Area: Adult Health/Renal

Reference
Lewis S, Heitkemper M, Dirksen S: *Medical-surgical nursing: assessment and management of clinical problems,* ed 6, St Louis, 2004, Mosby, p 1233.

---

77. A nurse is performing an admission assessment on a client with a diagnosis of Ménière disease. The nurse asks the client which question that would elicit information specific to the attacks that occur with this disease?

1 "Do you have a feeling of fullness in your ear?"

Answer: 1

Rationale: Ménière disease results from a disturbance in the fluid of the endolymphatic system. The cause of the disturbance is unknown. Attacks may be preceded by a feeling of fullness in the ear, or by tinnitus. Headaches are not associated with this disorder. Options 3 and 4 also are unrelated to Ménière disease.

Test-Taking Strategy: Focus on the disease and recall that this disorder is associated with the ear. This will

2 "Are you having any head-aches?"

3 "Do you have any visual problems?"

4 "Do you have difficulty sleeping at night?"

direct you to option 1, because this is the only option that relates to the ear. Review characteristics of Ménière disease and the various test-taking strategies if you had difficulty with this question.

Level of Cognitive Ability: Application
Client Needs: Physiological Integrity
Integrated Process: Nursing Process/Assessment
Content Area: Adult Health/Ear

Reference

Lewis S, Heitkemper M, Dirksen S: *Medical-surgical nursing: assessment and management of clinical problems,* ed 6, St Louis, 2004, Mosby, p 466.

---

78. A nurse administers a fatal dose of morphine sulfate to a client. During the subsequent investigation of the error, it is determined that the nurse did not assess the client's respiratory rate before administering the medication. Failure to adequately assess the client is addressed under which function of the Nurse Practice Act?

1 Defining the specific educational requirements for licensure in the state

2 Describing the scope of practice of licensed and unlicensed care providers

3 Recommending specific terms of incarceration for nurses who violate the law

4 Identifying the process for disciplinary action if standards of care are not met

Answer: 4

Rationale: In this situation, acceptable standards of care were not met (the nurse failed to adequately assess the client before administering a medication). Option 4 refers specifically to the situation described in the question, whereas options 1, 2, and 3 do not.

Test-Taking Strategy: Note the relation between the words *failure to adequately assess the client* in the question and *standards of care are not met* in option 4. Review the legal implications related to medication errors and the various test-taking strategies if you had difficulty with this question.

Level of Cognitive Ability: Analysis
Client Needs: Safe, Effective Care Environment
Integrated Process: Nursing Process/Assessment
Content Area: Leadership/Management

Reference

Harkreader H, Hogan MA: *Fundamentals of nursing: caring and clinical judgment,* ed 2, Philadelphia, 2004, WB Saunders, pp 22–23.

---

79. A nurse is providing instructions to a client with glaucoma about prescribed treatment measures for the disorder. The nurse tells the client that the goal of treatment is

1 Maintaining intraocular pressure at a reduced level

2 Producing mydriasis in the eyes

3 Increasing the formation of aqueous humor

4 Promoting dilation of the pupil of the eyes

Answer: 1

Rationale: The goal of treatment of the client with glaucoma is to maintain intraocular pressure at a reduced level to prevent further damage to intraocular structures. Medications are used to create miosis (constriction of the pupil) and to reduce formation of the aqueous humor by the ciliary body.

Test-Taking Strategy: Eliminate options 2 and 4 first because they are similar. Next, recalling that glaucoma is a condition that is characterized by increased intraocular pressure will assist in eliminating option 3. Also note that option 1 is the umbrella (global) option. Review instructions for the client with glaucoma and the various test-taking strategies if you had difficulty with this question.

Level of Cognitive Ability: Application
Client Needs: Physiological Integrity
Integrated Process: Teaching/Learning
Content Area: Adult Health/Eye

Reference

Lewis S, Heitkemper M, Dirksen S: *Medical-surgical nursing: assessment and management of clinical problems,* ed 6, St Louis, 2004, Mosby, p 457.

---

80. A nurse is reviewing the laboratory results of a client with bladder cancer and bone metastasis and notes that the calcium level is 15 mg/dL. Which of the following nursing actions is most appropriate?
    1 Notify the physician
    2 Document the findings
    3 Increase calcium-containing foods in the diet
    4 File the report in the client's record

Answer: 1

Rationale: Hypercalcemia is a serum calcium level greater than 11 mg/dL. It most often occurs in clients who have bone metastasis, and it is a late manifestation of extensive malignancy. The presence of cancer in the bone causes the bone to release calcium into the bloodstream. Hypercalcemia is an oncological emergency, and the physician should be notified. Options 2, 3, and 4 are incorrect.

Test-Taking Strategy: Eliminate options 2 and 4 first because they are similar actions. From the remaining options, knowing that the calcium level identified in the question indicates an increased level will assist in eliminating option 3. Remember, the physician is notified if a life-threatening or emergency situation occurs. Review the normal calcium level and the various test-taking strategies if you had difficulty with this question.

Level of Cognitive Ability: Application
Client Needs: Physiological Integrity
Integrated Process: Nursing Process/Implementation
Content Area: Adult Health/Oncology

Reference

Ignatavicius D, Workman M: *Medical-surgical nursing: critical thinking for collaborative care,* ed 4, Philadelphia, 2002, WB Saunders, p 441.

---

81. A nurse notes swelling and excessive bleeding on the dressing of a client who underwent enucleation. On the basis of this finding, which nursing action is most appropriate?
    1 Document the finding
    2 Reinforce the dressing
    3 Mark the amount of staining with a black pen and continue to monitor the drainage
    4 Notify the surgeon

Answer: 4

Rationale: Postoperative nursing care includes observing the dressing and reporting any swelling or excessive bleeding. The nurse would notify the surgeon if the client is bleeding. Although the nurse would document the findings and may reinforce the dressing until the surgeon arrives, these actions are not the most appropriate. Option 3 delays necessary intervention to the client who is bleeding.

Test-Taking Strategy: Note the words *most appropriate* and *excessive bleeding on the dressing.* Remember, the physician is notified if the client experiences an emergency or life-threatening occurrence. Review care to the client after enucleation and the various test-taking strategies if you had difficulty with this question.

Level of Cognitive Ability: Application
Client Needs: Physiological Integrity
Integrated Process: Nursing Process/Implementation
Content Area: Adult Health/Eye

Reference

Lewis S, Heitkemper M, Dirksen S: *Medical-surgical nursing: assessment and management of clinical problems*, ed 6, St Louis, 2004, Mosby, p 461.

---

82. A nurse is observing a nursing assistant talking to a client that is hearing impaired. The nurse would intervene if which of the following were performed by the nursing assistant during communication with the client?

1   The nursing assistant is facing the client when speaking
2   The nursing assistant is speaking clearly to the client
3   The nursing assistant is speaking directly into the impaired ear
4   The nursing assistant is speaking in a normal tone

Answer: 3

Rationale: When communicating with a hearing-impaired client, the nurse should speak in a normal tone to the client and should not shout. The nurse should talk directly to the client while facing the client and speaking clearly. If the client does not seem to understand what is said, the nurse should express the statement differently. Moving closer to the client and toward the better ear may facilitate communication, but the nurse should avoid talking directly into the impaired ear.

Test-Taking Strategy: Note the keywords *the nurse would intervene*. These words indicate a false response question and indicate that you are looking for the option that indicates an incorrect action by the nursing assistant. Noting the words *directly into the impaired ear* will direct you to option 3. Review care to the hearing-impaired client and the various test-taking strategies if you had difficulty with this question.

Level of Cognitive Ability: Application
Client Needs: Safe, Effective Care Environment
Integrated Process: Nursing Process/Implementation
Content Area: Leadership/Management

Reference

Harkreader H, Hogan MA: *Fundamentals of nursing: caring and clinical judgment*, ed 2, Philadelphia, 2004, WB Saunders, pp 989–990.

---

83. A nurse is developing a plan of care for a manic client and formulates a nursing diagnosis of Disturbed Thought Processes. Which activity related to this nursing diagnosis would the nurse provide for the client initially?

1   Writing
2   Playing cards with another client
3   Playing checkers with another client
4   Playing a board game with another client

Answer: 1

Rationale: When the client is manic, solitary activities requiring a short attention span or mild physical exertion activities such as writing, painting, finger-painting, woodworking, or walks with the staff are best initially. Solitary activities minimize stimuli, and mild physical activities release tension constructively. When less manic, the client may join one or two other clients in quiet, nonstimulating activities. Competitive games should be avoided because they can stimulate aggression and cause increased psychomotor activity.

Test-Taking Strategy: Note the similarity between options 2, 3, and 4 in that they all involve activities with another individual. Option 1 is the only solitary activity that will minimize stimuli. Review care to the manic client and the various test-taking strategies if you had difficulty with this question.

Level of Cognitive Ability: Application
Client Needs: Psychosocial Integrity
Integrated Process: Nursing Process/Planning
Content Area: Mental Health

Reference
Varcarolis E: *Foundations of psychiatric mental health nursing,* ed 4, Philadelphia, 2002, WB Saunders, pp 498–499.

---

84. Select all nursing interventions to be included in a plan of care for a client with schizophrenia who is experiencing disturbed thought processes.

____ Schedule frequent 1-hour sessions with the client.
____ Demonstrate an attitude of caring and concern.
____ Set goals for the client.
____ Help the client identify the difference between reality and internal thought processes.
____ Establish a nurse–client relationship contract mutually agreed on by the nurse and client.

Answer:

____ Schedule frequent 1-hour sessions with the client.
_X_ Demonstrate an attitude of caring and concern.
____ Set goals for the client.
_X_ Help the client identify the difference between reality and internal thought processes.
_X_ Establish a nurse–client relationship contract mutually agreed on by the nurse and client.

Rationale: The establishment of a trusting relationship is the basis for development of an open communication with the client. The nurse would schedule brief (5- to 10-minute), frequent contacts with the client, because the client with disturbed thought processes cannot tolerate extended, intrusive interactions and functions best in a structured environment. Demonstrating an attitude of caring and concern is basic to any nurse–client relationship. The nurse should establish mutual goals with the client and should help the client identify reality.

Test-Taking Strategy: Focus on the client situation and look for keywords in the interventions. Eliminate the intervention that reads, "Schedule frequent 1-hour sessions with the client" because of the words *1-hour.* Also eliminate the intervention that reads "Set goals for the client," because basic and fundamental principles of a nurse–client relationship indicate that goals should be mutually set between the nurse and client. Review care to the client experiencing disturbed thought processes and the various test-taking strategies if you had difficulty with this question.

Level of Cognitive Ability: Application
Client Needs: Psychosocial Integrity
Integrated Process: Nursing Process/Planning
Content Area: Mental Health

Reference
Stuart G, Laraia M: *Principles and practice of psychiatric nursing,* ed 7, St Louis, 2001, Mosby, p 433.

85. A client has received electroconvulsive therapy (ECT). The nurse implements which of the following activities first in the posttreatment area when the client awakens?
1. Monitors the client's vital signs
2. Discusses the treatment
3. Provides frequent reassurance to the client
4. Encourages the client to eat

Answer: 1

Rationale: The nurse first monitors vital signs, and then reviews the ECT treatment with the client. The nursing interventions outlined in options 2, 3, and 4 follow accordingly. In addition, the nurse would assess for the return of a gag reflex before encouraging the client to eat.

Test-Taking Strategy: Note the keyword *first*. Use the ABCs—airway, breathing, and circulation—to direct you to option 1. Review care to the client receiving ECT and the test-taking strategies for answering prioritizing questions if you had difficulty with this question.

Level of Cognitive Ability: Application
Client Needs: Physiological Integrity
Integrated Process: Nursing Process/Implementation
Content Area: Mental Health

Reference
Stuart G, Laraia M: *Principles and practice of psychiatric nursing,* ed 7, St Louis, 2001, Mosby, p 614.

---

86. A client is admitted to the emergency department with reports of severe, radiating chest pain. Admission orders include oxygen by nasal cannula at 4 L/min; troponins, creatine phosphokinase (CPK), and isoenzymes; a chest radiograph; and a 12-lead electrocardiogram (ECG). List in order of priority the actions that the nurse would take. (Number 1 is the first action.)
___ Obtain the 12-lead ECG.
___ Call the laboratory to order the stat blood work.
___ Call radiology to order the chest radiograph.
___ Apply oxygen to the client.

Answer: 2, 3, 4, 1

Rationale: The initial action is to apply oxygen, because the client may be experiencing myocardial ischemia. The ECG can provide evidence of cardiac damage and the location of myocardial ischemia and would be obtained next. The nurse then would obtain blood work, because it can assist in determining the choice of treatment. Although the chest radiograph may show cardiac enlargement, it does not influence the immediate treatment.

Test-Taking Strategy: Note the keyword *priority*. Remember that the immediate goal of therapy is to prevent myocardial ischemia. Use the ABCs—airway, breathing, and circulation—and the procedures for determining treatment to answer this question. Review care to the client with chest pain and the test-taking strategies for answering prioritizing questions if you had difficulty with this question.

Level of Cognitive Ability: Application
Client Needs: Physiological Integrity
Integrated Process: Nursing Process/Implementation
Content Area: Delegating/Prioritizing

Reference
Lewis S, Heitkemper M, Dirksen S: *Medical-surgical nursing: assessment and management of clinical problems,* ed 6, St Louis, 2004, Mosby, p 828.

---

87. A registered nurse is observing a nursing student auscultating the breath sounds of a client. The registered nurse would intervene if the

Answer: 1

Rationale: The client ideally should sit up and breathe slowly and deeply through the mouth. The diaphragm of the stethoscope, which is warmed before use, is placed directly on the client's skin, not over a gown or clothing.

nursing student did which of the following?
1   Asked the client to lie flat on the right side and then on the left side
2   Asked the client to breathe slowly and deeply through the mouth
3   Placed the stethoscope directly on the client's skin
4   Used the diaphragm of the stethoscope

Test-Taking Strategy: Note the keywords *registered nurse would intervene.* These words indicate a false response question and indicate that you are looking for the option that indicates an incorrect action by the nursing student. Noting the words *lie flat* will direct you to option 1. Review the procedure for auscultating breath sounds and the various test-taking strategies if you had difficulty with this question.

Level of Cognitive Ability: Application
Client Needs: Safe, Effective Care Environment
Integrated Process: Nursing Process/Implementation
Content Area: Leadership/Management

Reference
Potter P, Perry A: *Fundamentals of nursing,* ed 6, St Louis, 2005, Mosby, p 720.

---

88. A registered nurse is observing a licensed practical nurse insert a nasal trumpet airway into a client. The registered nurse would intervene if the licensed practical nurse did which of the following?
1   Checked the nose for septal deviation
2   Used a nasal trumpet that is slightly larger than the nares
3   Lubricated the nasal trumpet with a water-soluble, lubricant jelly containing a local anesthetic
4   Inserted the nasal trumpet while gently following the contour of the nasopharyngeal passageway

Answer: 2
Rationale: The nurse would select a nasal trumpet airway that is slightly smaller than the nares and slightly larger than the suction catheter to be used to suction the client. Options 1, 3, and 4 are correct actions for inserting a nasal trumpet airway.

Test-Taking Strategy: Note the keywords *registered nurse would intervene.* These words indicate a false response question and indicate that you are looking for the option that indicates an incorrect action by the licensed practical nurse. Noting the words *slightly larger than the nares* and visualizing this procedure will direct you to option 2. Review the procedure for inserting a nasal trumpet and the various test-taking strategies if you had difficulty with this question.

Level of Cognitive Ability: Application
Client Needs: Safe, Effective Care Environment
Integrated Process: Nursing Process/Implementation
Content Area: Leadership/Management

Reference
Harkreader H, Hogan MA: *Fundamentals of nursing: caring and clinical judgment,* ed 2, Philadelphia, 2004, WB Saunders, p 876.

---

89. A nurse is caring for a client who is being treated with an intravenous bolus of lidocaine hydrochloride (Xylocaine). The nurse monitors which of the following most closely?
1   Respiratory status and blood pressure
2   Urinary pH and urinary output
3   Radial pulse and peripheral pulses
4   Temperature and radial pulse

Answer: 1
Rationale: The nurse needs to monitor the client's respiratory status, blood pressure, and apical pulse while the client is being treated with an intravenous bolus of lidocaine hydrochloride. The urinary pH, urinary output, peripheral pulses, and temperature are nonspecific with this medication. It is best to monitor the apical pulse in this client.

Test-Taking Strategy: Note the keywords *most closely.* Use the ABCs—airway, breathing, and circulation. This will direct you to option 1. Review the characteristics of this medication and the test-taking strategies for answering prioritizing questions if you had difficulty with this question.

Level of Cognitive Ability: Application
Client Needs: Physiological Integrity
Integrated Process: Nursing Process/Assessment
Content Area: Pharmacology

Reference
Hodgson B, Kizior R: *Saunders nursing drug handbook 2004,* Philadelphia, 2004, WB Saunders, p 601.

---

90. A nurse is caring for a child who sustained a head injury from a fall. The nurse avoids which of the following in the care of the child?
    1   Elevating the head of the bed
    2   Restricting oral fluids
    3   Coughing and deep breathing
    4   Performing neurological assessments

Answer: 3

Rationale: A child with a head injury is at risk for increased intracranial pressure (ICP). Elevating the head of the bed decreases fluid retention in cerebral tissue and promotes drainage. Fluids may be restricted to reduce the chance of fluid overload and resultant increased ICP. Hypoxia and Valsalva maneuver associated with coughing both acutely increase intracranial pressure. Neurological assessments should be performed to monitor for increased ICP.

Test-Taking Strategy: Note the keyword *avoids* and recall that a head injury places the child at risk for increased ICP. From this point, identify the option that would cause an increase in ICP. This will direct you to option 3. Review care to the child who sustained a head injury and the various test-taking strategies if you had difficulty with this question.

Level of Cognitive Ability: Application
Client Needs: Physiological Integrity
Integrated Process: Nursing Process/Implementation
Content Area: Child Health

Reference
Wong D, Hockenberry M: *Wong's nursing care of infants and children,* ed 7, St Louis, 2003, Mosby, p 1658.

---

91. A client with a diagnosis of sickle cell crisis is being admitted to the hospital. The nurse anticipates that which priority intervention will be prescribed?
    1   Oxygen administration
    2   Red blood cell transfusions
    3   Laboratory studies
    4   Genetic counseling

Answer: 1

Rationale: Oxygen, intravenous fluids, and pain medication are the primary interventions for treating sickle cell crisis. Red blood cell transfusions may also be prescribed, as well as laboratory studies, but they are not the priority in the care of the client. Genetic counseling is recommended, but not during the acute phase of illness.

Test-Taking Strategy: Note the keyword *priority.* Using Maslow's Hierarchy of Needs theory, you can eliminate option 4 first, because this option addresses a psychosocial, not a physiological, need. From the remaining options, use the ABCs—airway, breathing, and circulation—to direct you to option 1. Review care to the client in sickle cell crisis and the test-taking strategies for questions that require prioritizing if you had difficulty with this question.

Level of Cognitive Ability: Analysis
Client Needs: Physiological Integrity
Integrated Process: Nursing Process/Planning
Content Area: Delegating/Prioritizing

Reference
Ignatavicius D, Workman M: *Medical-surgical nursing: critical thinking for collaborative care,* ed 4, Philadelphia, 2002, WB Saunders, p 840.

---

92. A nurse is planning the client assignments for the day. Which of the following clients would the nurse assign to the nursing assistant?
1   A client scheduled for discharge to home
2   A client on strict bed rest
3   A postoperative client who had an emergency appendectomy
4   A client scheduled for a cardiac catheterization

Answer: 2

Rationale: The nurse is legally responsible for client assignments and must assign tasks based on the guidelines of nursing practice acts and the job descriptions of the employing agency. A client scheduled for discharge to home, a postoperative client who had an emergency appendectomy, and a client scheduled for a cardiac catheterization have both physiological and psychosocial needs that require care by a licensed nurse. The nursing assistant has been trained to care for a client on bed rest. The nurse provides instructions to the nursing assistant, but the tasks required are within the role description of a nursing assistant.

Test-Taking Strategy: Note that the question asks for the assignment to be delegated to the nursing assistant. When asked questions related to delegation, think about the role description of the employee and the needs of the client. This will direct you to option 2. Review the principles for planning client assignments and the test-taking strategies for answering delegation questions if you had difficulty with this question.

Level of Cognitive Ability: Application
Client Needs: Safe, Effective Care Environment
Integrated Process: Nursing Process/Implementation
Content Area: Delegating/Prioritizing

Reference
Potter P, Perry A: *Fundamentals of nursing,* ed 6, St Louis, 2005, Mosby, p 379.

---

93. A client receiving a blood transfusion suddenly exhibits signs of a blood transfusion reaction. List in order of priority the actions that the nurse will take. (Number 1 is the first nursing action.)
____   Document the occurrence.
____   Stop the blood transfusion.

Answer: 5, 1, 2, 4, 3

Rationale: If a transfusion reaction is suspected, the transfusion is stopped; then normal saline is infused pending further physician orders. This maintains a patent intravenous access line and aids in maintaining the client's intravascular volume. The physician and blood bank are notified immediately. The nurse would monitor the client's vital signs and urine output, recheck the blood bag's identifying numbers and tags, treat symptoms per

___ Maintain a patent intravenous line with normal saline solution.

___ Send the blood bag and tubing to the blood bank for examination.

___ Monitor the client's vital signs and urine output.

physician's orders, send the blood bag and tubing to the blood bank for examination, collect required blood and urine samples, and document the occurrence on the transfusion report and in the client's chart.

Test-Taking Strategy: The best strategy to use to answer this question is to visualize the occurrence. Stopping the blood is the first action; then, because the intravenous line needs to remain patent, normal saline solution needs to be infused. Next, use the ABCs—airway, breathing, and circulation—to determine that the client's vital signs need to be monitored. From the remaining interventions, select documentation last, because all interventions, including that the nurse sent the blood bag and tubing to the blood bank for examination, need to be documented. Review interventions for when a transfusion reaction occurs and the test-taking strategies for answering prioritizing questions if you had difficulty with this question.

Level of Cognitive Ability: Application
Client Needs: Physiological Integrity
Integrated Process: Nursing Process/Implementation
Content Area: Delegating/Prioritizing

Reference
Lewis S, Heitkemper M, Dirksen S: *Medical-surgical nursing: assessment and management of clinical problems,* ed 6, St Louis, 2004, Mosby, p 747.

---

94. A nurse reviews the serum laboratory study results for a client taking chlorothiazide (Diuril). The nurse monitors for which most frequent medication side effect?
    1   Hyperphosphatemia
    2   Hypocalcemia
    3   Hypernatremia
    4   Hypokalemia

Answer: 4
Rationale: The client taking a potassium-wasting diuretic such as chlorothiazide should be monitored for decreased potassium levels. Other fluid and electrolyte imbalances that occur with use of this medication include hyponatremia, hypercalcemia, hypomagnesemia, and hypophosphatemia.

Test-Taking Strategy: Focus on the name of the medication and recall that most thiazide diuretic medication names end with *-zide.* Remember that thiazide diuretics are potassium-wasting, and hypokalemia is a concern. Review the characteristics of this medication and the test-taking strategies for answering pharmacology questions if you had difficulty with this question.

Level of Cognitive Ability: Application
Client Needs: Physiological Integrity
Integrated Process: Nursing Process/Assessment
Content Area: Pharmacology

Reference
Hodgson B, Kizior R: *Saunders nursing drug handbook 2004,* Philadelphia, 2004, WB Saunders, p 202.

95. A client is taking amiloride hydrochloride (Midamor) daily. The nurse gives the client which of the following instructions regarding the use of this medication?
1   Take the dose in the morning with breakfast.
2   Take the dose on an empty stomach.
3   Take the dose between lunch and dinner.
4   Take the dose at bedtime.

Answer: 1

Rationale: Amiloride is a potassium-sparing diuretic used to treat edema or hypertension. A daily dose should be taken in the morning to avoid nocturia. The dose should be taken with food to increase bioavailability.

Test-Taking Strategy: Eliminate options 2, 3, and 4 because they are similar in that they all indicate taking the medication dose without food. Review this medication and the test-taking strategies for answering pharmacology questions if you had difficulty with this question.

Level of Cognitive Ability: Application
Client Needs: Physiological Integrity
Integrated Process: Teaching/Learning
Content Area: Pharmacology

Reference
Hodgson B, Kizior R: *Saunders nursing drug handbook 2004,* Philadelphia, 2004, WB Saunders, p 41.

96. A client is prescribed tolbutamide (Orinase) once daily. The nurse observes for which intended effect of this medication?
1   Decreased blood pressure
2   Decreased blood glucose
3   Weight loss
4   Resolution of infection

Answer: 2

Rationale: Tolbutamide is an oral hypoglycemic agent that is taken in the morning. It is not used to decrease blood pressure, enhance weight loss, or treat infection.

Test-Taking Strategy: Note the keywords *intended effect.* Focus on the name of the medication and recall that most second-generation sulfonylurea medication names end with *-mide.* Remember that sulfonylureas are used to treat diabetes mellitus. Review the characteristics of this medication and the test-taking strategies for answering pharmacology questions if you had difficulty with this question.

Level of Cognitive Ability: Analysis
Client Needs: Physiological Integrity
Integrated Process: Nursing Process/Evaluation
Content Area: Pharmacology

Reference
Hodgson B, Kizior R: *Saunders nursing drug handbook 2004,* Philadelphia, 2004, WB Saunders, p 995.

97. A nurse is providing instructions to a client about quinapril hydrochloride (Accupril). The nurse tells the client
1   To take the medication with food only
2   To rise slowly from a lying to a sitting position
3   To discontinue the medication if nausea occurs
4   That a therapeutic effect will be seen immediately

Answer: 2

Rationale: Quinapril hydrochloride is an angiotensin-converting enzyme (ACE) inhibitor used in the treatment of hypertension. The client should be instructed to rise slowly from a lying to a sitting position and to permit the legs to dangle from the bed momentarily before standing to reduce the hypotensive effect. The medication may be given without regard to food. The client should be instructed to take a noncola, carbonated beverage and salted crackers or dry toast if feeling nauseous. A full therapeutic effect may take place in 1 to 2 weeks.

Test-Taking Strategy: Eliminate option 1 because of the absolute word *only* and option 4 because of the word *immediately*. Next, focus on the name of the medication, recall that most ACE inhibitor medication names end with *-pril,* and recall that these medications are used to treat hypertension. This will direct you to option 2. Review the characteristics of this medication and the test-taking strategies for answering pharmacology questions if you had difficulty with this question.

Level of Cognitive Ability: Application
Client Needs: Physiological Integrity
Integrated Process: Teaching/Learning
Content Area: Pharmacology

Reference
Hodgson B, Kizior R: *Saunders nursing drug handbook 2004,* Philadelphia, 2004, WB Saunders, p 862.

---

98. The nurse notes that a client is receiving ganciclovir sodium (Cytovene). The nurse suspects that the client is receiving this medication for the treatment of
  1   Cytomegalovirus retinitis
  2   Pancreatitis
  3   Urolithiasis
  4   Nephrotic syndrome

Answer: 1

Rationale: Ganciclovir sodium is an antiviral medication used to treat cytomegalovirus retinitis (CMV) in immuno-compromised clients, to treat CMV gastrointestinal infections and pneumonitis, and to prevent CMV disease in transplant clients. It is not used to treat pancreatitis, urolithiasis, or nephrotic syndrome.

Test-Taking Strategy: Focus on the name of the medication. Recalling that most antiviral medications names contain the letters *vir* will direct you to option 1. Review this medication and the test-taking strategies for answering pharmacology questions if you had difficulty with this question.

Level of Cognitive Ability: Analysis
Client Needs: Physiological Integrity
Integrated Process: Nursing Process/Analysis
Content Area: Pharmacology

Reference
Hodgson B, Kizior R: *Saunders nursing drug handbook 2004,* Philadelphia, 2004, WB Saunders, p 457.

---

99. A nurse is planning to teach a client how to mix Regular and NPH insulin in the same syringe. Which of the following instructions is included in the plan of care?
  1   Take all of the air out of the bottle before mixing.
  2   Draw up the Regular insulin first into the syringe.
  3   Keep both bottles stored in the refrigerator for 1 month.
  4   Shake the NPH insulin bottle in the hands before mixing.

Answer: 2

Rationale: Before mixing different types of insulin, the bottle should be rotated for at least 1 minute between both hands. This resuspends the insulin and helps warm the medication. The nurse should not shake the bottles. Shaking causes foaming and bubbles to form, which may trap particles of insulin and alter the dosage. Insulin may be maintained at room temperature. Additional bottles of insulin should be stored in the refrigerator for future use. Regular insulin is drawn up before NPH insulin. Air does not need to be removed from the insulin bottle.

Test-Taking Strategy: Visualize the procedure as you carefully read each option. When answering questions that relate to mixing insulin remember the letters *RN*—draw the *R*egular insulin into the syringe before the *N*PH insulin. Review the procedures for administering insulin and the test-taking strategies for answering pharmacology questions if you had difficulty with this question.

Level of Cognitive Ability: Application
Client Needs: Physiological Integrity
Integrated Process: Nursing Process/Planning
Content Area: Pharmacology

Reference
Hodgson B, Kizior R: *Saunders nursing drug handbook 2004,* Philadelphia, 2004, WB Saunders, p 537.

---

100. A client has been taking lansoprazole (Prevacid). The nurse monitors the client for the relief of which of the following symptoms?
1 Constipation
2 Diarrhea
3 Flatulence
4 Heartburn

Answer: 4
Rationale: Lansoprazole is a gastric pump inhibitor (proton pump inhibitor). Its intended effect is relief of gastric irritation pain, often referred to as heartburn. The medication does not relieve constipation, diarrhea, or flatulence.

Test-Taking Strategy: Focus on the keywords *relief of.* Note the name of the medication and recall that most proton pump inhibitor medication names end with *-zole.* This will direct you to option 4. Review this medication and the test-taking strategies for answering pharmacology questions if you had difficulty with this question.

Level of Cognitive Ability: Analysis
Client Needs: Physiological Integrity
Integrated Process: Nursing Process/Evaluation
Content Area: Pharmacology

Reference
Hodgson B, Kizior R: *Saunders nursing drug handbook 2004,* Philadelphia, 2004, WB Saunders, p 583.

---

101. A physician has written an order for ranitidine (Zantac) once daily. The nurse schedules administration of the medication
1 At bedtime
2 With dinner
3 After lunch
4 Just before breakfast

Answer: 1
Rationale: Ranitidine should be taken at bedtime when given as a single daily dose. This allows for its prolonged effect and the greatest protection of gastric mucosa around the clock. The other options are incorrect.

Test-Taking Strategy: Note the similarity in options 2, 3, and 4 in that these times indicate administration of the medication with food. Review the characteristics of this medication and the test-taking strategies for answering pharmacology questions if you had difficulty with this question.

Level of Cognitive Ability: Application
Client Needs: Physiological Integrity

Integrated Process: Nursing Process/Implementation
Content Area: Pharmacology

Reference

Hodgson B, Kizior R: *Saunders nursing drug handbook 2004,* Philadelphia, 2004, WB Saunders, p 873.

---

102. A client reports to the emergency department stating that his "heart is skipping beats." After diagnostic studies, it is determined that the client is experiencing isolated premature ventricular contractions (PVCs) and has no underlying cardiac disease. The nurse provides dietary instructions to the client and tells him that which item is acceptable to consume?
    1   Coffee
    2   Tea
    3   Cola
    4   Apple juice

Answer: 4

Rationale: Clients experiencing a cardiac dysrhythmia such as PVCs should not consume caffeinated beverages because of the vasoconstriction effect associated with caffeine. Options 1, 2, and 3 are items that contain caffeine.

Test-Taking Strategy: Note the similarity among options 1, 2, and 3 in that they contain caffeine. Review the treatment for PVCs and the various test-taking strategies if you had difficulty with this question.

Level of Cognitive Ability: Application
Client Needs: Health Promotion and Maintenance
Integrated Process: Teaching/Learning
Content Area: Adult Health/Cardiovascular

Reference

Ignatavicius D, Workman M: *Medical-surgical nursing: critical thinking for collaborative care,* ed 4, Philadelphia, 2002, WB Saunders, p 675.

---

103. A client is admitted to the hospital with chest pain, and myocardial infarction is suspected. The client tells the nurse that the chest pain has returned, and the nurse administers one 0.4-mg nitroglycerin tablet sublingually as prescribed. What does the nurse do next before administering another sublingual nitroglycerin tablet if the pain is not relieved?
    1   Notify the physician
    2   Check the client's blood pressure
    3   Place the client in Trendelenburg position
    4   Encourage the client to breathe deeply

Answer: 2

Rationale: Nitroglycerin tablets are administered as follows: one tablet every 5 minutes, not exceeding three tablets for chest pain, as long as the client maintains a systolic blood pressure of 100 mm Hg or greater. The nurse would check the client's blood pressure before administering a second nitroglycerin tablet. The physician is notified if the chest pain is not relieved after administering three tablets. If there is a sudden decrease in blood pressure, the client is placed in the Trendelenburg (head-lowered) position, and the physician is notified. Deep breathing will not relieve the chest pain that occurs as a result of myocardial infarction.

Test-Taking Strategy: Note the keyword *next.* Use the ABCs—airway, breathing, and circulation. This will direct you to option 2. Checking the blood pressure is a means of checking the client's circulatory status. Review care to the client experiencing chest pain and the test-taking strategies for answering pharmacology questions if you had difficulty with this question.

Level of Cognitive Ability: Application
Client Needs: Physiological Integrity
Integrated Process: Nursing Process/Implementation
Content Area: Delegating/Prioritizing

Reference

Hodgson B, Kizior R: *Saunders nursing drug handbook 2004,* Philadelphia, 2004, WB Saunders, p 745.

104. An emergency department nurse is caring for a client with a suspected myocardial infarction who is experiencing chest pain unrelieved by nitroglycerin. The nurse administers 5 mg morphine sulfate intravenously as prescribed by the physician to treat the chest pain. After administration of morphine sulfate, the nurse takes which priority action?

1 Places the call bell at the client's side and instructs the client to call the nurse if the chest pain is not relieved
2 Monitors the respirations and blood pressure
3 Monitors urinary output
4 Places the client in a supine (head-lowered) position

Answer: 2

Rationale: Morphine sulfate is administered to control pain in cardiac clients. After administration, the nurse must monitor the client's heart rhythm and vital signs, especially the client's respirations. Signs of morphine sulfate toxicity include respiratory depression and hypotension. The client is placed in a supine (head-lowered) position only if a sudden decrease in blood pressure occurs; otherwise, a semi-Fowler to high-Fowler position is maintained. Urinary output is not directly related to the administration of this medication. The client with a suspected myocardial infarction would not be left alone.

Test-Taking Strategy: Note the keyword *priority*. Use the ABCs—airway, breathing, and circulation—to direct you to option 2. Review this medication and the test-taking strategies for answering prioritizing questions if you had difficulty with this question.

Level of Cognitive Ability: Application
Client Needs: Physiological Integrity
Integrated Process: Nursing Process/Implementation
Content Area: Adult Health/Cardiovascular

Reference
Hodgson B, Kizior R: *Saunders nursing drug handbook 2004,* Philadelphia, 2004, WB Saunders, p 689.

---

105. A nurse has just finished suctioning the tracheostomy of a client. The nurse evaluates the effectiveness of the procedure by checking which of the following items?

1 Respiratory rate
2 Oxygen saturation level
3 Breath sounds
4 Capillary refill

Answer: 3

Rationale: After suctioning a client with or without an artificial airway, the breath sounds are auscultated to determine the extent to which the airways have been cleared of respiratory secretions. The other methods are not as precise indicators as breath sounds for this purpose.

Test-Taking Strategy: Note that this question is an evaluation type of question. Focus on the issue: the effectiveness of suctioning. Also, recall that the purpose of suctioning is to clear the airways of secretions. This will direct you to option 3. Review the procedure for suctioning and the various test-taking strategies if you had difficulty with this question.

Level of Cognitive Ability: Analysis
Client Needs: Physiological Integrity
Integrated Process: Nursing Process/Evaluation
Content Area: Adult Health/Respiratory

Reference
Harkreader H, Hogan MA: *Fundamentals of nursing: caring and clinical judgment,* ed 2, Philadelphia, 2004, WB Saunders, p 867.

106. A nurse is carrying out emergency care measures for a postoperative client who is suspected of having a pulmonary embolism. The nurse implements which of the following physician orders first?
1   Obtains an arterial blood gas specimen
2   Applies oxygen
3   Starts an intravenous line
4   Obtains an electrocardiogram

Answer: 2

Rationale: The client needs immediate oxygen as a result of hypoxemia, which is most often accompanied by respiratory distress and cyanosis. The client should have an intravenous line for administration of emergency medications such as morphine sulfate. An electrocardiogram is useful in determining the presence of possible right ventricular hypertrophy, and an arterial blood gas specimen is drawn to assess oxygenation, respiratory, and metabolic status. All of the interventions listed are appropriate, but the client needs the oxygen first.

Test-Taking Strategy: Note the keyword *first.* Use the ABCs—airway, breathing, and circulation. This will direct you to option 2. Review care to the client experiencing pulmonary embolism and the test-taking strategies for answering prioritizing questions if you had difficulty with this question.

Level of Cognitive Ability: Application
Client Needs: Physiological Integrity
Integrated Process: Nursing Process/Implementation
Content Area: Delegating/Prioritizing

Reference
Lewis S, Heitkemper M, Dirksen S: *Medical-surgical nursing: assessment and management of clinical problems,* ed 6, St Louis, 2004, Mosby, p 940.

---

107. A nurse is collecting data about a client's cigarette-smoking habit. The client admits to smoking 1.5 packs/day for the last 10 years. The nurse documents that the client has a smoking history of how many pack-years?
Answer: _____

Answer: 15

Rationale: The standard method for quantifying smoking history is to multiply the number of packs smoked per day by the number of years of smoking. The number is recorded as the number of pack-years. The calculation for the number of pack-years for the client who has smoked 1.5 packs/day for 10 years is: 1.5 packs × 10 years = 15.0 pack-years.

Test-Taking Strategy: Focus on the information in the question. This question requires simple multiplication of the number of packs of cigarettes smoked per day by the number of years of smoking. Use a calculator to multiply; then verify your answer before documenting it. Review respiratory assessment procedures and the various test-taking strategies if you had difficulty with this question.

Level of Cognitive Ability: Comprehension
Client Needs: Health Promotion and Maintenance
Integrated Process: Nursing Process/Assessment
Content Area: Adult Health/Respiratory

Reference
Lewis S, Heitkemper M, Dirksen S: *Medical-surgical nursing: assessment and management of clinical problems,* ed 6, St Louis, 2004, Mosby, p 552.

108. A neonate is diagnosed with imperforate anus. The parents ask the nurse to describe this abnormality. The nurse bases the response on which characteristic of the disorder?
1 Absence of the anus in its normal position in the perineum
2 Invagination of a section of the intestine into the distal bowel
3 The infrequent and difficult passage of dry stools
4 The presence of fecal incontinence

Answer: 1

Rationale: Imperforate anus (anal atresia, anal agenesis) is the incomplete development or absence of the anus in its normal position in the perineum. Option 2 describes intussusception. Option 3 describes constipation. Option 4 describes encopresis. Constipation can affect any child at any time, although it peaks at 2 to 3 years of age. Encopresis generally affects preschool and school-age children.

Test-Taking Strategy: Noting the relation between the disorder *imperforate anus* and *absence of the anus* in option 1 will direct you to this option. Also, noting that the question addresses a neonate will direct you to the correct option. Review the characteristics of this disorder and the various test-taking strategies if you had difficulty with this question.

Level of Cognitive Ability: Application
Client Needs: Physiological Integrity
Integrated Process: Teaching/Learning
Content Area: Maternity/Postpartum

Reference
Wong D, Hockenberry M: *Wong's nursing care of infants and children,* ed 7, St Louis, 2003, Mosby, pp 466, 469.

---

109. A nurse is called by a group of neighbors to the scene of a house fire where a person escaped but sustained burns to the face and neck and is having slight trouble breathing. The nurse takes which priority action while waiting for emergency medical services to arrive?
1 Places a wet towel over the victim's face and places the client in a supine position
2 Keeps the client standing and supports the client while he leans up against a tree for support
3 Assists the client to a comfortable position and monitors for airway patency
4 Places the client in a supine position and begins rescue breathing

Answer: 3

Rationale: The client requires continuous monitoring by the nurse to ensure that the client's condition does not deteriorate, and to provide assistance if it does. Although the client is having only slight trouble breathing and is managing his own airway at this time, inhalation injury could cause laryngeal edema and subsequent airway obstruction. A supine position can make breathing more difficult for the client and can enhance edema development. Option 2 does nothing to assist the client and could cause added fatigue if the client becomes weak or has difficulty standing. Option 4 is unnecessary if the client is already breathing.

Test-Taking Strategy: Focus on the data in the question and use the ABCs—airway, breathing, and circulation. This will direct you to option 3. Review care to the burn client and the test-taking strategies for answering prioritizing questions if you had difficulty with this question.

Level of Cognitive Ability: Application
Client Needs: Physiological Integrity
Integrated Process: Nursing Process/Implementation
Content Area: Adult Health/Integumentary

Reference
Lewis S, Heitkemper M, Dirksen S: *Medical-surgical nursing: assessment and management of clinical problems,* ed 6, St Louis, 2004, Mosby, p 521.

110. A mental health nurse is performing an admission interview with a depressed client who has suicidal ideation. After the interview, which nursing intervention is carried out first?

1   Isolate the client from other client's in the nursing unit
2   Provide the client with diversional activities
3   Communicate the client's risk for suicide to all team members
4   Develop a plan of activities for the client

Answer: 3

Rationale: The first priority intervention for the suicidal individual is to communicate the risk for suicide to all team members. The plan of activities (options 2 and 4) would take second priority. Client isolation is inappropriate. The client should be placed on 1:1 supervision if the client is suicidal.

Test-Taking Strategy: Note the keyword *first.* Eliminate options 2 and 4 first because they are similar. From the remaining options, the priority item is communication to other members of the health care team, with the ultimate aim to increase client safety. Review care to the client with suicidal ideation and the test-taking strategies for answering prioritizing questions if you had difficulty with this question.

Level of Cognitive Ability: Application
Client Needs: Safe, Effective Care Environment
Integrated Process: Nursing Process/Implementation
Content Area: Mental Health

Reference
Varcarolis E: *Foundations of psychiatric mental health nursing,* ed 4, Philadelphia, 2002, WB Saunders, p 642.

---

111. A nurse is caring for a client with pancreatic cancer who is scheduled for a radical pancreaticoduodenectomy. The nurse would best meet the psychosocial needs of the client by

1   Giving the client time to be alone to think about the outcome of the surgery
2   Ensuring that the client has been visited by a member of the clergy
3   Giving the client information about the surgery
4   Exploring the meaning of the surgery with the client

Answer: 4

Rationale: The nurse should explore the meaning of the surgery from the client's perspective in terms of pain, body image changes, fear, and dying. It is then possible for the nurse to work effectively with the client. Option 4 is a direct action by the nurse that can best meet the client's need because it addresses the client's feelings. Options 1, 2, and 3 do not address the client's feelings.

Test-Taking Strategy: Note the keyword *best.* Use therapeutic communication techniques and the nursing process to answer the question. Only option 4 addresses both assessment and the client's feelings. Review therapeutic communication techniques and the test-taking strategies for answering prioritizing questions if you had difficulty with this question.

Level of Cognitive Ability: Application
Client Needs: Psychosocial Integrity
Integrated Process: Caring
Content Area: Adult Health/Oncology

Reference
Lewis S, Heitkemper M, Dirksen S: *Medical-surgical nursing: assessment and management of clinical problems,* ed 6, St Louis, 2004, Mosby, p 1141.

112. An antepartum client at 32 weeks of gestation positioned herself supine on the examination table to await the obstetrician. The nurse enters the examination room and the client says, "I'm feeling a little lightheaded and sick to my stomach." The nurse recognizes that the client may be experiencing vena cava syndrome (hypotensive syndrome) and takes which immediate action?

1 Gives the client an emesis basin

2 Places a cool cloth on the client's forehead

3 Places a folded towel or sheet under the client's right hip

4 Calls the obstetrician to see the client immediately

Answer: 3

Rationale: Lying supine (on the back) applies additional gravitational pressure on the abdominal blood vessels (iliac vessels, inferior vena cava, and ascending aorta), increasing compression and impeding blood flow and cardiac output. This results in hypotension, dizziness, nausea, pallor, clammy (cool, damp) skin, and sweating. Raising one hip higher than the other reduces the pressure on the vena cava, restoring the circulation and relieving the symptoms. Although an emesis basin and a cool cloth placed on the forehead may be helpful, these are not the immediate actions. It is not necessary to call the obstetrician immediately unless the client's symptoms are unrelieved after repositioning.

Test-Taking Strategy: Note the keyword *immediate*. Focus on the information in the question and the goals of care; that is, think about what complications you want to prevent. Remember that if a question requires you to prioritize, and one of the options relates to positioning a client, that option may be the correct one. Review care to the client experiencing vena cava syndrome and the test-taking strategies for answering prioritizing questions if you had difficulty with this question.

Level of Cognitive Ability: Application
Client Needs: Physiological Integrity
Integrated Process: Nursing Process/Implementation
Content Area: Delegating/Prioritizing

Reference
Lowdermilk D, Perry A: *Maternity & women's health care,* ed 8, St Louis, 2004, Mosby, p 536.

---

113. A postoperative client is angry after an argument on the telephone with her son and tells the nurse about her conversation. Which statement by the nurse would be most therapeutic?

1 "All mothers have arguments with their children."

2 "That's not very kind of your son. Doesn't he realize that you are trying to recuperate from surgery?"

3 "You seem quite upset."

4 "You need to focus your energy on building your strength."

Answer: 3

Rationale: Option 3 provides an opportunity for the client to share further and discuss feelings. Option 1 is a stereotypical comment. Options 2 and 4 seem to console the client, but they indicate that the nurse has taken "a side" in the argument, which is nontherapeutic.

Test-Taking Strategy: Use therapeutic communication techniques. Remember to address the client's concerns or feelings and elicit further information from the client. This will direct you to option 3. Review therapeutic communication techniques and the test-taking strategies for answering communication questions if you had difficulty with this question.

Level of Cognitive Ability: Application
Client Needs: Psychosocial Integrity
Integrated Process: Communication and Documentation
Content Area: Mental Health

Reference
Harkreader H, Hogan MA: *Fundamentals of nursing: caring and clinical judgment,* ed 2, Philadelphia, 2004, WB Saunders, pp 251, 255–257.

114. A client who had a mitral valve replacement is having a slow recovery. The client states, "I need to get better so that I can go hunting this season. If I'm not going to get better, I would be better off dead." Which of the following responses by the nurse would be most helpful?
1   "Can you tell me more about the way you feel?"
2   "Try to be a bit more positive."
3   "There are plenty of hunting seasons ahead of you. Let's focus on what you need to do now to get better."
4   "I know what you are saying. My husband is an avid hunter."

Answer: 1
Rationale: Option 1 encourages the client to share his or her fears. All of the incorrect options represent a block to communication, because they do not acknowledge the client's feelings or concerns and they put the client's feelings on hold.

Test-Taking Strategy: Use therapeutic communication techniques. Option 1 addresses the client's feelings, is nonjudgmental, and promotes further communication. Remember, the client's feelings are the priority. Review therapeutic communication techniques and the test-taking strategies for answering communication questions if you had difficulty with this question.

Level of Cognitive Ability: Application
Client Needs: Psychosocial Integrity
Integrated Process: Communication and Documentation
Content Area: Adult Health/Cardiovascular

Reference
Harkreader H, Hogan MA: *Fundamentals of nursing: caring and clinical judgment,* ed 2, Philadelphia, 2004, WB Saunders, pp 251, 255–257.

---

115. Levothyroxine sodium (Synthroid) is prescribed for a client with hypothyroidism. The nurse tells the client that this medication will result in
1   Decreased body temperature
2   Reduced gastric acid production
3   Increased energy level
4   Faster weight gain

Answer: 3
Rationale: Levothyroxine sodium is a synthetically prepared thyroid hormone that increases body metabolism and the client's energy level. It promotes weight loss and increases body temperature. It does not affect gastric acid production.

Test-Taking Strategy: Note that the question indicates the client's diagnosis. Also, recall that many thyroid hormone medications contain the letters *thy* in their name. Remember, if the medication is used to treat the hypothyroidism, the medication effects must be the opposite of the disease symptoms. This will direct you to option 3. Review the characteristics of this medication and the test-taking strategies for answering pharmacology questions if you had difficulty with this question.

Level of Cognitive Ability: Application
Client Needs: Physiological Integrity
Integrated Process: Teaching/Learning
Content Area: Adult Health/Endocrine

Reference
Hodgson B, Kizior R: *Saunders nursing drug handbook 2004,* Philadelphia, 2004, WB Saunders, p 596.

---

116. A client is admitted to the hospital after a high-voltage electrical injury. The client has dark-colored urine, and urinalysis results are positive for myoglobin. The nurse places

Answer: 1
Rationale: To prevent myoglobin from precipitating in the renal tubules, fluid intake is increased orally or by the intravenous route to maintain an adequate urine output of 30 to 50 mL or 0.5 mL/kg per hour in an adult client. There

highest priority on which of the following nursing actions?

1 Monitoring the urine output and examining the urine for color, odor, and the presence of particulate matter
2 Obtaining a nasogastric tube and lubricant from the supply area in preparation for insertion
3 Ambulating the client frequently
4 Reassuring the client that the injury will resolve without residual effects

are no data in the question indicating that a nasogastric tube is needed. Even so, this action is not the priority. A client with an acute injury would not be ambulated frequently. Option 4 is incorrect because it provides false reassurance.

Test-Taking Strategy: Note the keyword *priority.* Also note the relation between the abnormal urine sample finding in the question and in option 1. Also, option 3 can be eliminated because of the word *frequently.* Option 4 can be eliminated using Maslow's Hierarchy of Needs theory because it is unrelated to a physiological need. Review care to the client who sustained a high-voltage electrical injury and the test-taking strategies for answering prioritizing questions if you had difficulty with this question.

Level of Cognitive Ability: Application
Client Needs: Physiological Integrity
Integrated Process: Nursing Process/Implementation
Content Area: Adult Health/Integumentary

Reference
Ignatavicius D, Workman M: *Medical-surgical nursing: critical thinking for collaborative care,* ed 4, Philadelphia, 2002, WB Saunders, p 1567.

---

117. A woman is treated in the emergency department for a broken clavicle and a black eye. The woman reports that she sustained the injury from falling off of a step stool while trying to change window curtains. If the nurse suspects physical abuse by the client's husband, which statement would best encourage the client to share this information with the nurse?

1 "At times I see women who have been hurt by their husbands. Have you been hurt by anyone?"
2 "Your black eye sure doesn't seem as though it could have happened by accident."
3 "That black eye looks awfully painful. Did your husband hit you?"
4 "If your husband is abusing you, you can take him to court or get a restraining order."

Answer: 1
Rationale: The best approach to asking a woman about violence is to approach the client in a caring and nonthreatening manner. Options 2 and 3 are confrontational, and option 4 assumes that the client desires a restraining order. Option 2 also is incorrect because it is a judgmental statement that is likely to put the client on the defensive. Only option 1 allows the client the right to reject or accept further intervention by the nurse, and it is a caring response.

Test-Taking Strategy: Use therapeutic communication techniques. Option 1 is the only therapeutic statement, is supportive and displays caring, and provides the client the opportunity to talk about the situation if she so desires. Review care to the client suspected of abuse and the test-taking strategies for answering communication questions if you had difficulty with this question.

Level of Cognitive Ability: Application
Client Needs: Psychosocial Integrity
Integrated Process: Caring
Content Area: Mental Health

Reference
Varcarolis E: *Foundations of psychiatric mental health nursing,* ed 4, Philadelphia, 2002, WB Saunders, p 696.

118. A nurse is caring for a woman who has just undergone an emergency cesarean section. In preparing to discuss postoperative and home care measures, the nurse would first

1 Determine the client's ability to take in and process information

2 Make referrals to community agencies and support groups as needed

3 Provide comprehensive information about recovery and child care

4 Provide routine information according to standard teaching protocols

Answer: 1

Rationale: The residual physical and psychological effects of an emergency cesarean section can interfere with the client's ability to concentrate and learn new information. Therefore, the nurse should first determine the client's anxiety level, level of consciousness, and ability to take in and process information. Teaching is likely to be ineffective if the client is not able to process information.

Test-Taking Strategy: Note the keyword *first*. Use the nursing process and teaching and learning principles to answer the question. Recalling that assessment is the first step in the nursing process will direct you to option 1. Review home care measures for the client after an emergency cesarean section and the test-taking strategies for answering prioritizing questions if you had difficulty with this question.

Level of Cognitive Ability: Application
Client Needs: Health Promotion and Maintenance
Integrated Process: Nursing Process/Implementation
Content Area: Maternity/Postpartum

Reference
Lowdermilk D, Perry A: *Maternity & women's health care*, ed 8, St Louis, 2004, Mosby, pp 461, 1021.

---

119. A client is scheduled for electroconvulsive therapy. The client says to the nurse, "I'm so afraid that it will hurt and will make me worse off than I am." The nurse makes which best statement to the client?

1 "Can you tell me what you understand about the procedure?"

2 "Those are very normal fears, but please be assured that everything will be okay."

3 "Try not to worry. This is a well-known and easy procedure for the doctor."

4 "Your fears are a sign that you really should have this procedure."

Answer: 1

Rationale: Option 1 is a therapeutic communication technique that explores the client's feelings, determines the level of client understanding about the procedure, and displays caring. Option 2 does not address the client's fears and puts the client's feelings on hold. Option 3 diminishes the client's feelings by directing attention away from the client and to the doctor's importance. Option 4 demeans the client and does not encourage further sharing by the client.

Test-Taking Strategy: Use therapeutic communication techniques and remember to focus on the client's feelings and concerns. Option 1 is the only option that addresses the client's feelings, encourages client verbalization, and displays caring. Review therapeutic communication techniques and the test-taking strategies for answering communication questions if you had difficulty with this question.

Level of Cognitive Ability: Application
Client Needs: Psychosocial Integrity
Integrated Process: Caring
Content Area: Mental Health

Reference
Harkreader H, Hogan MA: *Fundamentals of nursing: caring and clinical judgment*, ed 2, Philadelphia, 2004, WB Saunders, pp 251, 255–257.

120. A 16-year-old client who underwent emergency surgery for a ruptured appendix refuses to allow the nurse to change the abdominal dressing. The client states: "Go away. There is nothing wrong with this dressing." Which of the following is the best nursing response?

1 "I promise to do this really quickly, and then I will leave you alone."

2 "I'll draw the curtain and expose only the area on your abdomen that is needed. Can I go ahead with that?"

3 "You can refuse the dressing change at this time, but your friends can't visit you until it is done."

4 "Please don't be upset with me. I am just doing my job."

Answer: 2

Rationale: The primary developmental need of the hospitalized teenager is maintenance of privacy, modesty, and control. The correct option strives to meet these needs. Options 1 and 4 do not address the client's concerns, and option 3 contains a threat.

Test-Taking Strategy: Note the keywords *16-year-old client.* Remember the developmental issues of the adolescent when answering this question. Also, use therapeutic communication techniques. Option 2 is the only option that focuses on the client's feelings and needs. Review therapeutic communication techniques and the test-taking strategies for answering communication questions if you had difficulty with this question.

Level of Cognitive Ability: Application
Client Needs: Health Promotion and Maintenance
Integrated Process: Communication and Documentation
Content Area: Child Health

References
Harkreader H, Hogan MA: *Fundamentals of nursing: caring and clinical judgment,* ed 2, Philadelphia, 2004, WB Saunders, pp 251, 255–257.
Wong D, Hockenberry M: *Wong's nursing care of infants and children,* ed 7, St Louis, 2003, Mosby, pp 149, 812–817.

121. A nurse is teaching a client with left-sided weakness how to safely use a cane. The nurse tells the client to hold the cane with the

1 Left hand and 6 inches lateral to the left foot

2 Left hand, placing the cane in front of the left foot

3 Right hand and 6 inches lateral to the right foot

4 Right hand, placing the cane in front of the right foot

Answer: 3

Rationale: The client is taught to hold the cane on the opposite side of the weakness to provide support for the weak side. A client with left-sided weakness would hold the cane in the right hand. The cane is placed 6 inches lateral to the fifth toe. Options 1, 2, and 4 are incorrect.

Test-Taking Strategy: Visualize the procedure for walking with a cane. Recalling that the cane is held at the client's side, not in front, helps you to eliminate options 2 and 4 first. Knowing that the correct method is to have the cane positioned on the stronger side helps you to eliminate option 1. Review the procedure for teaching a client how to use a cane and the various test-taking strategies if you had difficulty with this question.

Level of Cognitive Ability: Application
Client Needs: Safe, Effective Care Environment
Integrated Process: Teaching/Learning
Content Area: Adult Health/Musculoskeletal

Reference
Harkreader H, Hogan MA: *Fundamentals of nursing: caring and clinical judgment,* ed 2, Philadelphia, 2004, WB Saunders, p 793.

122. A nurse is caring for a client 1 day after gastrectomy. The client has a nasogastric (NG) tube, and the nurse notes that the tube is draining brown-tinged secretions. Which of the following is the most appropriate nursing intervention?
1   Notify the physician immediately
2   Document the findings
3   Reposition the client
4   Irrigate the NG tube

Answer: 2

Rationale: After gastrectomy, drainage from the NG tube is normally bloody for 24 hours after the procedure, then changes to brown-tinged, and then to yellow or clear. The nurse would document this finding. There is no need to notify the physician immediately because this finding is expected. Although the client is repositioned in the post-operative period, this action is unrelated to the data in the question. After gastrectomy, an NG tube should not be irrigated without specific orders from the physician.

Test-Taking Strategy: Focus on the keywords *1 day after gastrectomy.* Recalling that the gastrointestinal drainage would be brown-tinged at this time will direct you to option 2. Review the expected findings after gastrectomy and various test-taking strategies if you had difficulty with this question.

Level of Cognitive Ability: Application
Client Needs: Physiological Integrity
Integrated Process: Nursing Process/Implementation
Content Area: Adult Health/Gastrointestinal

Reference
Phipps W, Monahan F, Sands J, Marek J, Neighbors M: *Medical-surgical nursing: health and illness perspectives,* ed 7, St Louis, 2003, Mosby, p 1048.

---

123. A clinic nurse has provided instructions to the mother of a child with a urinary tract infection. Which statement by the mother indicates a need for further instructions?
1   "I should wipe my child from front to back after urination or a bowel movement."
2   "I should increase my child's fluid intake."
3   "I should encourage my child to hold the urine and to urinate at least four times a day."
4   "I should avoid the use of bubble baths with my child."

Answer: 3

Rationale: The parents should be taught to wipe the child from front to back after urination or a bowel movement to avoid moving bacteria from the anus to the urethra. Fluid intake including water should be encouraged. The child should be encouraged to avoid holding urine and to urinate at least four times a day; also, the bladder should be emptied with each void to prevent residual urine. Bubble baths are avoided secondary to possible urethral irritation.

Test-Taking Strategy: Note the keywords *need for further instructions.* This is a false response question. Therefore, you are looking for the option that indicates that further teaching needs to be done. Careful reading of the options and applying principles related to prevention of urinary tract infections will direct you to option 3. Review client instructions related to a urinary tract infection and the various test-taking strategies if you had difficulty with this question.

Level of Cognitive Ability: Analysis
Client Needs: Health Promotion and Maintenance
Integrated Process: Nursing Process/Evaluation
Content Area: Child Health

Reference
Wong D, Hockenberry M: *Wong's nursing care of infants and children,* ed 7, St Louis, 2003, Mosby, p 1268.

124. The nurse notes that a new postoperative client is experiencing tachycardia and tachypnea. The nurse takes the client's blood pressure and notes that it is 88/60 mm Hg. The nurse takes which immediate action?
    1 Checks the hourly urine output
    2 Checks the intravenous (IV) site for infiltration
    3 Elevates the client's feet, keeping the head slightly elevated
    4 Turns the client on the right side

Answer: 3

Rationale: The client is exhibiting signs of shock and requires emergency intervention. Placing the client flat or with the head elevated 30 degrees and elevating the feet increases venous return, and subsequently blood pressure. The nurse then can verify the client's volume status by checking the urine output and whether the IV is infusing. The nurse should obtain all this information quickly, and then call the physician. Turning the client on the right side will not assist the client in this situation.

Test-Taking Strategy: Focus on the information in the question and note the keyword *immediate*. After determining that this is an emergency situation, look for the option that supports the ABCs—airway, breathing, and circulation. Because only option 3 supports the client's immediate physiological needs, the nurse should take this action immediately. Review care to the postoperative client and the test-taking strategies for answering prioritizing questions if you had difficulty with this question.

Level of Cognitive Ability: Application
Client Needs: Physiological Integrity
Integrated Process: Nursing Process/Implementation
Content Area: Adult Health/Cardiovascular

Reference
Ignatavicius D, Workman M: *Medical-surgical nursing: critical thinking for collaborative care,* ed 4, Philadelphia, 2002, WB Saunders, p 780.

125. The nurse tells a client scheduled to have a lumbar puncture that he will be placed in a knee-chest position for the procedure. When the client asks the nurse why this position is necessary, the nurse responds that it
    1 Provides for greater client comfort
    2 Prevents leakage of fluid from the brain
    3 Allows for a smaller needle to be used
    4 Increases the spacing between the vertebrae

Answer: 4

Rationale: The anatomy of the vertebral column is such that curving the structure provides for more open spacing in the L3-L5 area. The choice of the size of the needle for puncture is not dependent on position. Also, client position is not related to leakage of cerebrospinal fluid. Pillows and support of the nursing staff aid in client comfort.

Test-Taking Strategy: Note the issue: the purpose of a knee-chest position. Visualizing this position will direct you to the correct option. Review this procedure and the various test-taking strategies if you had difficulty with this question.

Level of Cognitive Ability: Application
Client Needs: Physiological Integrity
Integrated Process: Teaching/Learning
Content Area: Adult Health/Neurological

Reference
Lewis S, Heitkemper M, Dirksen S: *Medical-surgical nursing: assessment and management of clinical problems,* ed 6, St Louis, 2004, Mosby, p 1487.

126. A client comes to the hospital emergency department and verbalizes reports of severe right lower abdominal pain characteristic of appendicitis. The client does not have any health insurance. The nurse understands that legally the hospital must

1 Refer the client to the nearest public hospital

2 Have a physician see the client before admission

3 Provide uncompensated care in emergency situations

4 Respect the family's requests to admit their family member to the hospital

Answer: 3

Rationale: Federal law and many state laws require that hospitals must provide emergency care. The client can be transferred only after the client has been medically screened and stabilized. The client must give consent for the transfer, and there must be a facility that will accept the client. Options 1, 2, and 4 do not fully address the legal requirements for emergency care.

Test-Taking Strategy: Note the keywords *does not have any health insurance* and the word *legally*. Noting that the situation presented is an emergency situation will direct you to option 3. Option 3 is the option that addresses the legal scope of providing emergency care. Review the legal issues related to providing emergency care and the various test-taking strategies if you had difficulty with this question.

Level of Cognitive Ability: Comprehension
Client Needs: Safe, Effective Care Environment
Integrated Process: Nursing Process/Planning
Content Area: Leadership/Management

References
Lauritsen-Christen B, Odea-Kockrow E: *Foundations of nursing,* ed 4, St Louis, 2003, Mosby, pp 13, 22.
Potter P, Perry A: *Fundamentals of nursing,* ed 6, St Louis, 2005, Mosby, p 43.

---

127. While caring for a client in labor, the nurse suspects an umbilical cord prolapse. The nurse would immediately

1 Adjust the bed to the Trendelenburg position

2 Encourage the woman to push with each contraction

3 Set up for an emergency cesarean section

4 Calmly reassure the woman and her partner that all possible measures are being taken

Answer: 1

Rationale: Adjusting the bed into Trendelenburg position uses gravity to reverse the direction of the pressure, keeping the presenting part off the umbilical cord. In addition, the knee-chest, or modified Sims', position can be used. Pushing with contractions is contraindicated because it will push the presenting part against the cord. Not all prolapsed cords require a cesarean section. The nurse would reassure the client and her partner after placing the client in the Trendelenburg position.

Test-Taking Strategy: Note the keyword *immediately* and visualize the situation. Eliminate option 4 first using Maslow's Hierarchy of Needs theory, because it does not address a physiological need. From the remaining options, select the option that addresses the physiological safety of the primary client (the fetus). Also, remember, in a prioritizing question, if repositioning is indicated in one of the options, that option may be the correct one. Review immediate interventions for umbilical cord prolapse and the test-taking strategies for answering prioritizing questions if you had difficulty with this question.

Level of Cognitive Ability: Application
Client Needs: Physiological Integrity

Integrated Process: Nursing Process/Implementation
Content Area: Maternity/Intrapartum

Reference

Lowdermilk D, Perry A: *Maternity & women's health care*, ed 8, St Louis, 2004, Mosby, p 1028.

---

128. A nurse hears a cardiac monitor alarm sound, rushes to the client, and notes a straight line on the monitor screen. The nurse's takes which action first?
1 Calls a code
2 Turns up the amplitude on the monitor
3 Checks the client
4 Confirms the rhythm using a different cardiac lead

Answer: 3

Rationale: If the monitor alarm sounds, the nurse should first check the clinical status of the client to determine whether the problem is an actual dysrhythmia or a malfunction of the monitoring system. Options 1, 2, and 4 are not the first actions.

Test-Taking Strategy: Note the keyword *first*. Use the steps of the nursing process. Remember, assessment is the first step, so check the client first. Review care to the client on a cardiac monitor and the test-taking strategies for answering prioritizing questions if you had difficulty with this question.

Level of Cognitive Ability: Application
Client Needs: Physiological Integrity
Integrated Process: Nursing Process/Implementation
Content Area: Adult Health/Cardiovascular

Reference

Lewis S, Heitkemper M, Dirksen S: *Medical-surgical nursing: assessment and management of clinical problems*, ed 6, St Louis, 2004, Mosby, pp 864–865.

---

129. A nurse is preparing to care for a woman victimized by physical abuse. The nurse would most appropriately plan to first
1 Talk to the woman about the fact that she might have provoked the abuse
2 Support the woman and facilitate access to a safe environment
3 Establish firm time lines for the woman to make necessary changes in her life situation
4 Reinforce that dealing with the psychological aspects is of the highest priority

Answer: 2

Rationale: The nurse must provide emotional support to the client and provide measures to ensure a safe environment. Option 1 fosters the notion that the client is at fault. In options 3 and 4, the nurse may be making unreasonable demands, which could cause further distress for the client.

Test-Taking Strategy: Note the keyword *first*. Use Maslow's Hierarchy of Needs theory to assist in directing you to option 2. Remember, if a physiological need does not exist in one of the options, then a safety need is the priority. Also, option 2 provides support to the client. Review care to the client victimized by physical abuse and the test-taking strategies for answering prioritizing questions if you had difficulty with this question.

Level of Cognitive Ability: Application
Client Needs: Safe, Effective Care Environment
Integrated Process: Caring
Content Area: Mental Health

Reference

Varcarolis E: *Foundations of psychiatric mental health nursing*, ed 4, Philadelphia, 2002, WB Saunders, p 696.

130. A nurse is assigned to care for a pregnant client with acquired immunodeficiency syndrome (AIDS). The nurse develops a plan of care for the client and includes which priority client goal in the plan?
1   The client will not have sexual relations during the remainder of the pregnancy
2   The client will not experience development of an opportunistic infection during the remainder of the pregnancy
3   The client knows about local AIDS support groups
4   The client moves through the grief process

Answer: 2

Rationale: AIDS is caused by the retrovirus human immunodeficiency virus (HIV), which invades T lymphocytes. This disables the body's ability to fight infection. Nursing goals are directed toward the prevention of infections. Sexual relations are not contraindicated if protective devices are used properly. Options 3 and 4 are the focus of interventions, not goals.

Test-Taking Strategy: Note the keyword *priority*. Focus on the issue: client goals; this will assist you in eliminating options 3 and 4. Option 1 is unrealistic and unnecessary if protective devices are properly used, and it may be a goal to which the client will not adhere. Also, use Maslow's Hierarchy of Needs theory and note that option 2 addresses a physiological need. Review care to the pregnant client with AIDS and the test-taking strategies for answering prioritizing questions if you had difficulty with this question.

Level of Cognitive Ability: Application
Client Needs: Safe, Effective Care Environment
Integrated Process: Nursing Process/Planning
Content Area: Adult Health/Immune

Reference
Lowdermilk D, Perry A: *Maternity & women's health care,* ed 8, St Louis, 2004, Mosby, p 203.

---

131. An older woman is admitted to the acute psychiatric unit with a diagnosis of moderate depression. The client is unclean, her hair is uncombed, and she is inappropriately dressed. She is accompanied by her adult daughter who is upset about her mother's lack of interest in her appearance. The nurse most appropriately alleviates the daughter's concern by telling her that
1   Hygiene is not important to those who are depressed
2   The nurse will assist her mother in meeting hygiene needs until she is able to resume self-care
3   Client self-esteem needs take priority over appearances
4   Group peer pressure on the unit will soon have her mother attending to her hygiene needs

Answer: 2

Rationale: Both the client and her family should know that the nurse will assist the client until the client can resume self-care activities. The client is experiencing psychomotor retardation and decreased energy at this time and requires assistance. Options 1, 3, and 4 will not alleviate the daughter's concern.

Test-Taking Strategy: Focus on the issue: alleviating the daughter's concern. Use Maslow's Hierarchy of Needs theory. Only option 2 addresses the client's physiological needs. Review care to the client with depression and the various test-taking strategies if you had difficulty with this question.

Level of Cognitive Ability: Application
Client Needs: Psychosocial Integrity
Integrated Process: Caring
Content Area: Mental Health

Reference
Varcarolis E: *Foundations of psychiatric mental health nursing,* ed 4, Philadelphia, 2002, WB Saunders, p 467.

132. An emergency department nurse prepares to care for a client with a suspected fracture of the right radial bone. The nurse would initially plan to do which of the following?

1 Obtain a radiograph of the right arm

2 Place a plastic cast on the right arm

3 Place the right arm in a sling and arrange for an orthopedic consultation

4 Check for distal pulses and the neurovascular status of the right arm

Answer: 4

Rationale: The initial intervention is to check for distal pulses and the neurovascular status of the affected extremity. A physician is responsible for obtaining a radiograph and applying a cast. It may be appropriate to place the extremity in a sling, but this is not the initial action.

Test-Taking Strategy: Note the keyword *initially.* Use both the steps of the nursing process and the ABCs—airway, breathing, and circulation—to answer the question. Option 4 addresses assessment and circulation. Review care to the client with a fracture and the test-taking strategies for answering prioritizing questions if you had difficulty with this question.

Level of Cognitive Ability: Application
Client Needs: Physiological Integrity
Integrated Process: Nursing Process/Planning
Content Area: Adult Health/Musculoskeletal

Reference
Phipps W, Monahan F, Sands J, Marek J, Neighbors M: *Medical-surgical nursing: health and illness perspectives,* ed 7, St Louis, 2003, Mosby, p 1478.

---

133. A nurse finds a client lying on the floor of his hospital room after sustaining a fall and hitting his head on the bedside table. The client's breathing is shallow, and a pulse is present. The nurse takes which action first?

1 Calls the doctor

2 Checks vital signs and level of consciousness

3 Calls a code

4 Calls the client's family

Answer: 2

Rationale: Because the client is breathing and has a pulse, the nurse needs to check the client before taking any other action. Level of consciousness and vital signs should be determined, particularly in a client who has sustained a head injury, and then the physician and family should be notified. Calling a code is not indicated at this time.

Test-Taking Strategy: Note the keyword *first.* Focus on the data in the question and note that the client is breathing and has a pulse. Next, use the steps of the nursing process. Only option 2 addresses assessment. Review care to the client who sustains a fall and the test-taking strategies for answering prioritizing questions if you had difficulty with this question.

Level of Cognitive Ability: Application
Client Needs: Physiological Integrity
Integrated Process: Nursing Process/Implementation
Content Area: Adult Health/Neurological

Reference
Lewis S, Heitkemper M, Dirksen S: *Medical-surgical nursing: assessment and management of clinical problems,* ed 6, St Louis, 2004, Mosby, p 1509.

---

134. A nurse is caring for a client who is dying. The nurse develops the plan of care understanding that which intervention would be inappropriate in the care of the client?

Answer: 1

Rationale: In planning care for the dying client, the nurse provides information and answers questions to the extent most helpful to the client and family. The nurse suggests making referrals to other disciplines and clergy based on an

1   Providing extremely thorough answers to each question asked by the client or family

2   Suggesting making referrals to other disciplines based on client's stated needs

3   Planning to balance the client's need for assistance with that for independence

4   Offering to contact the clergy to support the client's spiritual needs

identified need and tries to balance the client's need for assistance with the need to maintain some measure of independence. Also, it is important to spend time with the client.

Test-Taking Strategy: Note the keyword *inappropriate*. This indicates a false response question, and that you need to select the option that is an incorrect intervention. Eliminate options 2 and 4 first because they are similar. From the remaining options, note the exaggerated detail of response implied in option 1, which makes it inappropriate. Review the psychosocial needs of the dying client and the various test-taking strategies if you had difficulty with this question.

Level of Cognitive Ability: Comprehension
Client Needs: Psychosocial Integrity
Integrated Process: Caring
Content Area: Fundamental Skills

Reference
Ignatavicius D, Workman M: *Medical-surgical nursing: critical thinking for collaborative care,* ed 4, Philadelphia, 2002, WB Saunders, pp 111–113.

---

135. A nurse is preparing a client who will have spinal anesthesia for surgery. The nurse places highest priority on documenting and reporting which of the following items to the nurse on the next shift, who will care for the client after surgery?

1   Blood pressure of 126/78 mm Hg

2   Pulse rate of 78 beats/min

3   Voided 300 mL before surgery

4   Presence of weakness in the left lower extremity

Answer: 4

Rationale: It is important to document and report any preoperative weakness or impaired movement of a lower extremity in the client who is to have spinal anesthesia because it causes temporary paralysis of the lower extremities. Therefore, when the client's function returns, the preoperative weakness or impairment will not be misinterpreted as a complication of anesthesia. Options 1, 2, and 3 may be documented and reported, but they are not the highest priority.

Test-Taking Strategy: Note the keywords *spinal anesthesia* and *highest priority*. Note the relation between the words *spinal anesthesia* and option 4. Also note that the data in options 1, 2, and 3 are normal findings. Review care to the preoperative client and the test-taking strategies for answering prioritizing questions if you had difficulty with this question.

Level of Cognitive Ability: Analysis
Client Needs: Physiological Integrity
Integrated Process: Communication and Documentation
Content Area: Leadership/Management

Reference
Harkreader H, Hogan MA: *Fundamentals of nursing: caring and clinical judgment,* ed 2, Philadelphia, 2004, WB Saunders, pp 1211, 1217.

---

136. A client experiencing delusions of being poisoned is admitted to the hospital after not eating or drinking for several days. The client shows no evidence of dehydration and malnu-

Answer: 2

Rationale: The maintenance of safety is an important consideration when working with clients who have delusions. There are no data in the question to indicate that options 1, 3, and 4 require immediate attention.

trition at this time. The nurse prepares a plan of care for the client and includes which client need as the priority?

1　Physiological needs
2　Safety and security needs
3　Self-esteem needs
4　Love and belonging needs

Test-Taking Strategy: Note the keywords *priority* and *shows no evidence of dehydration and malnutrition.* Use Maslow's Hierarchy of Needs theory. Safety takes precedence if a physiological need does not exist. This will direct you to option 2. Review care to the client experiencing delusions and the test-taking strategies for answering prioritizing questions if you had difficulty with this question.

Level of Cognitive Ability: Application
Client Needs: Safe, Effective Care Environment
Integrated Process: Nursing Process/Planning
Content Area: Mental Health

References
Harkreader H, Hogan MA: *Fundamentals of nursing: caring and clinical judgment,* ed 2, Philadelphia, 2004, WB Saunders, pp 195–196.
Stuart G, Laraia M: *Principles and practice of psychiatric nursing,* ed 7, St Louis, 2001, Mosby, pp 422–424.

---

137. A nurse enters the room of a client with diabetes mellitus and finds the client difficult to arouse. The client's skin is cool and clammy, and the client's pulse rate is increased from the client's baseline. The nurse immediately

1　Prepares an intravenous insulin solution
2　Gives the client a glass of orange juice
3　Administers an intravenous bolus dose of 50% dextrose
4　Checks the client's capillary blood glucose

Answer: 4

Rationale: The client's signs and symptoms are consistent with hypoglycemia. The nurse must first obtain a blood glucose reading, and then report it to the physician for subsequent orders. The nurse would not give a client fluid or food if the client is not alert because of the risk for aspiration. The physician orders an intravenous bolus dose of 50% dextrose if needed. Option 1 is implemented as needed in the treatment of hyperglycemia.

Test-Taking Strategy: Note the keyword *immediately* and focus on the data in the question. Use the steps of the nursing process and note that only option 4 addresses assessment. Review care to the client experiencing hypoglycemia and the test-taking strategies for answering prioritizing questions if you had difficulty with this question.

Level of Cognitive Ability: Application
Client Needs: Physiological Integrity
Integrated Process: Nursing Process/Implementation
Content Area: Adult Health/Endocrine

Reference
Lewis S, Heitkemper M, Dirksen S: *Medical-surgical nursing: assessment and management of clinical problems,* ed 6, St Louis, 2004, Mosby, p 1292.

---

138. A home care nurse visits an older client who has hyperparathyroidism with severe osteoporosis. The nurse identifies which nursing diagnosis in the plan of care as the priority for this client?

1　Risk for Injury
2　Risk for Situational Low Self-esteem

Answer: 1

Rationale: The individual with hyperparathyroidism with severe osteoporosis is at risk for pathological fractures because of bone demineralization (option 1). Thus, home safety is a priority. No data in the question indicate that options 2, 3, and 4 are of concern.

Test-Taking Strategy: Focus on the client's diagnosis and note the keyword *priority.* Use Maslow's Hierarchy of

3   Social Isolation
4   Risk for Loneliness

Needs theory. Recall that if a physiological need is not identified in one of the options, then safety is the priority. Note that options 2, 3, and 4 are similar in that they address a psychosocial need. Review care to the client with hyperparathyroidism with severe osteoporosis and the test-taking strategies for answering prioritizing questions if you had difficulty with this question.

Level of Cognitive Ability: Analysis
Client Needs: Safe, Effective Care Environment
Integrated Process: Nursing Process/Analysis
Content Area: Adult Health/Endocrine

Reference

Lewis S, Heitkemper M, Dirksen S: *Medical-surgical nursing: assessment and management of clinical problems,* ed 6, St Louis, 2004, Mosby, pp 1324, 1709.

---

139. Oxygen through nasal cannula at 4 L/min is prescribed for a client admitted to the hospital. The nurse avoids which action in the care of the client?
1   Applying water-soluble lubricant to the nares
2   Instructing the client and family about the purpose of the oxygen
3   Humidifying the oxygen
4   Instructing the client to breath through the nose only

Answer: 4

Rationale: The nasal cannula provides for smaller concentrations of oxygen and can even be used with mouth breathers because movement of air through the oropharynx pulls oxygen from the nasopharynx. It is not necessary to instruct a client to breathe only through the nose. Options 1, 2, and 3 are correct interventions.

Test-Taking Strategy: Note the keyword *avoids*. This is a false response question, which indicates that you need to look for the incorrect nursing action. Noting that option 4 contains the absolute word *only* will direct you to this option. Review care to the client receiving oxygen and the various test-taking strategies if you had difficulty with this question.

Level of Cognitive Ability: Application
Client Needs: Physiological Integrity
Integrated Process: Nursing Process/Implementation
Content Area: Fundamental Skills

Reference

Ignatavicius D, Workman M: *Medical-surgical nursing: critical thinking for collaborative care,* ed 4, Philadelphia, 2002, WB Saunders, p 492.

---

140. A nurse notes that the client has a nursing diagnosis of Ineffective Airway Clearance documented in the plan of care. The nurse plans to use which of the following indicators as the best guide to determine when the client needs suctioning?
1   Apical heart rate
2   Respiratory rate
3   Inability to expectorate mucus
4   Arterial blood gas results

Answer: 3

Rationale: Suctioning is indicated when the client cannot expectorate mucus after using a variety of other assistive methods. The need for suctioning is best determined by listening for coarse gurgling or bubbling respirations, or by hearing abnormal breath sounds with auscultation. The other options could be affected by factors other than the accumulation of secretions.

Test-Taking Strategy: Focus on the issue: the need for suctioning; also note the nursing diagnosis. Note the relation of these items and option 3. Review suctioning procedures and the various test-taking strategies if you had difficulty with this question.

Level of Cognitive Ability: Analysis
Client Needs: Physiological Integrity
Integrated Process: Nursing Process/Planning
Content Area: Adult Health/Respiratory

Reference

Gulanick M, Myers J, Klopp A, Gradishar D, Galanes S, Puzas M: *Nursing care plans: nursing diagnosis and intervention,* ed 5, St Louis, 2003, Mosby, pp 10–11.

---

141. The nurse checks the stoma of a postoperative client who had a creation of a colostomy performed and notes that it is a dark, dusky color. The nurse takes which immediate action?

1 Changes the ostomy bag
2 Irrigates the colostomy
3 Orders a larger-sized ostomy bag
4 Notifies the surgeon

Answer: 4

Rationale: The color of a stoma should be a moist, beefy red. A dark, dusky stoma indicates ischemia, requiring notification of the surgeon. Options 1, 2, and 3 are incorrect actions.

Test-Taking Strategy: Note the keywords *immediate* and *dark, dusky color.* Recalling that a dark, dusky color indicates ischemia, and that if this occurs it presents an emergency situation, will direct you to option 4. Remember that if an emergency situation exists, the correct option may be the option that indicates physician notification. Review care to the client after creation of a colostomy and the test-taking strategies for answering prioritizing questions if you had difficulty with this question.

Level of Cognitive Ability: Application
Client Needs: Physiological Integrity
Integrated Process: Nursing Process/Implementation
Content Area: Adult Health/Gastrointestinal

Reference

Ignatavicius D, Workman M: *Medical-surgical nursing: critical thinking for collaborative care,* ed 4, Philadelphia, 2002, WB Saunders, p 1251.

---

142. A nurse witnesses a motor vehicle accident in which a pedestrian is hit by a car. The nurse suspects that the victim has a fractured leg. Which of the following is the most appropriate nursing action?

1 Stay with the victim and encourage the victim to remain still.
2 Assist the victim to get up and walk to the sidewalk, so that he is safe.
3 Leave the victim to call an ambulance.
4 Try to manually reduce the fracture.

Answer: 1

Rationale: The client with a suspected fracture is not moved unless it is dangerous to remain in that spot. The nurse should remain with the client and have someone else call for emergency help. A fracture is not reduced at the scene, and reduction is not performed by the nurse. The site of the fracture is immobilized to prevent further injury before moving the client.

Test-Taking Strategy: Note the keywords *most appropriate.* Focus on the issue: a fractured leg. Eliminate options 2 and 4 first because they could result in further injury to the client. From the remaining options, focus on the client's needs and remember that it is best for the nurse to remain with the client and have someone else call for emergency assistance. Review emergency interventions for a fracture and the various test-taking strategies if you had difficulty with this question.

Level of Cognitive Ability: Application
Client Needs: Physiological Integrity
Integrated Process: Nursing Process/Implementation
Content Area: Adult Health/Musculoskeletal

Reference
Lewis S, Heitkemper M, Dirksen S: *Medical-surgical nursing: assessment and management of clinical problems,* ed 6, St Louis, 2004, Mosby, p 1665.

---

143. A client with hypercholesterolemia is instructed to limit intake of dietary cholesterol. The nurse tells the client to select which of the following meat choices because it is lowest in fat?
  1 Lamb
  2 Pork spare ribs
  3 Broiled duck
  4 Baked goose

Answer: 1
Rationale: The best meat choices to decrease intake of cholesterol include lean cuts of beef with the fat trimmed, lamb, pork (except spare ribs), veal (except ground), skinless poultry, and shellfish. Meats that have larger amounts of cholesterol include prime grades of beef, pork spare ribs, goose, duck, organ meats (liver, brain, and kidney), sausage, bacon, luncheon meats, frankfurters, and caviar.

Test-Taking Strategy: Note the keywords *lowest in fat.* Eliminate options 3 and 4 first because they are similar food items. Next, eliminate option 2 because of its high fat content. Review dietary measures for the client with hypercholesterolemia and the various test-taking strategies if you had difficulty with this question.

Level of Cognitive Ability: Application
Client Needs: Health Promotion and Maintenance
Integrated Process: Teaching/Learning
Content Area: Adult Health/Cardiovascular

Reference
Williams S: *Basic nutrition & diet therapy,* ed 11, St Louis, 2001, Mosby, p 237.

---

144. A nurse provides dietary instructions to a client with hypertension. The nurse determines that the client understands the instructions if the client states that it is acceptable to eat which of the following food items?
  1 Hot dogs
  2 Turkey
  3 Salad with blue cheese dressing
  4 Corned beef hash

Answer: 2
Rationale: A client with hypertension needs to avoid foods that are high in sodium, such as bacon, hot dogs, luncheon meat, chipped or corned beef, kosher meat, smoked or salted meat or fish, peanut butter, and a variety of shellfish. Processed foods, canned foods, cheese, and many salad dressings also are high in sodium.

Test-Taking Strategy: Eliminate options 1 and 4 first because they are similar and because hot dogs and corned beef are highly processed meats and are high in sodium. Option 3 also is eliminated because blue cheese dressing is high in sodium. Review dietary instructions for the client with hypertension and the various test-taking strategies if you had difficulty with this question.

Level of Cognitive Ability: Analysis
Client Needs: Health Promotion and Maintenance
Integrated Process: Teaching/Learning
Content Area: Adult Health/Cardiovascular

Reference
Williams S: *Basic nutrition & diet therapy*, ed 11, St Louis, 2001, Mosby, p 366.

---

145. A nurse is assessing a client with a diagnosis of bulimia nervosa who has problems with nutrition. The nurse would obtain information from the client about which of the following first?
1 Feelings about self and body weight
2 Previous and current coping skills
3 Lack of control
4 Eating patterns, food preferences, and concerns about eating

Answer: 4

Rationale: The nurse first would identify the client's eating patterns, food preferences, and concerns about eating when caring for the client with bulimia nervosa. Obtaining information about the client's feelings about self and body weight, previous and current coping skills, and lack of control also would be obtained, but they are secondary to eating patterns and food preferences.

Test-Taking Strategy: Note the keyword *first*. Use Maslow's Hierarchy of Needs theory to prioritize. Option 4 is the only option that relates to a physiological need. Review care for the client with bulimia nervosa and the test-taking strategies for answering prioritizing questions if you had difficulty with this question.

Level of Cognitive Ability: Application
Client Needs: Physiological Integrity
Integrated Process: Nursing Process/Assessment
Content Area: Delegating/Prioritizing

Reference
Stuart G, Laraia M: *Principles and practice of psychiatric nursing*, ed 7, St Louis, 2001, Mosby, p 528.

---

146. A community health nurse is assisting residents involved in a hurricane and flood. Many of the older residents are emotionally despondent and refuse to evacuate their homes. With regard to rescue and relocation of the older residents, the nurse plans first to
1 Attend to emotional needs
2 Attend to nutritional and basic needs
3 Contact families
4 Arrange for transportation to shelters

Answer: 2

Rationale: Attending to people's basic needs of food, shelter, and clothing are the priority. Options 1, 3, and 4 may or may not be needed at a later date.

Test-Taking Strategy: Note the keyword *first* and use Maslow's Hierarchy of Needs theory. Option 2 addresses basic physiological needs. Options 1, 3, and 4 address psychosocial needs and may be appropriate at a later date. Review the nurse's role in the event of a disaster and the test-taking strategies for answering prioritizing questions if you had difficulty with this question.

Level of Cognitive Ability: Application
Client Needs: Physiological Integrity
Integrated Process: Nursing Process/Planning
Content Area: Delegating/Prioritizing

Reference
Clemen-Stone S, McGuire S, Eigsti D: *Comprehensive community family*, ed 6, St Louis, 2002, Mosby, p 163.

147. A nurse is preparing the parents of a neonate with respiratory distress syndrome for an initial visit to the neonatal intensive care unit. The nurse plans which action to best facilitate parent–neonate bonding?
1   Explains the equipment used and how it will assist their neonate
2   Encourages the parents to touch their neonate
3   Identifies specific care-taking tasks that may be assumed by the parents
4   Gives the parents literature to read about respiratory distress syndrome

Answer: 2
Rationale: The best action that promotes bonding is to encourage the parents to touch their neonate. Options 1 and 3 may be frightening because of the newborn's condition and the unfamiliarity of high-risk neonate care practices. Option 4 is inappropriate. Asking parents to read literature does not enhance the parent–neonate bond.

Test-Taking Strategy: Focus on the issue: the action that will best facilitate parent–neonate bonding. Note the relation of the issue to option 2. Option 2 is the only option that addresses touch, which is directly related to bonding. Review parent–neonate bonding concepts and the various test-taking strategies if you had difficulty with this question.

Level of Cognitive Ability: Application
Client Needs: Psychosocial Integrity
Integrated Process: Caring
Content Area: Maternity/Postpartum

Reference
Lowdermilk D, Perry A: *Maternity & women's health care,* ed 8, St Louis, 2004, Mosby, pp 648, 729.

---

148. A nurse is preparing to care for a client admitted to the mental health unit with a diagnosis of dementia and notes a nursing diagnosis of Self-Care Deficit in the plan of care. The nurse plans for which outcome in caring for the client?
1   The client will be oriented to place by the time of discharge
2   The client will correctly identify objects in his or her room by the time of discharge
3   The client will be free of hallucinations by the time of discharge
4   The client will feed self with cueing within 24 hours

Answer: 4
Rationale: Option 4 identifies an outcome directly related to the client's ability to care for self. Options 1, 2, and 3 are not related to self-care deficit.

Test-Taking Strategy: Note the relation between the nursing diagnosis Self-Care Deficit and option 4. Also, use Maslow's Hierarchy of Needs theory. Option 4 is the only option that addresses a physiological need. Review care to the client with dementia and the various test-taking strategies if you had difficulty with this question.

Level of Cognitive Ability: Application
Client Needs: Physiological Integrity
Integrated Process: Nursing Process/Planning
Content Area: Mental Health

Reference
Gulanick M, Myers J, Klopp A, Gradishar D, Galanes S, Puzas M: *Nursing care plans: nursing diagnosis and intervention,* ed 5, St Louis, 2003, Mosby, p 133.

---

149. The nurse is called by a physical therapist to the room of a client experiencing a seizure. The nurse does which of the following to ensure the client's safety?
1   Wiggles a bite stick (airway) between the client's clenched teeth

Answer: 4
Rationale: Nursing management during a seizure includes easing the client to the floor, if out of bed, and loosening clothing such as a belt, tie, or collar. The client is turned to the side whenever possible to allow drainage of secretions from the mouth. A bite stick (airway) is never forced between the teeth of a client during a seizure; this could damage the teeth and gums. The client is not

2 Restrains the client to prevent bruising

3 Draws the curtain around the bedside area

4 Turns the client to the side if possible

restrained because the strong muscle contractions during seizure activity could cause injury. The curtain should be drawn, but it is done for privacy, not to prevent injury.

Test-Taking Strategy: Focus on the issue: client safety. Use the ABCs—airway, breathing, and circulation—to direct you to option 4. Also, eliminate options 1 and 2 because they could harm the client and option 3 because it relates to privacy, not safety. Review care to the client experiencing a seizure and the various test-taking strategies if you had difficulty with this question.

Level of Cognitive Ability: Application
Client Needs: Safe, Effective Care Environment
Integrated Process: Nursing Process/Implementation
Content Area: Adult Health/Neurological

Reference
Ignatavicius D, Workman M: *Medical-surgical: critical thinking for collaborative care*, ed 4, Philadelphia, 2002, WB Saunders, p 901.

---

150. A nurse is providing information about caring for the client to the family of a client with left-sided unilateral neglect. The nurse tells the family that it would be least helpful to do which of the following?

1 Approach the client from the right side

2 Encourage the client to scan the environment

3 Move the commode and chair to the left side

4 Place bedside articles on the left side

Answer: 1

Rationale: Unilateral neglect is an unawareness of the paralyzed side of the body, which increases the client's risk for injury. The nurse's role is to refocus the client's attention to the affected side. Personal care items, belongings, bedside chair, and commode are all placed on the affected side. The client is taught to scan the environment to become aware of that half of the body. The client should be approached on the affected side by family and staff as well.

Test-Taking Strategy: Note the keywords *least helpful* and that the client has *left-sided unilateral neglect*. Remember, options that are similar are not likely to be correct; therefore, eliminate options 3 and 4. From the remaining options, recall that unilateral neglect is an unawareness of the paralyzed side of the body, and that it is necessary to refocus the client's attention to the affected side. Review care to the client with unilateral neglect and the various test-taking strategies if you had difficulty with this question.

Level of Cognitive Ability: Application
Client Needs: Safe, Effective Care Environment
Integrated Process: Nursing Process/Implementation
Content Area: Adult Health/Neurological

Reference
Ignatavicius D, Workman M: *Medical-surgical nursing: critical thinking for collaborative care*, ed 4, Philadelphia, 2002, WB Saunders, p 986.

---

151. A nurse is reviewing the diagnostic tests prescribed for a client. The nurse notes that a lupus cell preparation (LE cell prep) has been ordered. The nurse determines that

Answer: 2

Rationale: The LE cell prep may be performed on a client suspected of having SLE, or to screen for progressive systemic sclerosis. However, it is primarily used to screen for SLE. The other options are not associated with this diagnostic test.

this test is used to screen primarily for which of following disorders?
1. Histoplasmosis
2. Systemic lupus erythematosus (SLE)
3. Human immunodeficiency virus (HIV)
4. Progressive systemic sclerosis

Test-Taking Strategy: Note the keyword *primarily*. Also note the relation between the word *lupus* in the question and in the correct option. Review the purpose of an LE cell prep and the various test-taking strategie if you had difficulty with this question.

Level of Cognitive Ability: Analysis
Client Needs: Physiological Integrity
Integrated Process: Nursing Process/Assessment
Content Area: Adult Health/Immune

Reference
Ignatavicius D, Workman M: *Medical-surgical: critical thinking for collaborative care,* ed 4, Philadelphia, 2002, WB Saunders, p 354.

---

152. A nurse is preparing to assist a physician in performing a liver biopsy. The nurse assists the client to which position for this test to be performed?
1. Right lateral side-lying
2. Right Sims' position
3. Prone with the hands crossed under the head
4. Supine with the right hand under the head

Answer: 4

Rationale: A supine position is assumed with the right hand placed under the head for a liver biopsy. The client also is asked to remain as still as possible during the test. Options 1, 2, and 3 are incorrect because the physician would not be able to access the liver.

Test-Taking Strategy: Think about the anatomic location of the liver. Recalling that the liver is located on the right side will direct you to option 4. Review this procedure and the various test-taking strategies if you had difficulty with this question.

Level of Cognitive Ability: Application
Client Needs: Physiological Integrity
Integrated Process: Nursing Process/Implementation
Content Area: Adult Health/Gastrointestinal

Reference
Ignatavicius D, Workman M: *Medical-surgical: critical thinking for collaborative care,* ed 4, Philadelphia, 2002, WB Saunders, p 1162.

---

153. A nurse assists a client with a diagnosis of obsessive–compulsive disorder prepare for bed. One hour later, the client calls the nurse and says he is feeling anxious; he asks the nurse to sit and talk for a while. The nurse takes which most appropriate initial action?
1. Asks the client if he would like an antianxiety medication
2. Tells the client that it is time for sleep and that they will talk tomorrow
3. Sits and talks with the client
4. Asks a nursing assistant to sit with the client

Answer: 3

Rationale: The most appropriate initial nursing action is to sit and talk if the client is expressing anxiety. Antianxiety medication may be necessary, but this is not the initial nursing action. A nursing assistant may not be able to alleviate the client's anxiety. Option 2 is an inappropriate action and places the client's feelings on hold.

Test-Taking Strategy: Note the keyword *initial* and use therapeutic communication techniques. Recalling that it is best to address the client's feelings assists in directing you to option 3. Review care to the client with obsessive–compulsive disorder and the various test-taking strategies if you had difficulty with this question.

Level of Cognitive Ability: Application
Client Needs: Psychosocial Integrity
Integrated Process: Caring
Content Area: Mental Health

Reference
Stuart G, Laraia M: *Principles and practice of psychiatric nursing*, ed 7, St Louis, 2001, Mosby, pp 289–292.

154. A nurse is performing an admission interview with a client being admitted to the mental health unit and discovers that the client experienced a severe emotional trauma 1 month ago and is now experiencing paralysis of the right arm. The priority nursing action is to
1 Encourage the client to talk about his feelings
2 Assess the client for organic causes of the paralysis
3 Refer the client to group therapy
4 Encourage the client to move and use the arm

Answer: 2

Rationale: The priority action is to assess for any physiological cause of the paralysis. Although a component of the plan of care is to encourage the client to discuss his feelings, this is not the priority action. It is not appropriate to encourage the client to use the arm without ruling out a physiological cause of the paralysis. Although the client may be referred to group therapy, this also is not the priority action.

Test-Taking Strategy: Note the keyword *priority*. Use Maslow's Hierarchy of Needs theory, remembering that physiological needs are the first priority. Option 2 is the only option that addresses a physiological need. Review care to the mental health client who experiences physiological disorders and the test-taking strategies for answering prioritizing questions if you had difficulty with this question.

Level of Cognitive Ability: Application
Client Needs: Physiological Integrity
Integrated Process: Nursing Process/Implementation
Content Area: Mental Health

Reference
Stuart G, Laraia M: *Principles and practice of psychiatric nursing*, ed 7, St Louis, 2001, Mosby, p 309.

155. A nurse is developing a plan of care for a client admitted to the mental health unit with a diagnosis of obsessive–compulsive disorder who is experiencing severe anxiety. The nurse's priority in the plan of care for this client is to
1 Monitor for repetitive behavior
2 Demand active participation in care
3 Educate the client about self-care demands
4 Establish a trusting nurse–client relationship

Answer: 4

Rationale: The priority nursing action is to establish a trusting relationship with the client. Demanding anything from the client should never occur. The remaining options are appropriate components of the plan of care, but they are not the priority. A trusting nurse–client relationship needs to be established first.

Test-Taking Strategy: Focus on the keyword *priority* and note that the client is being admitted to the mental health unit. Recalling that a nurse–client relationship needs to be developed first assists in directing you to option 4. Review care to the client with obsessive–compulsive disorder and the test-taking strategies for answering prioritizing questions if you had difficulty with this question.

Level of Cognitive Ability: Application
Client Needs: Psychosocial Integrity
Integrated Process: Caring
Content Area: Mental Health

Reference
Stuart G, Laraia M: *Principles and practice of psychiatric nursing*, ed 7, St Louis, 2001, Mosby, p 289.

156. A community health nurse is teaching a group of women about breast cancer and the procedure for performing breast self-examination (BSE). Select all instructions that the nurse provides to the women.

_____ If you are menstruating, the best time to do a BSE is 2 to 3 days after your period ends.

_____ If you notice discharge from the nipple, there is no need to be concerned, because this is a common occurrence during menstruation.

_____ Stand before a mirror to inspect both breasts.

_____ Inspection should be done by pressing the hands firmly on the hips and bowing slightly toward the mirror as you pull your shoulders and elbows forward.

_____ If you are premenopausal, you may feel lumps in the breast, but these are normal because of hormonal changes that occur.

_____ Palpation can be done in the shower.

_____ To palpate the breasts, use three or four fingers, begin at the outer edge, press the flat part of your fingers in small circles, moving the circles slowly around the breast.

_____ It is not necessary to palpate the armpit area or the area between the breast and the armpit.

Answer:

__X__ If you are menstruating, the best time to do a BSE is 2 to 3 days after your period ends.

_____ If you notice discharge from the nipple, there is no need to be concerned, because this is a common occurrence during menstruation.

__X__ Stand before a mirror to inspect both breasts.

__X__ Inspection should be done by pressing the hands firmly on the hips and bowing slightly toward the mirror as you pull your shoulders and elbows forward.

_____ If you are premenopausal, you may feel lumps in the breast, but these are normal because of hormonal changes that occur.

__X__ Palpation can be done in the shower.

__X__ To palpate the breasts, use three or four fingers, begin at the outer edge, press the flat part of your fingers in small circles, moving the circles slowly around the breast.

_____ It is not necessary to palpate the armpit area or the area between the breast and the armpit.

Rationale: If the client is menstruating, the best time to do a BSE is 2 to 3 days after the period ends, because the breasts are less likely to be tender or swollen. Any lumps or nipple discharge is a concern and is always reported to the health care provider for further evaluation. Inspection is done by standing before a mirror, pressing the hands firmly on the hips, and bowing slightly toward the mirror as the client pulls the shoulders and elbows forward. Palpation can be done in the shower, and the client is taught to palpate the breasts using three or four fingers, beginning at the outer edge, pressing the flat part of the fingers in small circles, and moving the circles slowly around the breast. It is important to palpate the armpit area or the area between the breast and the armpit, and any masses or lumps noted in this area need to be reported.

Test-Taking Strategy: The best strategy to use to answer this question is to visualize the procedure. Also, recalling the anatomy of the breast and the characteristics of breast cancer will assist in answering this question. Review the procedure for BSE and the various test-taking strategies if you had difficulty with this question.

Level of Cognitive Ability: Application
Client Needs: Health Promotion and Maintenance
Integrated Process: Teaching/Learning
Content Area: Adult Health/Oncology

Reference
Potter P, Perry A: *Fundamentals of nursing,* ed 6, St Louis, 2005, Mosby, p 736.

157. A registered nurse is supervising a licensed practical nurse who is performing a pulse oximetry measurement on a client with peripheral vascular disease. The nurse determines that the licensed practical nurse is performing the procedure accurately if the nurse places the oximetry probe on which anatomic area?

1 Right index finger
2 Left thumb
3 One of the toes
4 Bridge of the nose

Answer: 4

Rationale: If the client has peripheral vascular disease, the pulse oximetry probe would be placed on the earlobe or bridge of the nose, because peripheral vasoconstriction or inadequate blood flow to the peripheral areas of the body will interfere with the oxygen saturation measurement. For the client with peripheral vascular disease, the pulse oximetry probe would be placed on the earlobe or bridge of the nose. Placing the probe on the anatomic areas noted in options 1, 2, and 3 will not provide an accurate measurement of the oxygen saturation level.

Test-Taking Strategy: Focus on the client's diagnosis: peripheral vascular disease. Recall the pathophysiology associated with this disease. Note that options 1, 2, and 3 are similar in that they indicate using a peripheral body area. Review the procedure for pulse oximetry measurement and the various test-taking strategies if you had difficulty with this question.

Level of Cognitive Ability: Analysis
Client Needs: Physiological Integrity
Integrated Process: Nursing Process/Analysis
Content Area: Leadership/Management

Reference
Potter P, Perry A: *Fundamentals of nursing,* ed 6, St Louis, 2005, Mosby, pp 651–652.

---

158. A nurse is reviewing the assessment data in the record of a client assigned to her care and notes documentation that the client has pallor. The nurse determines that this skin color variation is most likely caused by

1 An increased amount of bilirubin deposits in the tissues
2 An increased amount of deoxygenated hemoglobin associated with hypoxia
3 A reduced amount of oxyhemoglobin from decreased blood flow
4 An increased amount of melanin in the tissues

Answer: 3

Rationale: Pallor, a decrease in skin color, is caused by a decreased amount of oxyhemoglobin resulting from decreased blood flow. Some causes of pallor include anemia or shock. Pallor can best be assessed in the face, conjunctivae, nail beds, palms of the hands, or lips. A bluish discoloration (cyanosis) is caused by an increased amount of deoxygenated hemoglobin associated with hypoxia. A yellow-orange skin discoloration (jaundice) is caused by an increased amount of bilirubin deposits in the tissues. A tan-brown skin color is caused by an increased amount of melanin in the tissues.

Test-Taking Strategy: Focus on the issue: pallor. Recalling that pallor refers to a pale skin color will direct you to option 3. Also, noting the relation of the word *pallor* to the description in option 3 will direct you to this option. Review skin assessment findings and the various test-taking strategies if you had difficulty with this question.

Level of Cognitive Ability: Analysis
Client Needs: Physiological Integrity
Integrated Process: Nursing Process/Analysis
Content Area: Adult Health/Integumentary

Reference
Potter P, Perry A: *Fundamentals of nursing,* ed 6, St Louis, 2005, Mosby, p 689.

159. A nurse is performing a skin assessment on a client and checks the client's skin for turgor. The nurse grasps a fold of the client's skin in which body area to best assess turgor?
1 Back of the hand
2 Sternal area
3 Top of the foot
4 Sacral area

Answer: 2

Rationale: Turgor refers to the skin's elasticity. To assess the skin turgor, a fold of skin on the back of the forearm or sternal area is grasped with the fingertips and released. Normally, the skin lifts easily and snaps back immediately into its normal resting position. The back of the hand is not the best area to assess turgor because the skin normally is loose and thin in this area. The sacral area and foot and ankle area are sites to assess for edema.

Test-Taking Strategy: Focus on the issue: assessing skin turgor. Recalling that turgor refers to the skin's elasticity and visualizing each body area in the options will direct you to option 2. Review skin assessment techniques and the various test-taking strategies if you had difficulty with this question.

Level of Cognitive Ability: Application
Client Needs: Health Promotion and Maintenance
Integrated Process: Nursing Process/Assessment
Content Area: Adult Health/Integumentary

Reference
Potter P, Perry A: *Fundamentals of nursing,* ed 6, St Louis, 2005, Mosby, p 691.

---

160. The nurse notes documentation that a client has the presence of cherry angiomas located on the abdomen. On assessment of the client, the nurse would expect to note which characteristic of this skin lesion?
1 Ruby red papules
2 Thickened skin areas
3 Pinpoint-sized red or purple spots
4 Areas of redness that are warm to touch

Answer: 1

Rationale: Cherry angiomas are noted as ruby red papules. Areas of skin thickening are noted as senile keratosis. Pinpoint-sized red or purple spots are known as petechiae. Areas of redness that are warm to touch are noted as erythema.

Test-Taking Strategy: Focus on the issue: cherry angiomas. Note the relation between the word *cherry* in the question and the words *ruby red* in option 1. Review the characteristics of various skin lesions and the various test-taking strategies if you had difficulty with this question.

Level of Cognitive Ability: Analysis
Client Needs: Health Promotion and Maintenance
Integrated Process: Nursing Process/Assessment
Content Area: Adult Health/Integumentary

Reference
Potter P, Perry A: *Fundamentals of nursing,* ed 6, St Louis, 2005, Mosby, p 691.

---

161. A nurse reviews the assessment data on a client with a head injury and notes that the client's intracranial pressure reading is 10 mm Hg. On the basis of this finding, the nurse

Answer: 2

Rationale: The normal intracranial pressure readings are between 0 and 15 mm Hg, and pressures greater than 20 mm Hg are considered to be increased. Therefore, options 1, 3, and 4 are incorrect.

determines that the client's intracranial pressure reading

1   Is increased
2   Is normal
3   Needs to be reduced with aggressive treatment measures
4   Requires physician notification

Test-Taking Strategy: If you did not know the normal intracranial pressure reading, note that options 1, 3, and 4 are similar in that they indicate that the pressure is increased and requires action and treatment. Review the normal intracranial pressure reading and the various test-taking strategies if you had difficulty with this question.

Level of Cognitive Ability: Analysis
Client Needs: Physiological Integrity
Integrated Process: Nursing Process/Analysis
Content Area: Adult Health/Neurological

Reference
Phipps W, Monahan F, Sands J, Marek J, Neighbors M: *Medical-surgical nursing: health and illness perspectives,* ed 7, St Louis, 2003, Mosby, p 1330.

---

162. The nurse is performing a cardiovascular assessment on a client. The nurse palpates which anatomic area (see figure) to assess the popliteal pulse?

Answer: _____

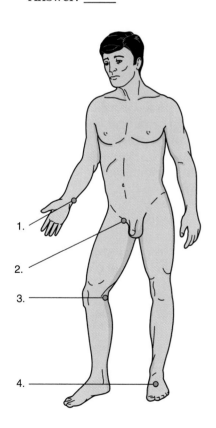

Answer: 3

Rationale: The popliteal pulse is located behind the knee. The ulnar pulse is located at the wrist. The femoral pulse is located in the groin area. The dorsalis pedis pulse is located on the top of the foot.

Test-Taking Strategy: Focus on the issue: the popliteal pulse. Use knowledge regarding anatomy of the body and pulse points to answer correctly. Review cardiovascular assessment techniques and the various test-taking strategies if you had difficulty with this question.

Level of Cognitive Ability: Application
Client Needs: Health Promotion and Maintenance
Integrated Process: Nursing Process/Assessment
Content Area: Adult Health/Cardiovascular

Reference
Phipps W, Monahan F, Sands J, Marek J, Neighbors M: *Medical-surgical nursing: health and illness perspectives,* ed 7, St Louis, 2003, Mosby, p 626.

163. The nurse notes documentation that a client's peripheral pulses are +3. The nurse determines that the pulses are
1   Full and brisk
2   Absent
3   Normal or average
4   Palpable, but diminished

Answer: 1

Rationale: Pulses are rated on a scale of 0 to +4 as follows: 0 = absent; +1 = palpable, but diminished; +2 = normal or average; +3 = full and brisk; and +4 = full and bounding, often visible.

Test-Taking Strategy: Note the keywords *peripheral pulses are +3*. Recalling that pulses are rated on a scale of 0 to +4 will assist in directing you to option 1. Review the rating scale for assessing pulses and the various test-taking strategies if you had difficulty with this question.

Level of Cognitive Ability: Analysis
Client Needs: Health Promotion and Maintenance
Integrated Process: Nursing Process/Analysis
Content Area: Adult Health/Cardiovascular

Reference
Phipps W, Monahan F, Sands J, Marek J, Neighbors M: *Medical-surgical nursing: health and illness perspectives,* ed 7, St Louis, 2003, Mosby, p 626.

---

164. A nurse is assessing the extent of pitting edema in a client with congestive heart failure. The nurse gently presses a finger on the client's ankle and notes a barely perceptible pit. The nurse interprets this finding as which measurement of pitting edema?
1   1+
2   2+
3   3+
4   4+

Answer: 1

Rationale: The level of pitting edema is rated on a scale of 1+ to 4+. A barely perceptible pit is rated as 1+. A deeper pit that rebounds in a few seconds is rated as 2+. A deep pit that rebounds in 10 to 20 seconds is rated as 3+. A deeper pit that rebounds in greater than 30 seconds is rated as 4+.

Test-Taking Strategy: Note the keywords *barely perceptible pit*. Recalling that the level of pitting edema is rated on a scale of 1+ to 4+, with 1+ indicating the least amount of edema, will direct you to option 1. Review the procedure for assessing edema and the various test-taking strategies if you had difficulty with this question.

Level of Cognitive Ability: Analysis
Client Needs: Health Promotion and Maintenance
Integrated Process: Nursing Process/Analysis
Content Area: Adult Health/Cardiovascular

Reference
Phipps W, Monahan F, Sands J, Marek J, Neighbors M: *Medical-surgical nursing: health and illness perspectives,* ed 7, St Louis, 2003, Mosby, p 627.

---

165. A nurse is preparing a list of discharge instructions for a client who had a permanent pacemaker inserted. Select all instructions that the nurse would place on the list.
____ Avoid lifting more than 25 pounds until cleared by the physician.

Answer:
____ Avoid lifting more than 25 pounds until cleared by the physician.
_X_ Monitor the insertion site for infection and bleeding.
____ The use of a cellular phone will never affect a pacemaker.
_X_ Avoid contact sports.

   ___ Monitor the insertion site for infection and bleeding.
   ___ The use of a cellular phone will never affect a pacemaker.
   ___ Avoid contact sports.
   ___ Notify the physician if the radial pulse is outside of the range programmed in the pacemaker.

    X   Notify the physician if the radial pulse is outside of the range programmed in the pacemaker.

Rationale: The client is instructed to avoid lifting more than 10 pounds (not 25 pounds) until cleared by the physician. The client is instructed to monitor the insertion site for infection and bleeding and to take the radial pulse and notify the physician if the radial pulse is outside of the range programmed in the pacemaker, because this may indicate pacemaker malfunction or battery depletion. Cellular phones should be used on the ear opposite the site of the pacemaker and should be carried away from the pacemaker site. Some cellular phones may not affect the pacemaker, and the client is instructed to check with the manufacturer of the cellular phone. Contact sports are avoided to prevent injury to the pacemaker site.

Test-Taking Strategy: Read each instruction carefully. The instruction that indicates to avoid lifting more than 25 pounds until cleared by the physician can be eliminated because of the excessive amount of weight. The instruction that indicates the use of a cellular phone will never affect a pacemaker can be eliminated because of the absolute word *never.* Review instructions for a client with a permanent pacemaker and the various test-taking strategies if you had difficulty with this question.

Level of Cognitive Ability: Application
Client Needs: Health Promotion and Maintenance
Integrated Process: Teaching/Learning
Content Area: Adult Health/Cardiovascular

Reference
Phipps W, Monahan F, Sands J, Marek J, Neighbors M: *Medical-surgical nursing: health and illness perspectives,* ed 7, St Louis, 2003, Mosby, p 627.

---

166. An emergency department nurse is assessing a client who sustained a blunt chest injury and suspects the presence of flail chest. Which specific characteristic finding would the nurse note in this condition?
1 Slow deep respirations
2 Asymmetric chest movement
3 Loss of consciousness
4 Anxiety

Answer: 2
Rationale: Flail chest is a thoracic injury resulting in paradoxical (asymmetric) motion of the chest wall segments. The client also exhibits severe chest pain; oscillation of the mediastinum; increasing dyspnea; rapid, shallow respirations; accessory muscle breathing; decreased breath sounds on auscultation; and cyanosis. Although the client may exhibit anxiety related to difficulty breathing, anxiety can occur in any respiratory disorder in which dyspnea is a problem. Loss of consciousness can occur with a head injury, or if the respiratory condition deteriorated significantly.

Test-Taking Strategy: Note the keywords *specific characteristic finding.* Also note the relation to the words *flail chest* in the question and the words *asymmetric chest movement* in the correct option. Review the characteristics of flail chest and the various test-taking strategies if you had difficulty with this question.

Level of Cognitive Ability: Analysis
Client Needs: Physiological Integrity
Integrated Process: Nursing Process/Assessment
Content Area: Adult Health/Respiratory

Reference
Phipps W, Monahan F, Sands J, Marek J, Neighbors M: *Medical-surgical nursing: health and illness perspectives,* ed 7, St Louis, 2003, Mosby, pp 605–606.

167. The nurse notes this cardiac rhythm (see figure) on the client's monitor. List in order of priority the actions that the nurse would take. (Number 1 is the first action.)
____ Defibrillate the client
____ Check for patency of the airway
____ Palpate for a carotid pulse
____ Check for breathing

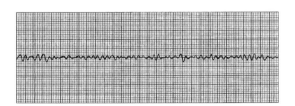

Answer: 4, 1, 3, 2

Rationale: Ventricular fibrillation is noted as an uncoordinated electrical activity of the heart. In this dysrhythmia, there is no identifiable P wave, QRS complex, or T wave. Immediate defibrillation is performed after assessment of the ABCs—airway, breathing, and circulation—of cardiopulmonary resuscitation (CPR).

Test-Taking Strategy: Note the keyword *priority.* Use the ABCs to determine the order of priority. Remember, immediate defibrillation is performed after assessment of the ABCs of CPR. Also, use the steps of the nursing process, noting that defibrillation is an action rather than an assessment. Review the care for the client on a cardiac monitor and the test-taking strategies for answering prioritizing questions if you had difficulty with this question.

Level of Cognitive Ability: Application
Client Needs: Physiological Integrity
Integrated Process: Nursing Process/Implementation
Content Area: Delegating/Prioritizing

Reference
Potter P, Perry A: *Fundamentals of nursing,* ed 6, St Louis, 2005, Mosby, p 1077.

168. A nurse is preparing to perform oropharyngeal suctioning on a client who has coughed, resulting in secretions in the mouth, and is unable to expectorate the secretions adequately. The nurse determines that there is a physician's order for the procedure and explains the procedure to the client. List in order of priority the actions that the nurse would take to perform this procedure safely. (Number 1 is the first action.)
____ Remove the client's oxygen mask.
____ Wash hands.
____ Attach the suction catheter to the connecting tubing.

Answer: 4, 1, 3, 2, 6, 5, 7

Rationale: The nurse always washes his or her hands before performing any procedure, and then dons a clean glove. A clean, rather than a sterile glove can be used in this procedure, because the oral cavity is not sterile. The nurse may also consider applying a mask or face shield, because suctioning may cause splashing of body fluids. The nurse then completes preparation by attaching the suction catheter to the connecting suction tubing. The nurse removes the oxygen mask just before implementing the procedure, so that the client is oxygenated as much as possible (remember, suctioning can deplete oxygen). The catheter then is inserted into the client's mouth until secretions are cleared. If the client is not tolerating the procedure, the catheter is removed and the oxygen mask is reapplied. The nurse then encourages the client to cough, because coughing moves secretions from the lower to upper airways into the mouth. At this point, suctioning is repeated if necessary. The oxygen mask then is reapplied.

____ Apply a clean, disposable glove to the dominant hand.

____ Encourage the client to cough.

____ Insert the catheter into the client's mouth and move the catheter around the mouth, pharynx, and gum line until secretions are cleared.

____ Place the oxygen mask on the client.

Test-Taking Strategy: The best strategy to use to answer this question is to first focus on the data in the question and then to visualize the procedure. Remember that hands are always washed first. Next, remember that any preparation activities are done before removing the client's oxygen mask, and that the client's oxygen is reapplied after completion of the procedure. Review the procedure for oropharyngeal suctioning and the test-taking strategies for answering prioritizing questions if you had difficulty with this question.

Level of Cognitive Ability: Application
Client Needs: Safe, Effective Care Environment
Integrated Process: Nursing Process/Implementation
Content Area: Delegating/Prioritizing

Reference
Potter P, Perry A: *Fundamentals of nursing,* ed 6, St Louis, 2005, Mosby, p 1103.

---

169. A nurse is assessing an adult client 1 hour after a right pulmonary wedge resection. The nurse notes the presence of 200 mL bloody drainage in the client's collection chamber of the chest tube drainage system. Which action by the nurse is most appropriate?

1 Irrigate the chest tube.

2 Decrease the amount of suction being applied.

3 Document the findings.

4 Contact the surgeon.

Answer: 3

Rationale: Between 100 and 300 mL fluid may drain in the pleural chest tube in an adult during the first 3 hours after insertion. This rate will decrease after 2 hours (500 to 1000 mL can be expected in the first 24 hours). Drainage is grossly bloody in the first several hours after surgery, and then changes to serous. Therefore, in this situation, the nurse would most appropriately document the findings. Decreasing the amount of suctioning being applied is inappropriate and would not be done without a physician's order. Chest tubes are never irrigated by the nurse. If excessive amounts or the continued presence of frank, bloody drainage occurs after the first several hours after surgery, these findings should be reported to the physician.

Test-Taking Strategy: Focus on the data in the question and note the keywords *1 hour after* and *200 mL bloody drainage.* Option 1 can be easily eliminated because the nurse would never irrigate a chest tube. Option 2 can be eliminated next because the amount of suction would not be decreased without a physician's order. From the remaining options, focusing on the keywords will direct you to option 3 by recalling that these findings are expected during this postoperative period. Review care to the client after right pulmonary wedge resection and the various test-taking strategies if you had difficulty with this question.

Level of Cognitive Ability: Application
Client Needs: Physiological Integrity
Integrated Process: Nursing Process/Implementation
Content Area: Adult Health/Respiratory

Reference
Potter P, Perry A: *Fundamentals of nursing,* ed 6, St Louis, 2005, Mosby, p 1120.

170. A nurse has provided instructions to a client with chronic obstructive pulmonary disease about the procedure for performing pursed lip breathing. The nurse observes the client perform the procedure and determines that he or she is performing it correctly if the client

1 Takes a deep breath and exhales quickly

2 Monitors inspiration time and ensures that expiration time is less than inspiration time

3 Lies on the side in a supine position to perform the procedure

4 Sits in an upright position, takes a deep breath, and exhales slowly

Answer: 4

Rationale: Pursed lip breathing involves deep inspiration and prolonged expiration through pursed lips to prevent alveolar collapse. While sitting up, the client is instructed to take a deep breath and to exhale slowly through pursed lips. Therefore, options 1, 2, and 3 are incorrect.

Test-Taking Strategy: Eliminate options 1 and 2 first because they are similar. From the remaining options, note the client's diagnosis and recall that clients with respiratory conditions are not positioned supine because this position affects respiratory status and will increase the work of breathing, resulting in dyspnea. Review the procedure for pursed lip breathing and the various test-taking strategies if you had difficulty with this question.

Level of Cognitive Ability: Analysis
Client Needs: Health Promotion and Maintenance
Integrated Process: Teaching/Learning
Content Area: Adult Health/Respiratory

Reference
Potter P, Perry A: *Fundamentals of nursing,* ed 6, St Louis, 2005, Mosby, p 1130.

---

171. Artificial rupture of the membranes is done to induce labor in a client. After this procedure, the nurse immediately

1 Cleans the client's perineal area

2 Places the client in a comfortable position

3 Informs the client that a wet feeling in the perineal area is normal and expected

4 Checks the fetal heart rate

Answer: 4

Rationale: Artificial rupture of the membranes may be done to augment or induce labor or to facilitate placement of internal monitors when fetal status indicates the need for some form of direct assessment. Because the umbilical cord can prolapse when the membranes rupture, the fetal heart rate and fetal pattern should be monitored immediately and for several minutes after the procedure to ascertain fetal well-being. Although options 1, 2, and 3 are appropriate, they are not the priority concern. In addition, in the preprocedural period, the client should be told that a wet feeling in the perineal area is normal and expected.

Test-Taking Strategy: Use the ABCs—airway, breathing, and circulation—to direct you to option 4. Also, use of the steps of the nursing process will direct you to option 4 because it is the only option that addresses assessment. Review care to the client after artificial rupture of the membranes and the test-taking strategies for answering prioritizing questions if you had difficulty with this question.

Level of Cognitive Ability: Application
Client Needs: Physiological Integrity
Integrated Process: Nursing Process/Implementation
Content Area: Maternity/Intrapartum

Reference
Lowdermilk D, Perry A: *Maternity & women's health care,* ed 8, St Louis, 2004, Mosby, pp 566–567.

172. A client in labor has been repositioned from side to side every 30 minutes. The client tells the nurse that she is tired of having to lie on her side and would like to lie on her back for a while. The nurse would most appropriately

1 Tell the client that the supine position is contraindicated during labor

2 Position the client supine and place a pillow under one hip to act as a wedge

3 Tell the client that the obstetrician will need to be called to obtain an order for lying in the supine position

4 Tell the client that bed rest lying on one side or the other is necessary

Answer: 2

Rationale: The client in labor should be assisted to change positions every 30 to 60 minutes. The side-lying (lateral) position is the preferred position because it promotes optimal uteroplacental and renal blood flow and increases fetal oxygenation. If the client wants to lie supine, the nurse may place a pillow under one hip as a wedge to prevent the uterus from compressing the aorta and vena cava. A physician's order is not needed to reposition this client.

Test-Taking Strategy: Eliminate options 1 and 4 first because they are similar. Next, eliminate option 3, recalling that a physician's order is not required to reposition this client. Review care to the client in labor and the various test-taking strategies if you had difficulty with this question.

Level of Cognitive Ability: Application
Client Needs: Physiological Integrity
Integrated Process: Nursing Process/Implementation
Content Area: Maternity/Intrapartum

Reference
Lowdermilk D, Perry A: *Maternity & women's health care*, ed 8, St Louis, 2004, Mosby, p 573.

---

173. A client in labor tells the nurse that she suddenly has a wet feeling in the vaginal area. The nurse quickly checks the client and notes the presence of a large amount of bright red blood. The nurse would immediately

1 Notify the obstetrician

2 Prepare the client for an emergency cesarean birth

3 Prepare to perform a vaginal examination

4 Insert an intravenous catheter

Answer: 1

Rationale: Vaginal bleeding (bright red, dark red, or in an amount in excess of that expected during normal cervical dilation) requires immediate notification of the obstetrician. This finding indicates the presence of an emergency situation and could have occurred as a result of placenta previa or placental separation. Although the nurse will prepare the client for an emergency cesarean section and insert an intravenous catheter, these are not the immediate actions. A vaginal examination is not performed on a pregnant client with vaginal bleeding.

Test-Taking Strategy: Note the keyword *immediately* and focus on the data in the question. Noting the words *large amount of bright red blood* will direct you to option 1. Remember, when an emergency situation is presented in the question, it is likely that the correct option will be to notify the health care provider. Review care to the client in labor, the test-taking strategies for answering prioritizing questions, and the strategies related to contacting the health care provider if you had difficulty with this question.

Level of Cognitive Ability: Application
Client Needs: Physiological Integrity
Integrated Process: Nursing Process/Implementation
Content Area: Maternity/Intrapartum

Reference
Lowdermilk D, Perry A: *Maternity & women's health care*, ed 8, St Louis, 2004, Mosby, p 581.

---

174. A client with a diagnosis of suspected food poisoning is admitted to the hospital because of dehydration. The nurse would expect to note which finding on assessment of this client?
1 Dry mucous membranes
2 Decreased pulse
3 Decreased respiratory rate
4 Increased urine output

Answer: 1

Rationale: A client with dehydration will have dry mucous membranes because of deficient fluid volume. The client also will have an increased depth and rate of respirations and an increased pulse rate. The deficient fluid volume is perceived by the body as decreased oxygen levels (hypoxia), and increased respiration and an increased pulse rate is an attempt to maintain oxygen delivery. Other assessment findings of deficient fluid volume are weight loss, poor skin turgor, decreased urine volume, concentrated urine with increased specific gravity, increased hematocrit, and altered level of consciousness.

Test-Taking Strategy: Focus on the issue: dehydration (deficient fluid volume). Note the relation between the issue and the assessment finding in option 1. Review the signs of dehydration and the various test-taking strategies if you had difficulty with this question.

Level of Cognitive Ability: Analysis
Client Needs: Physiological Integrity
Integrated Process: Nursing Process/Assessment
Content Area: Adult Health/Gastrointestinal

Reference
Ignatavicius D, Workman M: *Medical-surgical: critical thinking for collaborative care*, ed 4, Philadelphia, 2002, WB Saunders, p 163.

---

175. A nurse notes that a client's serum potassium level is 5.8 mEq/L. The nurse interprets that this is an expected finding in the client with which problem?
1 Diarrhea
2 Diabetes insipidus
3 Burn injury
4 Pulmonary edema being treated with loop diuretics

Answer: 3

Rationale: A serum potassium level greater than 5.1 mEq/L indicates hyperkalemia, and the nurse would report the result to the physician. Burn injuries are a cause of hyperkalemia. Other common causes of hyperkalemia include adrenal insufficiency (Addison disease), renal failure, and the use of potassium-sparing diuretics. The client with diarrhea or diabetes insipidus or the client being treated with loop diuretics is at risk for hypokalemia.

Test-Taking Strategy: Eliminate options 1, 2, and 4 because they are similar and all indicate that the client is experiencing body fluid losses, and thus a loss of potassium. Review the causes of hyperkalemia and the various test-taking strategies if you had difficulty with this question.

Level of Cognitive Ability: Analysis
Client Needs: Physiological Integrity
Integrated Process: Nursing Process/Analysis
Content Area: Adult Health/Integumentary

Reference
Ignatavicius D, Workman M: *Medical-surgical nursing: critical thinking for collaborative care,* ed 4, Philadelphia, 2002, WB Saunders, p 178.

---

176. A nurse is monitoring a client with hyperparathyroidism for signs of hypercalcemia. The nurse would expect to note which finding if hypercalcemia was present?

1 Hyperactive deep tendon reflexes

2 Positive Chvostek's sign

3 Diminished bowel sounds

4 Paresthesias

Answer: 3

Rationale: Signs of hypercalcemia include decreased gastrointestinal motility, muscle weakness, diminished or absent deep tendon reflexes, increased urine output, and increased heart rate and blood pressure. Options 1, 2, and 4 are signs of hypocalcemia.

Test-Taking Strategy: Eliminate options 1, 2, and 4 because they are similar and reflect a hyperactivity of the neuromuscular system. Review the signs of hypercalcemia and the various test-taking strategies if you had difficulty with this question.

Level of Cognitive Ability: Analysis
Client Needs: Physiological Integrity
Integrated Process: Nursing Process/Assessment
Content Area: Adult Health/Endocrine

Reference
Ignatavicius D, Workman M: *Medical-surgical nursing: critical thinking for collaborative care,* ed 4, Philadelphia, 2002, WB Saunders, p 188.

---

177. A nurse is reviewing the assessment findings and laboratory results of a child diagnosed with new-onset glomerulonephritis. Which of the following findings would the nurse most likely expect to note?

1 Increased creatinine levels

2 Hypotension

3 Low serum potassium

4 Tea-colored urine

Answer: 4

Rationale: Gross hematuria resulting in dark brown or smoky, tea-colored urine is a classic symptom of glomerulonephritis. Hypertension also is a common finding in glomerulonephritis. Blood urea nitrogen and creatinine levels are increased only when there is an 80% decrease in glomerular filtration rate and renal insufficiency is severe. A high potassium level results from inadequate glomerular filtration.

Test-Taking Strategy: Note that the child is experiencing a renal disorder. Also note the keywords *new-onset* and *most likely.* Recalling that the creatinine level increases only when there is an 80% decrease in glomerular filtration rate will assist in eliminating option 1. Next, eliminate options 2 and 3 knowing that hypertension, rather than hypotension, and hyperkalemia, rather than hypokalemia, will occur with this renal disorder. Review the clinical manifestations associated with glomerulonephritis and the various test-taking strategies if you had difficulty with this question.

Level of Cognitive Ability: Analysis
Client Needs: Physiological Integrity
Integrated Process: Nursing Process/Assessment
Content Area: Child Health

Reference
James S, Ashwill J, Droske S: *Nursing care of children: principles & practice,* ed 2, Philadelphia, 2002, WB Saunders, p 604.

178. A child newly diagnosed with type 1 diabetes mellitus who is receiving insulin suddenly experiences signs of a hypoglycemic reaction. The nurse would immediately give the child
1   A teaspoon of honey
2   A teaspoon of sugar
3   One-half cup of diet cola
4   8 oz skim milk

Answer: 4
Rationale: Hypoglycemia is immediately treated with 15 g carbohydrate. Glucose tablets or glucose gel may be administered. Other items used to treat hypoglycemia include one-half cup of fruit juice, one-half cup of regular (nondiet) soft drink, 8 oz skim milk, 6 to 10 hard candies, 4 cubes of sugar or 4 teaspoons of sugar, 6 saltines, 3 graham crackers, or 1 tablespoon honey or syrup. The items in options 1, 2, and 3 would not adequately treat hypoglycemia.

Test-Taking Strategy: Eliminate options 1 and 2 first because they are similar. From the remaining options, select option 4 because a diet cola does not contain the adequate amount of carbohydrate needed to treat hypoglycemia. Review the treatment measures for hypoglycemia and the various test-taking strategies if you had difficulty with this question.

Level of Cognitive Ability: Application
Client Needs: Physiological Integrity
Integrated Process: Nursing Process/Implementation
Content Area: Child Health

Reference
James S, Ashwill J, Droske S: *Nursing care of children: principles & practice,* ed 2, Philadelphia, 2002, WB Saunders, p 925.

179. A child with a diagnosis of pertussis (whooping cough) is admitted to the pediatric unit. As soon as the child arrives at the unit, the nurse would first
1   Place the child on a pulse oximeter
2   Weigh the child
3   Take the child's temperature
4   Administer the prescribed antibiotic

Answer: 1
Rationale: To adequately determine whether the child is getting enough oxygen, the child is placed on a pulse oximeter. The pulse oximeter then will provide ongoing information regarding the child's oxygen level. The child also is immediately placed on a cardiorespiratory monitor to provide early identification of periods of apnea and bradycardia. The nurse then would perform an assessment, including taking the child's temperature and weight and asking the parents about the child. An antibiotic may be prescribed, but the child's airway status needs to be assessed first.

Test-Taking Strategy: Note the keyword *first.* Focus on the child's diagnosis and use the ABCs—airway, breathing, and circulation. This will direct you to option 1. Review care to the child with pertussis and the test-taking strategies for answering prioritizing questions if you had difficulty with this question.

Level of Cognitive Ability: Application
Client Needs: Physiological Integrity
Integrated Process: Nursing Process/Implementation
Content Area: Delegating/Prioritizing

Reference
James S, Ashwill J, Droske S: *Nursing care of children: principles & practice*, ed 2, Philadelphia, 2002, WB Saunders, p 465.

180. A nurse is assessing a child with increased intracranial pressure who has been exhibiting decorticate posturing. On assessment, the nurse notes extension of the upper and lower extremities with internal rotation of the upper arms and wrists and the knees and feet. The nurse determines that the child's condition
  1 Has improved
  2 Indicates decreased intracranial pressure
  3 Indicates a deterioration in neurological function
  4 Is unchanged

Answer: 3

Rationale: In decorticate posturing, the nurse would note flexion of the upper extremities and extension of the lower extremities. In decerebrate posturing, the nurse would note extension of the upper and lower extremities with internal rotation of the upper arms and wrists and the knees and feet. The progression from decorticate to decerebrate posturing usually indicates deteriorating neurological function and warrants physician notification. Options 1, 2, and 4 are inaccurate interpretations.

Test-Taking Strategy: Eliminate options 1 and 2 first because they are similar. From the remaining options, recalling the significance of decerebrate posturing will direct you to option 3. Review the significance of posturing and the various test-taking strategies if you had difficulty with this question.

Level of Cognitive Ability: Analysis
Client Needs: Physiological Integrity
Integrated Process: Nursing Process/Analysis
Content Area: Child Health

Reference
James S, Ashwill J, Droske S: *Nursing care of children: principles & practice*, ed 2, Philadelphia, 2002, WB Saunders, p 950.

181. A nurse in the neonatal nursery is monitoring a neonate born to a mother with diabetes mellitus. The nurse determines that the neonate is at risk for which of the following conditions?
  1 Hypercalcemia
  2 Hypobilirubinemia
  3 Hyperglycemia
  4 Hypomagnesemia

Answer: 4

Rationale: The major neonatal complications of preexisting diabetes mellitus in the mother are hypoglycemia, hypocalcemia, hypomagnesemia, hyperbilirubinemia, and polycythemia. Congenital anomalies, macrosomia, birth trauma, perinatal asphyxia, respiratory distress syndrome, and cardiomyopathy also are problems seen in neonates of a mother with diabetes.

Test-Taking Strategy: Focusing on the mother's diagnosis will assist in eliminating option 3. From the remaining options, it is necessary to know the complications of the neonate of a mother with diabetes mellitus. Review the complications associated with the neonate born to a mother with diabetes mellitus and the various test-taking strategies if you had difficulty with this question.

Level of Cognitive Ability: Analysis
Client Needs: Physiological Integrity
Integrated Process: Nursing Process/Analysis
Content Area: Maternity/Postpartum

Reference
Lowdermilk D, Perry A: *Maternity & women's health care*, ed 8, St Louis, 2004, Mosby, p 1057.

---

182. A nurse is assessing a client in the fourth stage of labor and notes that the uterine fundus is firmly contracted and is midline at the level of the umbilicus. On the basis of this finding, the nurse would most appropriately
1   Massage the fundus
2   Contact the physician
3   Assist the mother to void
4   Record the findings

Answer: 4
Rationale: In the fourth stage of labor (first 1 or 2 hours after birth), the nurse assesses for uterine atony and checks the consistency and location of the uterine fundus. The uterine fundus should be firmly contracted, at or near the level of the umbilicus, and midline. Therefore, the nurse would record the finding. Because the finding is normal, options 1, 2, and 3 are not necessary. The nurse would massage the uterine fundus if it was soft and boggy. The physician would be contacted if the client experienced excessive bleeding. A full bladder may cause a displaced fundus and one that is above the level of the umbilicus.

Test-Taking Strategy: Use the process of elimination and focus on the data in the question. Recalling the normal location and consistency of the fundus will direct you to option 4. Review the expected findings in the fourth stage of labor if you had difficulty with this question.

Level of Cognitive Ability: Application
Client Needs: Physiological Integrity
Integrated Process: Nursing Process/Implementation
Content Area: Maternity/Postpartum

Reference
Murray S, McKinney E, Gorrie T: *Foundations of maternal-newborn nursing*, ed 3, Philadelphia, 2002, WB Saunders, p 779.

---

183. A client in the second trimester of pregnancy is admitted to the maternity unit with a diagnosis of abruptio placentae. The nurse expects to note which clinical manifestation associated with this disorder?
1   Painless vaginal bleeding
2   Soft, relaxed uterus with normal tone
3   Uterine hypertonicity
4   Nontender uterus

Answer: 3
Rationale: In abruptio placentae, abdominal pain, uterine tenderness, and uterine hypertonicity are present. Uterine tenderness accompanies placental abruption, especially with a central abruption in which blood becomes trapped behind the placenta. The abdomen will feel hard and boardlike on palpation as the blood penetrates the myometrium and causes uterine irritability. Excessive uterine activity with poor relaxation between contractions is present. Observation of the fetal monitoring often reveals loss of variability and late decelerations, uterine hyperstimulation and increased resting tone. Painless, bright red vaginal bleeding; a soft, relaxed uterus with normal tone; and a nontender uterus are signs of placenta previa.

Test-Taking Strategy: Eliminate options 1 and 4 first because they are similar. From the remaining options, note that option 3 indicates a sign opposite to the sign in option 2. This provides a clue that one of these options is correct. Recalling the signs of abruptio placentae will direct you to option 3. Review these signs and the various test-taking strategies if you had difficulty with this question.

Level of Cognitive Ability: Analysis
Client Needs: Physiological Integrity
Integrated Process: Nursing Process/Assessment
Content Area: Maternity/Antepartum

Reference
Lowdermilk D, Perry A: *Maternity & women's health care,* ed 8, St Louis, 2004, Mosby, pp 872, 876.

---

184. A nurse is performing an assessment on a client with severe preeclampsia. Which sign would indicate an improvement in the client's condition?
1   Protein in the urine is trace
2   Blood urea nitrogen level is 40 mg/dL
3   Blood pressure is 148/102 mm Hg
4   Client reports abdominal pain

Answer: 1
Rationale: Preeclampsia is considered mild when the diastolic blood pressure does not exceed 100 mm Hg; proteinuria is no more than 500 mg/day (trace to 1+); and symptoms such as headache, visual disturbances, or abdominal pain are absent. In addition, signs of kidney or liver involvement are absent. An increased blood urea nitrogen level indicates the presence of kidney damage as a result of the preeclampsia.

Test-Taking Strategy: Use the process of elimination, noting the keywords *severe preeclampsia* and *improvement in the client's condition.* Note the keyword *trace* in option 1. This is the only option that is not indicative of severe preeclampsia. Review the signs of mild and severe preeclampsia, the signs that indicate improvement, and the various test-taking strategies if you had difficulty with this question.

Level of Cognitive Ability: Analysis
Client Needs: Physiological Integrity
Integrated Process: Nursing Process/Evaluation
Content Area: Maternity/Antepartum

Reference
Murray S, McKinney E, Gorrie T: *Foundations of maternal-newborn nursing,* ed 3, Philadelphia, 2002, WB Saunders, pp 683–684.

---

185. A nurse develops a plan of care for a client newly diagnosed with Graves' disease. The nurse includes which of the following in the plan?
1   Provide a diet low in calories and protein
2   Keep the room temperature cool
3   Encourage frequent ambulation and other physical activities
4   Place extra blankets on the client's bed

Answer: 2
Rationale: Graves' disease is a form of hyperthyroidism and is characterized by a hypermetabolic state; the client benefits most from an environment that is restful both physically and mentally. Therefore, the client is encouraged to rest. To compensate for the hypermetabolic state, the client needs a diet that is high in calories and high in protein. These clients experience heat intolerance and diaphoresis and require a cool environment.

Test-Taking Strategy: Focus on the client's diagnosis. Recalling that Graves' disease is characterized by a hypermetabolic state will direct you to option 2. Review care to the client with Graves' disease and the various test-taking strategies if you had difficulty with this question.

Level of Cognitive Ability: Application
Client Needs: Physiological Integrity
Integrated Process: Nursing Process/Planning
Content Area: Adult Health/Endocrine

Reference
Black J, Hawks J: *Medical-surgical nursing: clinical management for positive outcomes,* ed 7, Philadelphia, 2005, WB Saunders, p 1199.

---

186. A nurse is caring for a client in the hospital with a diagnosis of acute pancreatitis. The nurse assists the client to which position that will decrease the abdominal pain?
  1   Prone
  2   Supine with the legs straight
  3   Side-lying with the head of the bed flat
  4   Upright in a sitting position with the trunk flexed

Answer: 4
Rationale: Correct positioning will assist in providing comfort to the client with acute pancreatitis. These positions include a side-lying position with the knees curled up to the chest and a pillow pressed against the abdomen or upright in a sitting position with the trunk flexed. Options 1, 2, and 3 are incorrect.

Test-Taking Strategy: Focus on the client's diagnosis and evaluate each of the options in terms of the amount of stretching or flexing of the abdominal wall that the action will cause. Also note that options 1, 2, and 3 are similar in that they are flat positions. Review the positions that will reduce pain in the client with acute pancreatitis and the various test-taking strategies if you had difficulty with this question.

Level of Cognitive Ability: Application
Client Needs: Physiological Integrity
Integrated Process: Nursing Process/Implementation
Content Area: Adult Health/Gastrointestinal

Reference
Black J, Hawks J: *Medical-surgical nursing: clinical management for positive outcomes,* ed 7, Philadelphia, 2005, WB Saunders, p 1294.

---

187. A client is diagnosed with viral hepatitis, and the nurse provides home care instructions to the client. The nurse determines that the client understands the instructions if the client makes which statement?
  1   "I need to remain in bed for the next 6 weeks."
  2   "I can take acetaminophen (Tylenol) for any discomfort."
  3   "I need to eat small, frequent meals that are low in fat and protein."
  4   "I need to limit my intake of alcohol."

Answer: 3
Rationale: Fatigue is a normal response to hepatic cellular damage. During the acute stage, rest is an essential intervention to reduce the liver's metabolic demands and increase its blood supply, but bed rest for 6 weeks is unnecessary. The client should avoid taking all medications, including acetaminophen (which is hepatotoxic), unless prescribed by the physician. The client needs to avoid all alcohol consumption. The client should consume small, frequent meals that are low in fat and protein to reduce the workload of the liver.

Test-Taking Strategy: Eliminate option 4 first recalling that the client needs to avoid (not limit) alcohol intake. Next, eliminate option 1 because of the words *next 6 weeks.* From the remaining options, recalling that acetaminophen is hepatotoxic will assist in eliminating option 2. Review instructions for the client with viral hepatitis and the various test-taking strategies if you had difficulty with this question.

Level of Cognitive Ability: Application
Client Needs: Physiological Integrity
Integrated Process: Teaching/Learning
Content Area: Adult Health/Gastrointestinal

Reference
Black J, Hawks J: *Medical-surgical nursing: clinical management for positive outcomes*, ed 7, Philadelphia, 2005, WB Saunders, p 1331.

---

188. The nurse teaches a client with gastroesophageal reflux disease (GERD) about the measures to prevent reflux while sleeping. The nurse determines that the client needs additional instructions if the client states:
  1 "I shouldn't eat anything at bedtime."
  2 "I should take an antacid at bedtime."
  3 "I should sleep flat on my right side."
  4 "Losing weight will decrease some of the stomach pressure."

Answer: 3
Rationale: Elevation of the head of the bed 6 to 8 inches will prevent nocturnal reflux. The client is instructed to avoid eating within 3 hours to bedtime to prevent nocturnal reflux. Antacids and histamine receptor antagonists may be prescribed for the client. Losing weight (if overweight) will decrease the gastroesophageal pressure gradient.

Test-Taking Strategy: Note the keywords *needs additional instructions*. These words indicate a false response question, and that you are looking for the option that is an incorrect client statement. Recalling that a backward flow of gastric contents occurs in this disorder will direct you to option 3. Review these client teaching points and the test-taking strategies for answering false response questions if you had difficulty with this question.

Level of Cognitive Ability: Analysis
Client Needs: Health Promotion and Maintenance
Integrated Process: Nursing Process/Evaluation
Content Area: Adult Health/Gastrointestinal

Reference
Black J, Hawks J: *Medical-surgical nursing: clinical management for positive outcomes*, ed 7, Philadelphia, 2005, WB Saunders, pp 732–733.

---

189. A cardiac monitor alarm sounds, and a nurse notes an unidentifiable rhythm on the monitor screen. The nurse takes which first action?
  1 Calls a code
  2 Calls the physician
  3 Obtains a rhythm strip from the monitor device
  4 Assesses the client

Answer: 4
Rationale: If a monitor alarm sounds, the nurse should first assess the clinical status of the client to see whether the problem is an actual dysrhythmia or a malfunction of the monitoring system. A dysrhythmia should not be mistaken for an unattached electrocardiogram wire. If the client is alert and the client's status is stable, the problem is likely an unattached cardiac lead or wire. Options 1, 2, and 3 are unnecessary if the client is stable. The nurse needs to determine the status of the client first.

Test-Taking Strategy: Note the keyword *first*. Use the steps of the nursing process, remembering that assessment is the first step. This will assist in eliminating options 1, 2, and 3. Review care to the client on a cardiac monitor and the test-taking strategies for answering prioritizing questions if you had difficulty with this question.

Level of Cognitive Ability: Application
Client Needs: Physiological Integrity
Integrated Process: Nursing Process/Implementation
Content Area: Adult Health/Cardiovascular

Reference

Ignatavicius D, Workman M: *Medical-surgical nursing: critical thinking for collaborative care,* ed 4, Philadelphia, 2002, WB Saunders, pp 656–658.

---

190. A client admitted to the hospital with chronic renal failure has returned to the nursing unit after a hemodialysis treatment. The nurse checks predialysis and postdialysis documentation of which parameters to determine the effectiveness of the procedure?
  1 Weight and blood urea nitrogen (BUN) level
  2 Blood pressure and weight
  3 Potassium and creatinine levels
  4 BUN and creatinine levels

Answer: 2

Rationale: After hemodialysis, the client's vital signs are monitored to determine whether the client is remaining hemodynamically stable and for comparison with predialysis measurements. The client's blood pressure and weight are expected to be reduced as a result of fluid removal. Laboratory studies are done as per protocol, but they are not necessarily done after the hemodialysis treatment has been ended.

Test-Taking Strategy: Focus on the issue: determining the effectiveness of hemodialysis. Also note that this question is an evaluation type of question. Remember that when options contain two parts, both parts need to be correct for the option to be correct. Knowing that weight is an important variable allows you to eliminate options 3 and 4. From the remaining options, recalling that vital signs reflect hemodynamic stability will direct you to option 2. Review the parameters that will determine the effectiveness of hemodialysis and the various test-taking strategies if you had difficulty with this question.

Level of Cognitive Ability: Analysis
Client Needs: Physiological Integrity
Integrated Process: Nursing Process/Evaluation
Content Area: Adult Health/Renal

Reference

Black J, Hawks J: *Medical-surgical nursing: clinical management for positive outcomes,* ed 7, Philadelphia, 2005, WB Saunders, p 961.

---

191. A client with chronic renal failure returns to the nursing unit after receiving his second hemodialysis treatment, and the nurse monitors the client closely for signs of disequilibrium syndrome. The nurse monitors for which sign of this syndrome?

Answer: 2

Rationale: Disequilibrium syndrome most often occurs in clients who are new to hemodialysis. It is characterized by headache, mental confusion, decreasing level of consciousness, nausea, vomiting, twitching, and possible seizure activity. It results from rapid removal of solutes from the body during hemodialysis and a greater residual concentration gradient in the brain because of the

1 Irritability
2 Mental confusion
3 Tachycardia
4 Hypothermia

blood–brain barrier. Water goes into cerebral cells because of the osmotic gradient, causing brain swelling and onset of symptoms. It is prevented by dialyzing for shorter times or at reduced blood flow rates. The signs in options 1, 3, and 4 are not associated with disequilibrium syndrome.

Test-Taking Strategy: Focusing on the name of the syndrome will assist in directing you to option 2. This is the only option that addresses a neurological sign. Review the signs of disequilibrium syndrome and the various test-taking strategies if you had difficulty with this question.

Level of Cognitive Ability: Analysis
Client Needs: Physiological Integrity
Integrated Process: Nursing Process/Analysis
Content Area: Adult Health/Renal

Reference
Black J, Hawks J: *Medical-surgical nursing: clinical management for positive outcomes,* ed 7, Philadelphia, 2005, WB Saunders, p 961.

---

192. A mother brings her child to the emergency department and reports that her son states that dirt flew into his eye during softball practice. The nurse takes which action first?
1 Assesses vision
2 Irrigates the eye with sterile saline
3 Removes the dirt
4 Places ice on the eye

Answer: 1

Rationale: If a surface foreign body injury occurs to the eye, the nurse would first assess visual acuity. The eye then will be assessed for corneal abrasions, followed by irrigating the eye with sterile normal saline to gently remove the particles. There is no reason to place ice on the eye in this case. Placing ice on the eye would be done if the client sustained an eye contusion.

Test-Taking Strategy: Use the steps of the nursing process. Option 1 is the only option that relates to assessment. Options 2, 3, and 4 relate to implementation. Review content related to initial treatment of eye injuries and the various test-taking strategies if you had difficulty with this question.

Level of Cognitive Ability: Application
Client Needs: Physiological Integrity
Integrated Process: Nursing Process/Implementation
Content Area: Child Health

Reference
Ignatavicius D, Workman M: *Medical-surgical nursing: critical thinking for collaborative care,* ed 4, Philadelphia, 2002, WB Saunders, p 1044.

---

193. The wife of a victim who sustained an eye injury calls the emergency department and speaks to a nurse. The wife reports that her husband was hit in the eye area by a piece of board while building a shed in the backyard. The nurse advises the wife to immediately

Answer: 1

Rationale: Treatment for a contusion ideally begins at the time of injury and includes applying ice to the site. The husband also should receive a thorough eye examination to rule out the presence of other injuries, but this is not the immediate action. Irrigating the eye with cool water may be implemented for injuries that involve a splash of

1 Apply ice to the affected eye
2 Call an ambulance
3 Irrigate the eye with cool water
4 Bring the husband to the emergency department

an irritant into the eye. It is not necessary to call an ambulance.

Test-Taking Strategy: Eliminate options 2 and 4 first because they are similar. From the remaining options, focusing on the type of injury sustained will direct you to option 1. Review initial treatment after an eye contusion and the various test-taking strategies if you had difficulty with this question.

Level of Cognitive Ability: Application
Client Needs: Physiological Integrity
Integrated Process: Nursing Process/Implementation
Content Area: Adult Health/Eye

Reference
Ignatavicius D, Workman M: *Medical-surgical nursing: critical thinking for collaborative care,* ed 4, Philadelphia, 2002, WB Saunders, p 1043.

---

194. A nurse employed in an eye clinic checks a client's intraocular pressure and notes that the pressure in the right eye is 16 mm Hg and the pressure in the left eye is 18 mm Hg. The nurse tells the client that
1 The pressure is increased in the left eye
2 The pressure is increased in the right eye
3 The pressure is normal in both eyes
4 The pressure in both eyes is low and requires treatment to increase it

Answer: **3**
Rationale: Normal intraocular pressure ranges from 8 to 21 mm Hg. Therefore, the client's intraocular pressure is normal. Options 1, 2, and 4 are incorrect.

Test-Taking Strategy: Focus on the data presented in the question. Note that options 1, 2, and 4 are similar and indicate abnormal findings. Review this normal finding and the various test-taking strategies if you had difficulty with this question.

Level of Cognitive Ability: Application
Client Needs: Health Promotion and Maintenance
Integrated Process: Nursing Process/Implementation
Content Area: Adult Health/Eye

Reference
Black J, Hawks J: *Medical-surgical nursing: clinical management for positive outcomes,* ed 7, Philadelphia, 2005, WB Saunders, p 1928.

---

195. A stapedectomy is performed on a client with otosclerosis. The nurse prepares the client for discharge and provides the client with which home care instruction?
1 To lie on the operative ear with the head of the bed flat
2 That acute vertigo is expected to occur
3 That it is all right to sneeze or blow his nose as he usually does
4 That plans for air travel need to be delayed for at least 1 month

Answer: **4**
Rationale: After stapedectomy, the client is instructed to lie on the nonoperative ear with the head of the bed elevated. The client also should avoid excessive exercise, straining, and activities that might lead to head trauma. If the client needs to blow his nose, it should be done gently, one nostril at a time, and the client should sneeze with the mouth open. The acute onset of vertigo needs to be reported to the physician. No airplane travel is allowed for 1 month.

Test-Taking Strategy: Focus on the surgical procedure and its location to direct you to option 4. Also, eliminate option 1 because of the words *lie on the operative ear with the head of the bed flat,* eliminate option 2 because of the words *acute vertigo,* and eliminate option 3 because of the words *as he usually does.* Review postoperative care after stapedectomy and the various test-taking strategies if you had difficulty with this question.

Level of Cognitive Ability: Application
Client Needs: Health Promotion and Maintenance
Integrated Process: Teaching/Learning
Content Area: Adult Health/Ear

Reference

Black J, Hawks J: *Medical-surgical nursing: clinical management for positive outcomes,* ed 7, Philadelphia, 2005, WB Saunders, p 1980.

---

196. A nurse provides instructions to a client about the measures to treat gout. The nurse determines that the client needs additional instructions if the client states that
1 The intake of red meats needs to be limited
2 Weight loss can help prevent an attack
3 Medication can help keep the uric acid level down
4 Fluid intake needs to be limited

Answer: 4

Rationale: Medication therapy is a component of management for clients with gout, and the physician normally prescribes a medication that will promote uric acid excretion or will reduce its production for clients with chronic gout. Fluid intake is important to promote uric acid excretion. Weight loss can reduce the incidence of attacks and reduce uric acid levels. A decrease in the intake of red meats and organ meats will assist in controlling uric acid levels.

Test-Taking Strategy: Note the keywords *needs additional instructions.* This indicates a false response question and directs you to look for the client statement that is incorrect. Recalling that in this disorder the client experiences an increased uric acid level and that measures need to be implemented to promote uric acid excretion will direct you to option 4. Review the management of gout and the test-taking strategies for answering false response questions if you had difficulty with this question.

Level of Cognitive Ability: Analysis
Client Needs: Health Promotion and Maintenance
Integrated Process: Nursing Process/Evaluation
Content Area: Adult Health/Musculoskeletal

Reference

Black J, Hawks J: *Medical-surgical nursing: clinical management for positive outcomes,* ed 7, Philadelphia, 2005, WB Saunders, p 608.

---

197. Buck's extension traction will be applied to the right leg of a client who sustained a right hip fracture. The nurse develops a plan of care for the client and includes which intervention in the plan?
1 Applying lanolin to the skin before applying the traction
2 Removing the traction weights once every 2 hours for 15 minutes

Answer: 4

Rationale: Buck's extension traction is a type of skin traction. It is important with skin traction to inspect the skin underneath at least once every 8 hours for irritation or inflammation. The nurse never releases the weights of traction unless specifically ordered to do so by the physician. Applying lanolin to the skin could make the skin area slippery, making it difficult to maintain the belt or boot used for the skin traction. There are no pins to care for with skin traction.

3 Cleaning the pin sites with half-strength hydrogen peroxide once per shift

4 Checking the skin integrity of the right leg at least every 8 hours

Test-Taking Strategy: Focus on the issue: Buck's extension traction. Recalling that Buck's extension traction is a skin traction will assist in eliminating option 3. Eliminate option 2 next because the nurse never removes weights without a specific order to do so. From the remaining options, use the steps of the nursing process. Option 4 addresses assessment. Review care to the client in Buck's traction and the various test-taking strategies if you had difficulty with this question.

Level of Cognitive Ability: Application
Client Needs: Physiological Integrity
Integrated Process: Nursing Process/Planning
Content Area: Adult Health/Musculoskeletal

Reference
Ignatavicius D, Workman M: *Medical-surgical: critical thinking for collaborative care,* ed 4, Philadelphia, 2002, WB Saunders, p 1136.

---

198. A client diagnosed with acquired immunodeficiency syndrome (AIDS) is admitted to the hospital. The nurse develops a plan of care and determines that which intervention is the priority?

1 Discussing the ways that the client contracted the AIDS virus

2 Identifying the ways that AIDS can be contracted by others

3 Instituting measures to prevent infection in the client

4 Providing emotional support to the client

Answer: 3
Rationale: The client with AIDS has inadequate immune bodies and is at risk for infection. The priority nursing intervention would be to protect the client from infection. The nurse also would provide emotional support to the client, but this is not the priority from the options provided. Discussing the ways that the client contracted the AIDS virus and the ways others can contract AIDS are not appropriate priority interventions.

Test-Taking Strategy: Note the keyword *priority.* Eliminate options 1 and 2 first because they are similar. Also, use Maslow's Hierarchy of Needs theory. Remember that physiological needs are the priority. This will direct you to option 3. Review the priority needs of a client with AIDS and the test-taking strategies for answering prioritizing questions if you had difficulty with this question.

Level of Cognitive Ability: Application
Client Needs: Physiological Integrity
Integrated Process: Nursing Process/Planning
Content Area: Adult Health/Immune

Reference
Ignatavicius D, Workman M: *Medical-surgical nursing: critical thinking for collaborative care,* ed 4, Philadelphia, 2002, WB Saunders, p 367.

---

199. A client arrives at the emergency department with reports of hives, itching, and difficulty swallowing and states that "my throat feels as though it is closing off." The client states that he was visiting a relative who has two cats and two dogs and

Answer: 1
Rationale: The initial action of the nurse would be to maintain a patent airway. Once airway is established, the client would receive a subcutaneous injection of epinephrine. Intravenous corticosteroids and intravenous fluids may also be prescribed. The application of ice to the throat will not relieve the symptoms.

believes that he is allergic to cats. The nurse ensures that the client has a patent airway, and then prepares the client for which initial intervention?

1 Administration of a subcutaneous injection of epinephrine (Adrenalin)
2 Administration of an intravenous glucocorticoid
3 Administration of normal saline solution
4 The application of ice to the throat

Test-Taking Strategy: Note the keyword *initial.* Use the ABCs—airway, breathing, and circulation—to direct you to option 1. Remember, once airway is established, the client will receive epinephrine. Review care to the client who experiences an allergic reaction and the various test-taking strategies if you had difficulty with this question.

Level of Cognitive Ability: Application
Client Needs: Physiological Integrity
Integrated Process: Nursing Process/Planning
Content Area: Adult Health/Immune

References
Black J, Hawks J: *Medical-surgical nursing: clinical management for positive outcomes,* ed 7, Philadelphia, 2005, WB Saunders, p 2325.

---

200. A client with a spinal cord injury suddenly reports a severe, pounding headache. The nurse quickly checks the client and notes that the client is diaphoretic, has an increased blood pressure, and has a decreased heart rate. The nurse suspects that the client is experiencing autonomic dysreflexia, elevates the head of the client's bed, and immediately

1 Notifies the physician
2 Checks to see whether the client has an order for an antihypertensive medication
3 Increases the rate of intravenous fluids
4 Checks the client's bladder for distention and the rectum for impaction

Answer: 4

Rationale: Autonomic dysreflexia is an acute emergency that occurs as a result of exaggerated autonomic responses to stimuli that are innocuous in healthy individuals. It occurs after spinal shock has resolved. A number of stimuli may trigger this response including a distended bladder (the most common cause); distension or contraction of the visceral organs, especially the bowel (from constipation, impaction); or stimulation of the skin. When autonomic dysreflexia occurs, the client is immediately placed in a sitting position to decrease the blood pressure. The nurse then would perform a rapid assessment to identify and alleviate the cause. The client's bladder is emptied immediately through a urinary catheter; the rectum is checked for the presence of a fecal mass; and the skin is examined for areas of pressure, irritation, or broken skin. The physician is notified, and then the nurse documents the occurrence and the actions taken. Increasing the rate of intravenous fluids is an inappropriate action.

Test-Taking Strategy: Focus on the data in the question and note that the nurse has already elevated the head of the client's bed and checked the client's blood pressure. Next, recalling that autonomic dysreflexia occurs as a result of exaggerated autonomic responses to stimuli and that the stimuli needs to be removed quickly will direct you to option 4. Review immediate interventions to treat autonomic dysreflexia and the various test-taking strategies if you had difficulty with this question.

Level of Cognitive Ability: Application
Client Needs: Physiological Integrity
Integrated Process: Nursing Process/Implementation
Content Area: Adult Health/Neurological

Reference
Black J, Hawks J: *Medical-surgical nursing: clinical management for positive outcomes,* ed 7, Philadelphia, 2005, WB Saunders, p 2229.

201. A client who is recovering from a cerebrovascular accident (CVA) has residual dysphagia. To assist in assessing the client's swallowing ability, the nurse would do which of the following?

1. Ask the client to swallow some water
2. Ask the client to swallow a teaspoon of applesauce
3. Ask the client to produce an audible cough
4. Ask the client to suck on a piece of hard candy

Answer: 3

Rationale: To assess the client's readiness and ability to swallow, the nurse would assess the client's level of consciousness (client needs to be alert), check for a gag reflex (gag reflex must be present), have the client produce an audible cough (client must be able to produce an audible cough), and ask the client to produce a voluntary swallow (client must be able to do this). The nurse would not give the client a liquid or food item and would not ask the client to suck on a piece of hard candy or any other item because of the risk for aspiration.

Test-Taking Strategy: Eliminate options 1, 2, and 4 because they are similar and would place the client at risk for aspiration. Also, use the ABCs—airway, breathing, and circulation—to direct you to option 3. Review care of the client with residual dysphagia and the various test-taking strategies if you had difficulty with this question.

Level of Cognitive Ability: Application
Client Needs: Safe, Effective Care Environment
Integrated Process: Nursing Process/Implementation
Content Area: Adult Health/Neurological

Reference
Black J, Hawks J: *Medical-surgical nursing: clinical management for positive outcomes,* ed 7, Philadelphia, 2005, WB Saunders, p 697.

---

202. A nurse is developing a plan of care for a client who is experiencing homonymous hemianopia after a cerebrovascular accident (CVA). The nurse documents interventions that will promote a safe environment knowing that in this disorder

1. The client is unable to carry out a skilled act such as dressing in the absence of paralysis
2. The client has lost the ability to recognize familiar objects through the senses
3. The client has paralysis of the sympathetic nerves of the eye, causing sinking of the eyeball
4. The client has a visual loss in the same half of the visual field of each eye

Answer: 4

Rationale: Homonymous hemianopsia is a visual loss in the same half of the visual field of each eye, so the client has only half of normal vision. Option 1 describes apraxia. Option 2 describes agnosia. Option 3 describes Horner syndrome.

Test-Taking Strategy: Focus on the issue: homonymous hemianopia. Use medical terminology noting that *hemi* means "half" and *op* refers to the "eye." This will direct you to option 4. Review care for the client with homonymous hemianopia and the various test-taking strategies if you had difficulty with this question.

Level of Cognitive Ability: Application
Client Needs: Safe, Effective Care Environment
Integrated Process: Nursing Process/Planning
Content Area: Adult Health/Neurological

Reference
Black J, Hawks J: *Medical-surgical nursing: clinical management for positive outcomes,* ed 7, Philadelphia, 2005, WB Saunders, p 2114.

---

203. A nurse is providing home care instructions about measures to control a right-sided hand tremor to

Answer: 2

Rationale: If the client has a tremor, the client is instructed to use both hands to accomplish a task. The a client with Parkinson disease. The nurse tells the client to

1 Use the right hand only to perform tasks
2 Squeeze a rubber ball with the right hand
3 Use the left hand only to perform tasks
4 Sleep on the unaffected side

client also is instructed to hold change in a pocket or to squeeze a rubber ball with the affected hand. The client should sleep on the side that has the tremor to control it.

Test-Taking Strategy: Eliminate options 1 and 3 first because of the absolute word *only.* From the remaining options, visualize each and think about each effect in terms of controlling the tremor. This will direct you to option 2. Review client teaching points for Parkinson disease and the various test-taking strategies if you had difficulty with this question.

Level of Cognitive Ability: Application
Client Needs: Health Promotion and Maintenance
Integrated Process: Teaching/Learning
Content Area: Adult Health/Neurological

Reference
Black J, Hawks J: *Medical-surgical nursing: clinical management for positive outcomes,* ed 7, Philadelphia, 2005, WB Saunders, p 2174.

---

204. A nurse answers the call bell of a client who has an internal cervical radiation implant. The client states that she thinks that the implant fell out. The nurse checks the client and sees the implant lying in the bed. The nurse immediately uses the long-handled forceps to pick up the implant and places the implant into the lead container (pig) that is in the client's room. Which action would the nurse take next?

1 Contact the radiation therapist and radiation safety officer
2 Call a security officer and ask the officer to send someone to guard the client's room until the situation is resolved
3 Call for a transport personnel to deliver the lead container (pig) to the radiation department
4 Ask another nurse to assist in reinserting the implant

Answer: 1

Rationale: A lead container (called a pig) and a pair of long-handled forceps should be kept in the client's room at all times during internal radiation therapy. If the implant becomes dislodged, the nurse should pick up the implant with long-handled forceps and place it in the lead container. The radiation therapist and radiation safety officer are notified immediately of the situation so that they can retrieve and secure the radiation source. The physician also is called after taking action to maintain the safety of the client and others. The nurse does not reinsert a radiation implant device. Options 2 and 3 are incorrect and can expose individuals to the radiation.

Test-Taking Strategy: Note the keyword *next.* Option 4 can be eliminated first because inserting a radiation device is not a nursing activity. Recalling that the nurse needs to protect himself or herself and others from exposure to radiation will assist in eliminating options 2 and 3. In addition, these options are similar. Review the measures related to a dislodged implant and the various test-taking strategies if you had difficulty with this question.

Level of Cognitive Ability: Application
Client Needs: Safe, Effective Care Environment
Integrated Process: Nursing Process/Implementation
Content Area: Adult Health/Oncology

Reference
Black J, Hawks J: *Medical-surgical nursing: clinical management for positive outcomes,* ed 7, Philadelphia, 2005, WB Saunders, p 363.

205. A female client who has undergone placement of a sealed radiation implant asks the nurse whether she can take a walk with her husband to the clients' lounge at the end of the hall. The nurse makes which most appropriate response to the client?

  1 "Yes, it is fine to take a walk to the clients' lounge."

  2 "Yes, as long as there are no other clients in the lounge. Let me check for you."

  3 "It is really a far walk. Are you sure that you are up to it?"

  4 "Because of the treatment you are receiving, you need to remain in your room."

Answer: 4

Rationale: The client with a sealed radiation implant needs to remain in a private room (with a private bath) to prevent exposure of radiation to others. Therefore, options 1, 2, and 3 are incorrect.

Test-Taking Strategy: Eliminate options 1, 2, and 3 because they are similar and indicate that the client is able to leave the room. Review care to the client with a radiation implant and the various test-taking strategies if you had difficulty with this question.

Level of Cognitive Ability: Application
Client Needs: Safe, Effective Care Environment
Integrated Process: Nursing Process/Implementation
Content Area: Adult Health/Oncology

Reference
Black J, Hawks J: *Medical-surgical nursing: clinical management for positive outcomes,* ed 7, Philadelphia, 2005, WB Saunders, p 363.

---

206. A nurse is teaching a nursing assistant how to measure a carotid pulse. The nurse tells the nursing assistant to measure the pulse on only one side of the client's neck primarily

  1 So that the client will not feel a sense of choking

  2 Because it will provide a more accurate determination of the quality of the pulse

  3 Because the pulse rate will be easier to count

  4 To prevent dizziness and a decrease in heart rate

Answer: 4

Rationale: Applying pressure to both carotid arteries at the same time is contraindicated. Excess pressure to the baroreceptors in the carotid vessels could cause the heart rate and blood pressure to reflexively decrease and cause syncope. In addition, the manual pressure could interfere with the flow of blood to the brain.

Test-Taking Strategy: Note the keyword *primarily.* Note that option 4 describes the greatest danger to the client. Review the function and location of baroreceptors in the carotid vessels and the various test-taking strategies if you had difficulty with this question.

Level of Cognitive Ability: Application
Client Needs: Physiological Integrity
Integrated Process: Teaching/Learning
Content Area: Leadership/Management

Reference
Black J, Hawks J: *Medical-surgical nursing: clinical management for positive outcomes,* ed 7, Philadelphia, 2005, WB Saunders, p 1482.

---

207. A client being treated for respiratory failure has the following arterial blood gas (ABG) results: pH, 7.30; $Paco_2$, 58 mm Hg; PaO_2, 75 mm Hg; HCO_3^-, 27 mEq/L. The nurse interprets that the client has which of the following acid–base disturbances?

  1 Metabolic acidosis

  2 Metabolic alkalosis

  3 Respiratory acidosis

  4 Respiratory alkalosis

Answer: 3

Rationale: Acidosis is defined as a pH less than 7.35, whereas alkalosis is defined as a pH greater than 7.45. In a respiratory condition, an opposite effect will be seen between the pH and the $Paco_2$. In respiratory acidosis, the pH is decreased and the $Paco_2$ is increased. The normal HCO_3^- is 22 to 27 mm Hg. Metabolic acidosis is present when the HCO_3^- is less than 22 mEq/L, whereas metabolic alkalosis is present when the HCO_3^- is greater than 27 mEq/L. This client's ABGs are consistent with respiratory acidosis.

Test-Taking Strategy: Focus on the client's diagnosis and recall that this client will have difficulty exchanging oxygen and carbon dioxide. This will assist in eliminating options 1 and 2. From the remaining options, remember that the pH is decreased with acidosis. This will direct you to option 3. Review the steps related to reading blood gas values and the various test-taking strategies if you had difficulty with this question.

Level of Cognitive Ability: Analysis
Client Needs: Physiological Integrity
Integrated Process: Nursing Process/Analysis
Content Area: Adult Health/Respiratory

Reference

Black J, Hawks J: *Medical-surgical nursing: clinical management for positive outcomes,* ed 7, Philadelphia, 2005, WB Saunders, p 252.

---

208. A client with type 1 diabetes mellitus has a blood glucose level of 554 mg/dL. The nurse calls the physician to report the level and monitors the client closely for which acid–base imbalance?
1 Respiratory acidosis
2 Respiratory alkalosis
3 Metabolic acidosis
4 Metabolic alkalosis

Answer: 3

Rationale: Diabetes mellitus can lead to metabolic acidosis. When the body does not have sufficient circulating insulin, the blood glucose level increases. At the same time, the cells of the body use all available glucose. The body then breaks down glycogen and fat for fuel. The byproducts of fat metabolism are acidotic and can lead to the condition known as diabetic ketoacidosis.

Test-Taking Strategy: Note the client's diagnosis. This tells you that the primary problem is metabolic in nature, not respiratory. Therefore, eliminate options 1 and 2. From the remaining options, recalling the complications associated with diabetes mellitus will assist in directing you to option 3. Review these complications and the various test-taking strategies if you had difficulty with this question.

Level of Cognitive Ability: Analysis
Client Needs: Physiological Integrity
Integrated Process: Nursing Process/Analysis
Content Area: Adult Health/Endocrine

Reference

Black J, Hawks J: *Medical-surgical nursing: clinical management for positive outcomes,* ed 7, Philadelphia, 2005, WB Saunders, p 252.

---

209. A client has made an appointment to have an annual Papanicolaou smear done. The nurse who schedules the appointment tells the client that
1 The test is very uncomfortable, but a local anesthetic will be injected into the vaginal area

Answer: 4

Rationale: A Papanicolaou smear cannot be performed during menstruation. The test usually is painless, but it may be slightly uncomfortable with placement of the speculum, or while a cervical scraping is obtained. A local anesthetic is not injected into the vaginal area. The client is instructed to avoid sexual intercourse, douching, or using vagina hygiene sprays or deodorants for 2 to 3 days before the test.

2 If the client is menstruating, douching will be required right before the test

3 A vaginal hygiene spray should be used for 2 consecutive days before the scheduled test

4 Sexual intercourse needs to be avoided for 2 to 3 days before the test

Test-Taking Strategy: Eliminate option 1 first because of the words *very uncomfortable.* From the remaining options, thinking about the test and its purpose will direct you to option 4. Review client preparation for a Papanicolaou test and the various test-taking strategies if you had difficulty with this question.

Level of Cognitive Ability: Application
Client Needs: Health Promotion and Maintenance
Integrated Process: Teaching/Learning
Content Area: Adult Health/Oncology

Reference
Black J, Hawks J: *Medical-surgical nursing: clinical management for positive outcomes,* ed 7, Philadelphia, 2005, WB Saunders, p 997.

---

210. A client with a diagnosis of multiple myeloma is admitted to the hospital. On assessment, the nurse asks the client which question that specifically relates to a clinical manifestation of this disorder?
1 "Are you having any bone pain?"
2 "Do you have diarrhea?"
3 "Have you noticed an increase in appetite?"
4 "Do you have feelings of anxiety and nervousness, together with difficulty sleeping?"

Answer: 1
Rationale: Multiple myeloma is characterized by an abnormal proliferation of plasma B cells. These cells infiltrate the bone marrow and produce abnormal and excessive amounts of immunoglobulin. The most common presenting symptom is bone pain. Hypercalcemia occurs as a result of release of calcium from the deteriorating bone tissue; subsequently, the client experiences confusion, somnolence, constipation, nausea, and thirst.

Test-Taking Strategy: Focus on the client's diagnosis and use medical terminology to answer the question. Also, recalling the pathophysiology of multiple myeloma and the effects it produces on the body will direct you to option 1. Review the manifestations associated with multiple myeloma and the various test-taking strategies if you had difficulty with this question.

Level of Cognitive Ability: Analysis
Client Needs: Physiological Integrity
Integrated Process: Nursing Process/Assessment
Content Area: Adult Health/Oncology

Reference
Black J, Hawks J: *Medical-surgical nursing: clinical management for positive outcomes,* ed 7, Philadelphia, 2005, WB Saunders, p 2302.

---

211. A woman scheduled for an annual mammogram says to the nurse, "Is there a risk in the exposure to radiation?" The nurse makes which most appropriate response to alleviate the client's concern?
1 "There is no exposure at all to radiation."
2 "The machine does not use radiation to visualize the breast."

Answer: 4
Rationale: Mammography uses the smallest dose of radiation possible, and the long-term effects of an annual mammogram are considered to be harmless. Options 1, 2, and 3 are incorrect.

Test-Taking Strategy: Eliminate options 1, 2, and 3 because they are similar and indicate that radiation is not used for this procedure. Review this procedure and the various test-taking strategies if you had difficulty with this question.

3 "A fluoroscopic method is used to perform this test."
4 "This test uses the smallest dose of radiation possible, and the long-term effects are considered to be harmless."

Level of Cognitive Ability: Application
Client Needs: Psychosocial Integrity
Integrated Process: Nursing Process/Implementation
Content Area: Adult Health/Oncology

Reference
Black J, Hawks J: *Medical-surgical nursing: clinical management for positive outcomes,* ed 7, Philadelphia, 2005, WB Saunders, p 1002.

---

212. The nurse provides preprocedural instructions to a client who is scheduled for an excision of a skin lesion and biopsy in 1 week. Which statement by the client indicates a need for further instructions?
1 "I may need to avoid taking aspirin or aspirin products for 2 days before the procedure."
2 "I can eat a light meal before this procedure."
3 "I know that I won't have to sign a consent to have this procedure performed because it is being done on my skin."
4 "I know that I have to take antibiotics because I had a heart valve replaced one year ago."

Answer: 3
Rationale: Depending on the size of the excision, the client may need to avoid taking aspirin or aspirin-containing products for 48 hours to avoid a prolonged postprocedure bleeding time. If the client is taking an anticoagulant, then the physician is contacted for specific instructions. If the client has a history of cardiac valve replacement, then prophylactic antibiotics are prescribed. The client can eat a light meal before the procedure to prevent syncope. An informed consent is obtained for any invasive procedure.

Test-Taking Strategy: Note the keywords *indicates a need for further instructions.* These words indicate that this is a false response question, and that you need to select the option that indicates an incorrect client statement. Careful reading of the options and recalling that an informed consent is needed for any invasive procedure will direct you to option 3. Review preprocedural care for a skin biopsy and the strategies for answering false response questions if you had difficulty with this question.

Level of Cognitive Ability: Analysis
Client Needs: Physiological Integrity
Integrated Process: Nursing Process/Evaluation
Content Area: Adult Health/Integumentary

Reference
Black J, Hawks J: *Medical-surgical nursing: clinical management for positive outcomes,* ed 7, Philadelphia, 2005, WB Saunders, p 1388.

---

213. A postoperative client who underwent pelvic surgery suddenly experiences development of dyspnea and tachypnea. The nurse suspects that the client has a pulmonary embolism and takes which action first?
1 Obtains an intravenous infusion pump to administer heparin
2 Increases the rate of the intravenous fluids infusing to prevent hypotension
3 Administers low-flow oxygen through nasal cannula
4 Obtains an ampule of bicarbonate to treat acidosis

Answer: 3
Rationale: Pulmonary embolism is a life-threatening emergency. Maintenance of cardiopulmonary stability is the first priority. Low-flow oxygen through nasal cannula is administered first. Some clients may require endotracheal intubation to maintain an adequate PaO_2. Hypotension is treated with fluids. Intravenous anticoagulation is initiated, and bicarbonate may be administered to correct acidosis. A perfusion scan among other tests may be performed, and the electrocardiogram is monitored for the presence of dysrhythmias. In addition, a urinary catheter may be inserted. However, the first nursing action is to administer oxygen.

Test-Taking Strategy: Note the keyword *first.* Use of the ABCs—airway, breathing, and circulation—will direct you to option 3. Review the immediate nursing actions when pulmonary embolism occurs and the test-taking strategies for answering prioritizing questions if you had difficulty with this question.

Level of Cognitive Ability: Application
Client Needs: Physiological Integrity
Integrated Process: Nursing Process/Implementation
Content Area: Delegating/Prioritizing

Reference

Black J, Hawks J: *Medical-surgical nursing: clinical management for positive outcomes,* ed 7, Philadelphia, 2005, WB Saunders, p 1832.

---

214. A nurse caring for a postoperative client after a bowel resection notes that the client is restless. The nurse takes the client's vital signs and notes that the client's pulse rate has increased and that the blood pressure has decreased significantly since the previous readings. The nurse suspects that the client is going into shock and immediately
    1 Checks the client's oxygen saturation level
    2 Increases the rate of flow of the oxygen being delivered
    3 Rechecks the vital signs to verify the findings
    4 Slows the rate of the intravenous (IV) fluid infusing

Answer: 2

Rationale: In addition to hypotension, manifestations of shock include tachycardia; restlessness and apprehension; and cold, moist, pale, or cyanotic skin. If a client shows signs of shock, the nurse would immediately administer oxygen or increase its rate of delivery. The nurse also would raise the client's legs above the level of the heart, increase the rate of IV fluids (unless contraindicated), notify the surgeon, administer medications as prescribed, and continue to assess the client and the client's response to interventions.

Test-Taking Strategy: Note the keyword *immediately.* Use the ABCs—airway, breathing, and circulation—to answer the question. This will direct you to option 2. Review the interventions for shock and the test-taking strategies for answering prioritizing questions if you had difficulty with this question.

Level of Cognitive Ability: Application
Client Needs: Physiological Integrity
Integrated Process: Nursing Process/Implementation
Content Area: Adult Health/Cardiovascular

Reference

Black J, Hawks J: *Medical-surgical nursing: clinical management for positive outcomes,* ed 7, Philadelphia, 2005, WB Saunders, p 303.

---

215. A client returns to the nursing unit from the postanesthesia care unit (PACU) after a transurethral resection of the prostate. The nurse does which of the following first?
    1 Checks the client's respirations
    2 Reads the nursing notes written by the PACU nurse
    3 Checks the color of the client's urine
    4 Checks the Foley catheter for patency

Answer: 1

Rationale: The first action of the nurse is to assess the patency of the airway. The nurse would observe the client and assess the breathing pattern. If the airway is not patent, immediate measures must be taken for the survival of the client. The nurse then performs an assessment of cardiovascular function, the condition of the surgical site, the tubes or drains for patency, and the function of the central nervous system. The PACU nurse normally provides a verbal report. Even so, reading the nursing notes would not be the first action.

Test-Taking Strategy: Note the keyword *first.* Use the ABCs—airway, breathing, and circulation. This will direct you to option 1. Airway patency is the priority. Review priority nursing assessments in the postoperative client and the test-taking strategies for answering prioritizing questions if you had difficulty with this question.

Level of Cognitive Ability: Application
Client Needs: Physiological Integrity
Integrated Process: Nursing Process/Implementation
Content Area: Adult Health/Renal

Reference
Black J, Hawks J: *Medical-surgical nursing: clinical management for positive outcomes,* ed 7, Philadelphia, 2005, WB Saunders, p 305.

216. A client is scheduled for a liver biopsy, and the nurse reviews the results of the laboratory tests prescribed for the client. The nurse would contact the physician if which laboratory result is noted?
    1 Platelets: 210,000/mm^3
    2 Thrombin time: 20 seconds
    3 Hematocrit: 40%
    4 Hemoglobin: 14 g/dL

Answer: 2
Rationale: The normal thrombin time is 10 to 15 seconds. A prolonged time indicates that the client is at risk for bleeding. Coagulation profile tests are performed before a liver biopsy to ensure that the client is not at risk for bleeding as a result of the procedure. The laboratory results in options 1, 3, and 4 are within reference range.

Test-Taking Strategy: Note that the client is scheduled for a liver biopsy. Recalling that bleeding is a concern after this procedure will direct you to option 2. Also, recalling the normal values for the laboratory studies identified in the options will direct you to option 2. Review these normal laboratory values and the various test-taking strategies if you had difficulty answering this question.

Level of Cognitive Ability: Analysis
Client Needs: Physiological Integrity
Integrated Process: Nursing Process/Analysis
Content Area: Adult Health/Gastrointestinal

Reference
Black J, Hawks J: *Medical-surgical nursing: clinical management for positive outcomes,* ed 7, Philadelphia, 2005, WB Saunders, pp 1186, 2266.

217. A client is tested for human immunodeficiency virus (HIV) with an enzyme-linked immunosorbent assay (ELISA) test, and the test result is positive. The client is very upset and asks the nurse if this means that he definitely has HIV. The nurse most appropriately tells the client that
    1 He definitely has HIV
    2 False-positive results are reported all of the time, and that he should not be worried

Answer: 3
Rationale: The normal result for an ELISA test is negative. If the ELISA test result is positive, a second test, the Western blot, is performed to confirm a positive HIV status. The other options are incorrect. In addition, the nurse would not tell a client that "he should not be worried." If testing is performed too early in the initial infection period, a false-negative result may occur.

Test-Taking Strategy: Use therapeutic communication techniques to eliminate options 1 and 2. Next, careful reading of option 4 will assist in eliminating this option. Remember, if testing is performed too early in the initial

3   Another test will be done to determine whether he has HIV

4   A positive ELISA means that the infection was diagnosed early in the initial infection period

infection period, a false-negative result may occur. Review interpretations of results of an ELISA test and the various test-taking strategies if you had difficulty with this question.

Level of Cognitive Ability: Application
Client Needs: Physiological Integrity
Integrated Process: Nursing Process/Implementation
Content Area: Adult Health/Immune

Reference
Black J, Hawks J: *Medical-surgical nursing: clinical management for positive outcomes,* ed 7, Philadelphia, 2005, WB Saunders, p 2382.

---

218. A CD4⁺ T-cell count is performed on a client who is human immunodeficiency virus (HIV)-positive. The results of the test indicate a CD4⁺ count of 700 mm³. The nurse interprets this test result to indicate

1   That infection is likely to develop

2   That the count is dangerously low

3   Improvement in the client's condition

4   The need for aggressive therapy with intravenous antibiotics

Answer: 3
Rationale: The average laboratory range for the CD4⁺ T-cell count is 500 to 1600 mm³. Therefore, option 3 is correct. Options 1, 2, and 4 are incorrect interpretations of this laboratory result.

Test-Taking Strategy: Eliminate options 1, 2, and 4 because they are similar and indicate that the laboratory result is low. If you had difficulty with this question, review the CD4⁺ T-cell count, the significance of its results, and the various test-taking strategies.

Level of Cognitive Ability: Analysis
Client Needs: Physiological Integrity
Integrated Process: Nursing Process/Analysis
Content Area: Adult Health/Immune

Reference
Black J, Hawks J: *Medical-surgical nursing: clinical management for positive outcomes,* ed 7, Philadelphia, 2005, WB Saunders, p 2379.

---

219. A nurse provides instructions to a client who is being discharged 24 hours after undergoing a percutaneous renal biopsy. Which statement by the client indicates a need to reinforce the instructions?

1   "I need to avoid any strenuous lifting for about two weeks."

2   "I shouldn't work out at the gym for about two weeks."

3   "I will call the physician if my urine becomes bloody."

4   "A fever is normal after this procedure."

Answer: 4
Rationale: After percutaneous renal biopsy, the client is instructed to report immediately fever, increasing pain levels (back, flank, or shoulder), bleeding from the puncture site, weakness, dizziness, grossly bloody urine, or dysuria. Activity should be restricted if blood is seen in the urine. The client also is instructed to avoid strenuous lifting, physical exertion, or trauma to the biopsy site for up to 2 weeks after discharge.

Test-Taking Strategy: Note the keywords *need to reinforce the instructions.* Eliminate options 1 and 2 first because they are similar. From the remaining options, recall the complications of this procedure. This will direct you to option 4. Review client instructions after a percutaneous renal biopsy and the various test-taking strategies if you had difficulty with this question.

Level of Cognitive Ability: Analysis
Client Needs: Health Promotion and Maintenance

Integrated Process: Nursing Process/Evaluation
Content Area: Adult Health/Renal

Reference
Black J, Hawks J: *Medical-surgical nursing: clinical management for positive outcomes,* ed 7, Philadelphia, 2005, WB Saunders, p 803.

---

220. A nurse has instructed a nursing assistant in the procedure for collecting a 24-hour urine specimen from a client. The nurse determines that the nursing assistant understands the directions if the nursing assistant states to

1 Save the first urine specimen collected at the start time
2 Keep the specimen at room temperature
3 Discard the last voided specimen at the end of the collection time
4 Ask the client to void, discard the specimen, and note the start time

Answer: 4
Rationale: Because a 24-hour urine specimen is a timed quantitative determination, the test must be started with an empty bladder. Therefore, the first urine is discarded. Fifteen minutes before the end of the collection time, the client should be asked to void, and this specimen is added to the collection. The urine collection should be refrigerated or placed on ice to prevent changes in urine composition.

Test-Taking Strategy: Note that options 1 and 4 are opposite, which is an indication that one of them is likely to be the correct option. Recalling that the 24-hour urine specimen is a timed quantitative determination will assist in directing you to option 4. Review the procedure for collecting a 24-hour urine specimen and the various test-taking strategies if you had difficulty with this question.

Level of Cognitive Ability: Analysis
Client Needs: Safe, Effective Care Environment
Integrated Process: Teaching/Learning
Content Area: Leadership/Management

Reference
Potter P, Perry A: *Fundamentals of nursing,* ed 6, St Louis, 2005, Mosby, p 1335.

---

221. A client has undergone cardiac catheterization using the right femoral artery for access. The nurse determines that the client is experiencing a complication of the procedure if which of the following is noted?

1 Blood pressure of 118/76 mm Hg
2 Pallor and coolness of the right leg
3 Urine output of 40 mL/hr
4 Respirations of 18 breaths/min

Answer: 2
Rationale: Potential complications after cardiac catheterization include allergic reaction to the dye, cardiac dysrhythmias, and a number of vascular complications, including hemorrhage, thrombosis, or embolism. The nurse detects these complications by monitoring for signs and symptoms of allergic reaction, decreased urine output, hematoma or hemorrhage at the insertion site, or signs of decreased circulation to the affected leg. Options 1, 3, and 4 are normal findings.

Test-Taking Strategy: Note the keywords *experiencing a complication.* This tells you that the correct option is an abnormal piece of assessment data. Eliminate options 1, 3, and 4 because they are normal findings. Pallor and coolness indicate thrombosis or hematoma and should be further assessed and reported. Review the signs of complications after a cardiac catheterization if you had difficulty with this question.

Level of Cognitive Ability: Analysis
Client Needs: Physiological Integrity
Integrated Process: Nursing Process/Analysis
Content Area: Adult Health/Cardiovascular

Reference

Black J, Hawks J: *Medical-surgical nursing: clinical management for positive outcomes,* ed 7, Philadelphia, 2005, WB Saunders, p 103.

---

222. A nurse reviews a client's urinalysis report. The nurse determines that which finding is abnormal?
  1 Opacity is clear
  2 Specific gravity is 1.018
  3 Ketones are negative
  4 Protein is positive

Answer: 4

Rationale: The urine has a normal pH range of 4.5 to 8, and a specific gravity ranging from 1.002 to 1.035. Urine typically is screened for protein, glucose, ketones, bilirubin, casts, crystals, red blood cells, and white blood cells, all of which should be negative.

Test-Taking Strategy: Note the keyword *abnormal.* Noting the word *positive* in option 4 will direct you to this option. Review normal findings in a urinalysis and the various test-taking strategies if you had difficulty with this question.

Level of Cognitive Ability: Analysis
Client Needs: Physiological Integrity
Integrated Process: Nursing Process/Analysis
Content Area: Adult Health/Renal

Reference

Black J, Hawks J: *Medical-surgical nursing: clinical management for positive outcomes,* ed 7, Philadelphia, 2005, WB Saunders, p 97.

---

223. A registered nurse is reviewing with a licensed practical nurse the pre-procedural care for a client who is scheduled for a cardiac catheterization. The registered nurse determines that the licensed practical nurse needs supervision while preparing the client if the licensed practical nurse states that the client needs to be told that
  1 He may experience flushing feelings during the procedure
  2 The blood vessels and flow of blood will be assessed with this procedure
  3 The procedure takes about 4 hours
  4 There is little to no pain with catheter insertion because a local anesthetic is used

Answer: 3

Rationale: A cardiac catheterization is a diagnostic test that assesses the coronary arteries and the flow of blood through them. The procedure is done in a darkened cardiac catheterization room in the radiology department. A local anesthetic is used, so there is little to no pain with catheter insertion. The procedure may take up to 2 hours, during which time the client may feel various sensations such as a feeling of warmth or flushing with catheter passage and dye injection.

Test-Taking Strategy: Note the keywords *that the licensed practical nurse needs supervision.* These words indicate that this is a false response question, and that you need to select the incorrect statement by the licensed practical nurse. Recalling the purpose of the procedure will assist in eliminating option 2. Next, recalling that a dye is injected will assist in eliminating options 1 and 4. Also, noting the words *4 hours* in option 3 will direct you to this option. Review the procedure for a cardiac catheterization and the test-taking strategies for answering false response questions if you had difficulty with this question.

Level of Cognitive Ability: Analysis
Client Needs: Safe, Effective Care Environment
Integrated Process: Teaching/Learning
Content Area: Leadership/Management

Reference

Black J, Hawks J: *Medical-surgical nursing: clinical management for positive outcomes,* ed 7, Philadelphia, 2005, WB Saunders, p 103.

---

224. A registered nurse is reviewing the preprocedural care for a client scheduled to have an echocardiogram after a myocardial infarction. The registered nurse determines that the licensed practical nurse understands the preprocedural instructions if the licensed practical nurse states that the client needs to be told that

1 An allergy to iodine or shellfish is a contraindication to having the procedure

2 The procedure is painless and takes 30 to 60 minutes to complete

3 He cannot eat or drink anything for 4 hours before the procedure

4 He needs to sign an informed consent

Answer: 2

Rationale: Echocardiography uses ultrasound to evaluate the heart's structure and motion. It is a noninvasive, risk-free, pain-free test that involves no special preparation. It is commonly done at the bedside or on an outpatient basis. The client must lie quietly for 30 to 60 minutes while the procedure is being performed. Options 1, 3, and 4 are incorrect.

Test-Taking Strategy: Focus on the diagnostic test being performed. Recalling that echocardiography uses ultrasound and that ultrasound is noninvasive will assist in eliminating options 1, 3, and 4. Review this procedure and the various test-taking strategies if you had difficulty with this question.

Level of Cognitive Ability: Analysis
Client Needs: Safe, Effective Care Environment
Integrated Process: Teaching/Learning
Content Area: Leadership/Management

Reference

Black J, Hawks J: *Medical-surgical nursing: clinical management for positive outcomes,* ed 7, Philadelphia, 2005, WB Saunders, p 1590.

---

225. A nurse has provided instructions to a client scheduled for an exercise electrocardiogram (stress test) at 9:00 AM on the following day. The nurse determines that the client needs additional instructions if the client states:

1 "I should not go to the gym to lift weights today."

2 "Smoking is not allowed for at least 2 to 3 hours before the procedure."

3 "I can eat breakfast before the procedure as long as I eat by 8:00 AM."

4 "I should wear sneakers when I come for the test."

Answer: 3

Rationale: The client should wear rubber-soled, supportive shoes, such as sneakers for the procedure. The client also should wear light, loose, comfortable clothing. A shirt that buttons in front is helpful for electrocardiogram lead placement. The client should not eat or smoke for 2 to 3 hours before the test. No strenuous physical efforts should be made for at least 12 hours before testing.

Test-Taking Strategy: Note the key words *needs additional instructions.* This indicates that this is a false response question, and that you need to select the option that is an incorrect client statement. Recall what this test entails. Select the option that could interfere with testing and test results—that is, digestion. Review client teaching related to a stress test and the test-taking strategies for answering false response questions if you had difficulty with this question.

Level of Cognitive Ability: Analysis
Client Needs: Physiological Integrity
Integrated Process: Teaching/Learning
Content Area: Adult Health/Cardiovascular

Reference

Black J, Hawks J: *Medical-surgical nursing: clinical management for positive outcomes,* ed 7, Philadelphia, 2005, WB Saunders, p 1587.

---

226. A client has undergone pericardiocentesis to treat cardiac tamponade. The nurse monitors the client for which sign to determine whether the tamponade is recurring?
    1 Decreasing pulse
    2 Paradoxical pulse
    3 Facial flushing
    4 Increasing blood pressure

Answer: 2

Rationale: Cardiac tamponade is a life-threatening situation caused by the accumulation of fluid in the pericardium. The fluid accumulates rapidly and in sufficient quantity to compress the heart and restrict blood flow in and out of the ventricles. Hypotension, tachycardia, jugular vein distension, cyanosis of the lips and nails, dyspnea, muffled heart sounds, diaphoresis, and paradoxical pulse (a decrease in systolic arterial pulsation exceeding 10 mm Hg during inspiration) are indications of this emergency situation. The preferred emergency intervention is pericardiocentesis, a procedure in which fluid is aspirated from the pericardial sac. Options 1, 3, and 4 are not indications of cardiac tamponade.

Test-Taking Strategy: Note the keyword *recurring*. This tells you that the correct option is a symptom of the original problem, which is cardiac tamponade. Recalling the pathophysiology associated with cardiac tamponade will direct you to option 2. Review these signs and the various test-taking strategies if you had difficulty with this question.

Level of Cognitive Ability: Analysis
Client Needs: Physiological Integrity
Integrated Process: Nursing Process/Evaluation
Content Area: Adult Health/Cardiovascular

Reference

Black J, Hawks J: *Medical-surgical nursing: clinical management for positive outcomes,* ed 7, Philadelphia, 2005, WB Saunders, p 1623.

---

227. A nurse is observing a nursing assistant measuring the blood pressure (BP) of a client. The nurse intervenes if which action that would interfere with accurate measurement of the BP is observed?
    1 Positioning the client's arm at heart level
    2 Exposing the extremity fully by removing constricting clothing
    3 Palpating the radial artery and placing the cuff of the sphyg-

Answer: 3

Rationale: When taking a blood pressure measurement the brachial artery is palpated, and the cuff of the sphygmomanometer is positioned 1 inch above this site of pulsation. Options 1, 2, and 4 are correct actions when measuring blood pressure.

Test-Taking Strategy: Note the keywords *nurse intervenes*. This indicates that this is a false response question, and that you need to select the option that indicates an incorrect action by the nursing assistant. Visualizing this procedure will assist in eliminating options 1, 2, and 4. Review the principles related to blood pressure measure-

momanometer 1 inch above the site of pulsation
4   Explaining the procedure to the client and asking the client to rest for 5 minutes

ment and the test-taking strategies for answering false response questions if you had difficulty with this question.

Level of Cognitive Ability: Analysis
Client Needs: Safe, Effective Care Environment
Integrated Process: Teaching/Learning
Content Area: Leadership/Management

Reference
Potter P, Perry A: *Fundamentals of nursing,* ed 6, St Louis, 2005, Mosby, pp 657–658.

---

228. A technician from the radiology department calls the nursing unit to report the results of a chest radiograph for a client with a chest tube. The technician reports that the client's affected lung is fully reexpanded. The nurse anticipates that the physician will prescribe which of the following?
1   Increasing the amount of suction in the suction control chamber of the chest tube drainage system
2   Adding fluid to the water seal chamber of the chest tube drainage system
3   Vigorous coughing and deep breathing every hour
4   Removal of the chest tube

Answer: 4
Rationale: When the client's lung is fully reexpanded, the chest tube will be removed. Options 1, 2, and 3 are incorrect.

Test-Taking Strategy: Note the keywords *lung is fully reexpanded.* Recall the purpose of a chest tube drainage system, and recall that if the lung is fully reexpanded, then the chest tube is no longer needed. Review assessment of a client with a chest tube and the various test-taking strategies if you had difficulty with this question.

Level of Cognitive Ability: Analysis
Client Needs: Physiological Integrity
Integrated Process: Nursing Process/Analysis
Content Area: Adult Health/Respiratory

Reference
Black J, Hawks J: *Medical-surgical nursing: clinical management for positive outcomes,* ed 7, Philadelphia, 2005, WB Saunders, p 1866.

---

229. A nurse is monitoring a client who had a pleural biopsy. The nurse determines that the client is experiencing a complication if the client exhibits
1   Capillary refill of 2 seconds
2   Warm, dry skin
3   Diaphoresis
4   Mild pain at the biopsy site

Answer: 3
Rationale: The nurse observes the client for dyspnea, excessive pain, pallor, or diaphoresis after pleural biopsy. These symptoms could indicate the presence of complications such as pneumothorax, hemothorax, or intercostal nerve injury. Mild pain is expected because the procedure itself is painful. Abnormal signs and symptoms should be reported to the physician. Options 1 and 2 are normal findings.

Test-Taking Strategy: Focus on the issue: a complication. Eliminate options 1 and 2 because they are normal findings. From the remaining options, noting the word mild in option 4 will assist in eliminating this option. Review the complications associated with a pleural biopsy and the various test-taking strategies if you had difficulty with this question.

Level of Cognitive Ability: Analysis
Client Needs: Physiological Integrity
Integrated Process: Nursing Process/Analysis
Content Area: Adult Health/Respiratory

Reference

Black J, Hawks J: *Medical-surgical nursing: clinical management for positive outcomes,* ed 7, Philadelphia, 2005, WB Saunders, p 1773.

---

230. A nurse has an order to discontinue a client's nasogastric tube. The nurse prepares the client and asks the client to take a deep breath and
1 Exhale rapidly
2 Hold the breath
3 Breathe normally
4 Bear down

Answer: 2

Rationale: On tube removal, the client is instructed to take and hold a deep breath. The client takes a deep breath because the airway will be temporarily obstructed during tube removal. Holding the breath helps to prevent aspiration. Bearing down and exhaling rapidly could inhibit tube removal by increasing intrathoracic pressure. Breathing normally could result in aspiration of gastric secretions during inhalation.

Test-Taking Strategy: Visualize this procedure. Eliminate options 1 and 4 because they are similar. From the remaining options, remember that holding the breath will prevent aspiration. Option 2 also relates to the ABCs—airway, breathing, and circulation. Review the procedure for removing a nasogastric tube and the various test-taking strategies if you had difficulty with this question.

Level of Cognitive Ability: Application
Client Needs: Physiological Integrity
Integrated Process: Nursing Process/Implementation
Content Area: Adult Health/Gastrointestinal

Reference

Potter P, Perry A: *Fundamentals of nursing,* ed 6, St Louis, 2005, Mosby, p 1407.

---

231. A nurse administers ondansetron (Zofran) to a client receiving chemotherapy. The nurse determines that the medication is effective if the client states
1 That pain is minimal
2 That he is not experiencing any nausea
3 That the intravenous site is not burning
4 That he feels sleepy

Answer: 2

Rationale: Ondansetron is an antiemetic that is used in the treatment of nausea and vomiting associated with chemotherapy, as well as postoperative nausea and vomiting. Options 1, 3, and 4 are unrelated to the intended effects of this medication.

Test-Taking Strategy: Note the keywords *medication is effective.* Focus on the data in the question and note that the client is receiving the medication during chemotherapy. Recalling that chemotherapy can cause nausea and vomiting will direct you to the correct option. Review the action of this medication and the test-taking strategies for answering pharmacology questions if you had difficulty with this question.

Level of Cognitive Ability: Analysis
Client Needs: Physiological Integrity
Integrated Process: Nursing Process/Evaluation
Content Area: Pharmacology

Reference

Hodgson B, Kizior R: *Saunders nursing drug handbook 2004,* Philadelphia, 2004, WB Saunders, p 755.

232. After the delivery of a neonate, a nurse performs an initial assessment and determines that the Apgar score is 9. This score indicates that the infant

1 Is adjusting well to extrauterine life
2 Requires some resuscitative intervention
3 Is having difficulty adjusting to extrauterine life
4 Requires vigorous resuscitation

Answer: 1

Rationale: One of the earliest indicators of successful adaptation by the neonate is the Apgar score. Scoring ranges from 0 to 10. A score of 8 to 10 indicates that the neonate is adjusting well to extrauterine life. A score of 5 to 7 often indicates a neonate who requires some resuscitative intervention. A score of less than 5 indicates neonates who are having difficulty adjusting to extrauterine life and require vigorous resuscitation.

Test-Taking Strategy: Recall that the Apgar score ranges from 0 to 10. Noting that the question addresses a score of 9 will direct you to option 1. Also note that options 2, 3, and 4 are similar. Review this assessment test and the various test-taking strategies if you had difficulty with this question.

Level of Cognitive Ability: Analysis
Client Needs: Physiological Integrity
Integrated Process: Nursing Process/Analysis
Content Area: Maternity/Intrapartum

Reference
Lowdermilk D, Perry A: *Maternity & women's health care,* ed 8, St Louis, 2004, Mosby, p 708.

---

233. A nurse is assigned to care for a client in labor who has a diagnosis of sickle cell anemia. The nurse administers oxygen to the client and implements which additional measure to prevent a sickling crisis from occurring?

1 Reassures the client
2 Maintains adequate hydration
3 Maintains strict asepsis
4 Monitors the temperature

Answer: 2

Rationale: Oxygen is administered continuously during labor to the client with sickle cell anemia to provide adequate oxygenation and to prevent sickling. Adequate hydration also is an important measure to prevent sickling of blood cells. Although options 1, 3, and 4 are appropriate nursing interventions, they are unrelated to preventing a sickling crisis.

Test-Taking Strategy: Eliminate options 3 and 4 first because they are similar and relate to preventing and monitoring for infection. From the remaining options, use Maslow's Hierarchy of Needs theory. Option 1 relates to a psychosocial need, whereas option 2 relates to a physiological need. Review care to the client in labor who has sickle cell anemia and the various test-taking strategies if you had difficulty with this question.

Level of Cognitive Ability: Application
Client Needs: Physiological Integrity
Integrated Process: Nursing Process/Implementation
Content Area: Maternity/Intrapartum

Reference
Lowdermilk D, Perry A: *Maternity & women's health care,* ed 8, St Louis, 2004, Mosby, p 921.

234. A nurse is preparing to perform fundal massage on a client with uterine atony. The nurse performs this procedure by
  1 Placing one hand just above the symphysis pubis and gently but firmly massaging the fundus in a circular motion
  2 Placing one hand just above the symphysis pubis and pushing on the uterus in a vertical position
  3 Placing one hand just below the symphysis pubis and massaging the fundus in a horizontal motion
  4 Placing one hand just below the symphysis pubis and massaging the fundus in a circular motion

Answer: 1
Rationale: When performing fundal massage, one hand is placed just above the symphysis pubis to support the lower uterine segment, whereas the fundus is gently but firmly massaged in a circular motion. Pushing on an uncontracted uterus could invert the uterus and cause massive hemorrhage.

Test-Taking Strategy: Eliminate option 2 first because of the word *pushing;* recall that pushing on an uncontracted uterus could invert the uterus and cause massive hemorrhage. Next, visualize the anatomy of the uterus. Eliminate options 3 and 4 because the hand is not placed below the symphysis pubis. Review the procedure for fundal massage and the various test-taking strategies if you had difficulty with this question.

Level of Cognitive Ability: Application
Client Needs: Physiological Integrity
Integrated Process: Nursing Process/Implementation
Content Area: Maternity/Postpartum

Reference
Murray S, McKinney E, Gorrie T: *Foundations of maternal-newborn nursing,* ed 3, Philadelphia, 2002, WB Saunders, p 776.

---

235. Immediately after the delivery of a neonate, the nurse prepares to assist in the delivery of the placenta. The most appropriate action to deliver the placenta is to
  1 Pull on the umbilical cord
  2 Instruct the mother to push during a uterine contraction
  3 Place traction on the umbilical cord and pull on the placenta as it enters the vaginal canal
  4 Separate the placenta from the uterine wall using the forceps, and then allow the placenta to deliver spontaneously

Answer: 2
Rationale: After the placenta separates, the mother is instructed to push during a uterine contraction. Pulling on the umbilical cord or placing traction on the umbilical cord may cause it to break, making the placenta harder to deliver. The placenta is not separated from the uterine wall using forceps. This may result in bleeding.

Test-Taking Strategy: Eliminate option 1 because of the word *pull* and eliminate option 3 because of the word *traction.* From the remaining options, eliminate option 4 recalling that the placenta is attached to the uterine wall, and unnatural separation will result in bleeding. Review the procedure for placental delivery and the various test-taking strategies if you had difficulty with this question.

Level of Cognitive Ability: Application
Client Needs: Physiological Integrity
Integrated Process: Nursing Process/Implementation
Content Area: Maternity/Intrapartum

Reference
Lowdermilk D, Perry A: *Maternity & women's health care,* ed 8, St Louis, 2004, Mosby, p 597.

---

236. A prenatal client tells the nurse that she is really worried about knowing how to care for her first-born child.

Answer: 4
Rationale: Deficient Knowledge indicates a lack of information or psychomotor skills concerning a skill, condition, or treatment. This nursing diagnosis best describes the

The nurse formulates which nursing diagnosis for this client?
1   Ineffective Coping
2   Dysfunctional Grieving
3   Situational Low Self-esteem
4   Deficient Knowledge

situation presented in the question. Situational Low Self-esteem represents temporary negative feelings about self in response to an event. Ineffective Coping implies that the person is unable to manage stressors adequately. Dysfunctional Grieving implies prolonged unresolved grief leading to detrimental activities.

Test-Taking Strategy: When a question asks to identify a nursing diagnosis, focus on the information in the question. Option 4 is the one that will focus on the mother's concern about *knowing how to care for her first-born child.* Review the defining characteristics of Deficient Knowledge and the various test-taking strategies if you had difficulty with this question.

Level of Cognitive Ability: Analysis
Client Needs: Health Promotion and Maintenance
Integrated Process: Nursing Process/Analysis
Content Area: Maternity/Antepartum

Reference
Gulanick M, Myers J, Klopp A, Galanes S, Gradishar D, Puzas M: *Nursing care plans: nursing diagnosis and intervention,* ed 5, St Louis, 2003, Mosby, p 103.

---

237. A nurse is monitoring the status of a client in labor who is experiencing hypotonic uterine dysfunction. The nurse interprets that which of the following findings would be least consistent with this type of dysfunctional labor?
1   The client initially makes normal progress into the active stage of labor, and then contractions weaken
2   Contractions weaken during the active stage of labor
3   Contractions become inefficient or stop during the active stage of labor
4   The client is having painful and frequent contractions that are ineffective in causing cervical or effacement progress

Answer: 4

Rationale: In hypotonic uterine dysfunction, the client initially makes normal progress into the active stage of labor, and then contractions weaken, become inefficient, or stop. Option 4 is characteristic of hypertonic uterine dysfunction.

Test-Taking Strategy: Note the keywords *least consistent.* These words indicate that this is a false response question, and that you need to identify the option that is not characteristic of hypotonic uterine dysfunction. Noting that options 1, 2, and 3 are similar and noting the word *hypotonic* in the question will direct you to option 4. Review the manifestations of hypotonic uterine dysfunction and the various test-taking strategies if you had difficulty with this question.

Level of Cognitive Ability: Analysis
Client Needs: Physiological Integrity
Integrated Process: Nursing Process/Analysis
Content Area: Maternity/Intrapartum

Reference
Lowdermilk D, Perry A: *Maternity & women's health care,* ed 8, St Louis, 2004, Mosby, p 997.

---

238. A client has just experienced a precipitate labor. The nurse notes that the mother is lying quietly in bed and is avoiding physical contact

Answer: 4

Rationale: Precipitate labor is defined as labor that lasts less than 3 hours from the onset of contractions to the time of birth. After a precipitate labor, the mother may

with her child. The nurse most appropriately
1   Requests a psychiatric consult
2   Contacts the physician
3   Encourages the mother to breast-feed the infant
4   Provides support to the mother

need help to process what has happened and time to assimilate it all. The mother may be exhausted, in pain, stunned by the rapid nature of the delivery, or simply following cultural norms. Providing support to the mother is the most appropriate and therapeutic action by the nurse. Options 1 and 2 are similar and do not enhance the therapeutic relationship. Option 3 is an appropriate nursing intervention, but the question does not indicate whether the mother has chosen to breast-feed.

Test-Taking Strategy: Eliminate options 1 and 2 first because they are similar. From the remaining options, note that there are no data that indicate that the mother is going to breast-feed. This will direct you to option 4. Review care to the client after precipitate labor and the various test-taking strategies if you had difficulty with this question.

Level of Cognitive Ability: Application
Client Needs: Psychosocial Integrity
Integrated Process: Caring
Content Area: Maternity/Postpartum

Reference
Lowdermilk D, Perry A: *Maternity & women's health care*, ed 8, St Louis, 2004, Mosby, p 1033.

---

239. A pregnant client experienced a uterine rupture with subsequent fetal death. After ensuring that the client is physiologically stable, the nurse uses which of the following approaches as the best first step to support the client psychologically?
1   Suggests that family members see and hold the dead infant if they wish
2   Assesses how the client perceived the event
3   Avoids talking about the dead fetus
4   Asks the client and partner about plans for future pregnancies

Answer: 2
Rationale: Because of anesthesia, anxiety, and the experience of a sudden, catastrophic event, the client may well have experienced a decreased ability to take in and process information. The nurse should first assess the client's perception of the event before deciding how to intervene. Option 1 may be helpful, but not as a first step. Options 3 and 4 are not helpful because they are not therapeutic; option 3 avoids the issue, and option 4 deals with issues the client may not be ready to face.

Test-Taking Strategy: Use the steps of the nursing process, remembering that assessment comes first. This will direct you to option 2. Review care to the pregnant client who experienced a crisis and the various test-taking strategies if you had difficulty with this question.

Level of Cognitive Ability: Application
Client Needs: Psychosocial Integrity
Integrated Process: Caring
Content Area: Maternity/Postpartum

Reference
Lowdermilk D, Perry A: *Maternity & women's health care*, ed 8, St Louis, 2004, Mosby, p 1165.

240. A pregnant client with a suspected diagnosis of placenta previa arrives at the health care clinic for an examination. The nurse prepares the client for the examination and tells the client that which of the following will be deferred until the diagnosis is confirmed?
1   Urine testing for glucose
2   Vaginal speculum examination
3   Vital sign measurement
4   Abdominal ultrasound

Answer: 2

Rationale: The placenta is implanted low in the uterus in placenta previa, and a vaginal speculum examination could cause disruption of the placenta and initiate severe hemorrhage. The abdominal ultrasound is used to confirm the diagnosis of placenta previa. There is no reason to defer urine testing or vital sign measurement.

Test-Taking Strategy: Note the keyword *deferred* and focus on the client's suspected diagnosis. Recalling that, in this condition, the placenta is implanted low in the uterus and that the client is at risk for hemorrhage will direct you to option 2. Review nursing care to the client with placenta previa and the various test-taking strategies if you had difficulty with this question.

Level of Cognitive Ability: Application
Client Needs: Physiological Integrity
Integrated Process: Nursing Process/Planning
Content Area: Maternity/Antepartum

Reference
Lowdermilk D, Perry A: *Maternity & women's health care,* ed 8, St Louis, 2004, Mosby, p 872.

---

241. A nurse is preparing to perform an assessment on a client with placenta previa and plans to assess which of the following first?
1   The client's compliance with activity limitations
2   The client's temperature
3   The fetal heart rate
4   The client's understanding of the treatment for placenta previa

Answer: 3

Rationale: A primary concern with placenta previa is a risk for fetal injury related to a potential decreased placental perfusion. Although all of the options may be assessed, assessing the fetal heart rate is the priority.

Test-Taking Strategy: Note the keyword *first.* Also note that options 1 and 4 are similar, and therefore can be eliminated. Use the ABCs—airway, breathing, and circulation—to direct you to option 3. Review care to the client with placenta previa and the test-taking strategies for answering prioritizing questions if you had difficulty with this question.

Level of Cognitive Ability: Application
Client Needs: Physiological Integrity
Integrated Process: Nursing Process/Assessment
Content Area: Delegating/Prioritizing

Reference
Lowdermilk D, Perry A: *Maternity & women's health care,* ed 8, St Louis, 2004, Mosby, p 873.

---

242. A nurse working in a prenatal clinic is reviewing the records of clients scheduled for prenatal visits. The nurse interprets that the client at greatest risk for abruptio placenta is the one who

Answer: 3

Rationale: Risk factors for abruptio placenta include maternal hypertension, smoking, and alcohol and/or cocaine use during pregnancy. Other risk factors include blunt external abdominal trauma, poor nutrition, and history of placental abruption.

1 Is 26 years old and is a primi-para

2 Rides an exercise bike for 30 minutes 3 times weekly

3 Has maternal hypertension

4 Takes folic acid supplements daily

Test-Taking Strategy: Note the keywords *at greatest risk.* Eliminate options 2 and 4 first because they are health-promoting behaviors. From the remaining options, select option 3 because hypertension can cause problems with placental perfusion. Review the risk factors related to abruptio placenta and the various test-taking strategies if you had difficulty with this question.

Level of Cognitive Ability: Analysis
Client Needs: Health Promotion and Maintenance
Integrated Process: Nursing Process/Assessment
Content Area: Maternity/Antepartum

Reference
Lowdermilk D, Perry A: *Maternity & women's health care,* ed 8, St Louis, 2004, Mosby, p 875.

---

243. A nurse is assessing the respiratory rate of a neonate. The nurse determines that the rate is normal if which of the following is noted?

1 10 breaths/min

2 15 breaths/min

3 25 breaths/min

4 40 breaths/min

Answer: 4

Rationale: The normal respiratory rate for a neonate ranges from 30 to 60 breaths/min.

Test-Taking Strategy: Focus on the issue: the respiratory rate of a neonate. Eliminate options 1 and 2 first because they are low rates. From the remaining options, focusing on the issue will direct you to option 4. Remember that the respiratory rate of a neonate is greater than that of an adult. Review the reference ranges for neonate vital signs and the various test-taking strategies if you had difficulty with this question.

Level of Cognitive Ability: Analysis
Client Needs: Physiological Integrity
Integrated Process: Nursing Process/Assessment
Content Area: Maternity/Postpartum

Reference
Lowdermilk D, Perry A: *Maternity & women's health care,* ed 8, St Louis, 2004, Mosby, p 713.

---

244. A newborn infant is diagnosed with esophageal atresia, and the parents ask the nurse to explain the diagnosis. The nurse tells the parents that in this condition

1 A portion of the stomach protrudes through part of the diaphragm

2 Abdominal contents herniate through an opening of the diaphragm

3 Gastric contents regurgitate back into the esophagus

4 The esophagus terminates before it reaches the stomach

Answer: 4

Rationale: Esophageal atresia and tracheoesophageal fistula are congenital malformations in which the esophagus terminates before it reaches the stomach or a fistula is present that forms an unnatural connection with the trachea, or both. Option 1 describes a hiatal hernia. Option 2 describes a congenital diaphragmatic hernia. Option 3 describes gastroesophageal reflux.

Test-Taking Strategy: Focus on the diagnosis: esophageal atresia. Note the relation between the word *atresia* and option 4. Review the characteristics of esophageal atresia and the various test-taking strategies if you had difficulty with this question.

Level of Cognitive Ability: Application
Client Needs: Physiological Integrity
Integrated Process: Nursing Process/Implementation
Content Area: Maternity/Postpartum

Reference
Lowdermilk D, Perry A: *Maternity & women's health care,* ed 8, St Louis, 2004, Mosby, p 1099.

---

245. A woman is examined in the prenatal clinic and reports morning sickness. Which of the following self-care measures will the nurse provide to the client?
1   Eat gas-forming foods only during the afternoon hours
2   Eat fried foods only during the afternoon and early evening hours
3   Eat a high-protein and high-fat snack before getting out of bed
4   Eat five to six small meals per day

Answer: 4
Rationale: Morning sickness is common during the first trimester of pregnancy and is associated with increased levels of human chorionic gonadotropin (hCG) and changes in carbohydrate metabolism. It most often occurs after waking up in the morning, although some women experience it throughout the day. There are several self-care measures that can be implemented to prevent or alleviate morning sickness. These measures include avoiding an empty or overloaded stomach; not smoking; eating a dry carbohydrate food item such as a dry cracker or toast before getting out of bed; eating five to six small meals per day; and avoiding fried, odorous, greasy, gas-forming, or spicy foods.

Test-Taking Strategy: Focus on the issue: morning sickness. Eliminate options 1 and 2 first because of the absolute word *only.* From the remaining options, eliminate option 3 because of the word *fat* in this option. Review measures to prevent or alleviate morning sickness and the various test-taking strategies if you had difficulty with this question.

Level of Cognitive Ability: Application
Client Needs: Health Promotion and Maintenance
Integrated Process: Teaching/Learning
Content Area: Maternity/Antepartum

Reference
Lowdermilk D, Perry A: *Maternity & women's health care,* ed 8, St Louis, 2004, Mosby, p 431.

---

246. A client in the third trimester of pregnancy is examined in the clinic and is reporting urinary frequency. Which of the following self-care measures will the nurse provide to the client?
1   Avoid emptying the bladder frequently
2   Perform Kegel exercises
3   Sip on small amounts of fluids during the day, restricting intake to 1000 mL
4   Avoid fluid intake after 6:00 PM

Answer: 2
Rationale: Urinary frequency may occur in the first trimester, and then again late in the third trimester, because of the pressure placed on the bladder by the enlarged uterus. Self-care measures for urinary frequency include emptying the bladder frequently (every 2 hours), drinking at least 2000 mL fluid per day, limiting fluid intake before bedtime (not avoiding fluid intake), performing Kegel exercises to strengthen the perineal muscles, and wearing a perineal pad. Options 1, 3, and 4 are incorrect and could lead to urinary stasis (option 1) and fluid volume deficit (options 3 and 4).

Test-Taking Strategy: Eliminate options 3 and 4 first because they are similar and could lead to fluid volume deficit. Eliminate option 1 next because it does not make sense to avoid emptying the bladder frequently. This action could lead to urinary stasis and could cause discomfort in the woman. Review measures that will assist with the discomfort of urinary frequency and the various test-taking strategies if you had difficulty with this question.

Level of Cognitive Ability: Application
Client Needs: Health Promotion and Maintenance
Integrated Process: Teaching/Learning
Content Area: Maternity/Antepartum

Reference
Lowdermilk D, Perry A: *Maternity & women's health care,* ed 8, St Louis, 2004, Mosby, p 431.

---

247. A client is examined in the prenatal clinic and is reporting ankle edema. The nurse assesses the client and notes that the edema is nonpitting, the client's blood pressure is within normal limits, and proteinuria is not present. The nurse provides home care instructions to the client and tells the client to
1 Restrict fluid intake
2 Stop wearing the support stockings prescribed by the obstetrician
3 Avoid exercising until the edema subsides
4 Rest periodically with the legs and hips elevated

Answer: 4
Rationale: Ankle edema is a common occurrence in the third trimester of pregnancy and is caused by decreased venous return from the feet because of gravity. It is a minor discomfort, and as long as the edema is nonpitting and hypertension and proteinuria are not present, it is not a cause for concern. Self-care measures include resting periodically with the legs and hips elevated; wearing supportive stockings or hose; drinking ample amounts of fluid; partaking in moderate exercise; and avoiding standing in one position or place for long periods.

Test-Taking Strategy: Eliminate option 1 first because of the word *restrict*. Restricting fluids can be detrimental to the fetus. Next, eliminate option 2 because the nurse would not tell a client to ignore the obstetrician's prescription. From the remaining options, use principles related to the effects of gravity to direct you to option 4. Review the measures to alleviate ankle edema and the various test-taking strategies if you had difficulty with this question.

Level of Cognitive Ability: Application
Client Needs: Health Promotion and Maintenance
Integrated Process: Teaching/Learning
Content Area: Maternity/Antepartum

Reference
Lowdermilk D, Perry A: *Maternity & women's health care,* ed 8, St Louis, 2004, Mosby, p 434.

---

248. A prenatal client reports heartburn, and the nurse provides instructions to the client regarding measures to alleviate the discomfort. Which statement by the client indicates a need for further instructions?

Answer: 3
Rationale: Heartburn is associated with regurgitation of gastric acid contents into the esophagus. Self-care measures for heartburn include eating small, frequent meals; avoiding fatty or spicy foods; remaining upright for 30 minutes after eating; and drinking approximately 2000 mL fluid per day.

1 "I need to eat small, frequent meals."

2 "I need to avoid fatty or spicy foods."

3 "I need to lie down after eating."

4 "I need to drink approximately 2000 mL fluid per day."

Test-Taking Strategy: Note the keywords *need for further instructions*. These words indicate that this is a false response question and that you need to select the option that indicates an incorrect client statement. Recalling that heartburn is associated with regurgitation of gastric acid contents into the esophagus will direct you to option 3. Review measures to relieve or prevent heartburn and the various test-taking strategies if you had difficulty with this question.

Level of Cognitive Ability: Analysis
Client Needs: Health Promotion and Maintenance
Integrated Process: Teaching/Learning
Content Area: Maternity/Antepartum

Reference
Lowdermilk D, Perry A: *Maternity & women's health care,* ed 8, St Louis, 2004, Mosby, p 432.

---

249. A nurse is performing an assessment on a client who is at 38 weeks' gestation and notes that the fetal heart rate (FHR) is 174 beats/min. On the basis of this finding, the most appropriate nursing action would be to

1 Document the finding

2 Notify the physician

3 Check the mother's heart rate

4 Tell the client that the fetal heart rate is normal

Answer: 2

Rationale: The FHR should be 110 to 160 beats/min at term. Because the FHR is increased from the reference range, the nurse would most appropriately notify the physician. The FHR would be documented, but option 2 is the most appropriate action. Options 3 and 4 are inappropriate actions based on the data in the question.

Test-Taking Strategy: Note the keywords *most appropriate*. Focus on the FHR noted in the question. Recalling that the normal FHR should be 110 to 160 beats/min at term will direct you to option 2. Remember, an abnormal finding in a pregnant client needs to be reported to the physician. Review the normal FHR and the test-taking strategies related to physician notification if you had difficulty with this question.

Level of Cognitive Ability: Application
Client Needs: Physiological Integrity
Integrated Process: Nursing Process/Implementation
Content Area: Maternity/Antepartum

Reference
Lowdermilk D, Perry A: *Maternity & women's health care,* ed 8, St Louis, 2004, Mosby, p 523.

---

250. A clinic nurse provides instructions to a woman in the second trimester of pregnancy regarding measures to relieve backache. Which statement by the client indicates an understanding of these measures?

1 "I will sleep on a soft mattress."

2 "I will avoid doing those pelvic tilt exercises."

Answer: 3

Rationale: Backache can occur because of the exaggerated lumbar and cervicothoracic curves caused by the change in the center of gravity from the enlarging abdomen. The client should be instructed to sleep on a firm mattress, to avoid fatigue, and to maintain good posture and body mechanics. Pelvic tilt exercises decrease strain to muscles of the abdomen and lower back caused by the added weight of the abdomen and the shift in the center of gravity. Wearing high-heeled shoes will add to the

3   "I will avoid getting tired, and I should work at maintaining a good posture."

4   "I will wear shoes with a heel of at least 2 inches."

strain on the muscles and will exaggerate the shift in the center of gravity.

Test-Taking Strategy: Note the keywords *understanding of these measures.* Focus on the issue: relieving backache. Also, thinking about the effects of each item in the options will direct you to option 3. Review measures to relieve backache and the various test-taking strategies if you had difficulty with this question.

Level of Cognitive Ability: Analysis
Client Needs: Health Promotion and Maintenance
Integrated Process: Teaching/Learning
Content Area: Maternity/Antepartum

Reference
Lowdermilk D, Perry A: *Maternity & women's health care,* ed 8, St Louis, 2004, Mosby, p 433.

---

251. A client with hypertension has been advised to eat foods that are low in sodium. The nurse tells the client that which food item is lowest in sodium?
1   Canned chicken noodle soup
2   Broccoli
3   Instant rice
4   Instant oatmeal

Answer: 2
Rationale: Fruits and vegetables (option 2) are lower in sodium because they do not contain physiologic saline. Highly processed or refined foods (options 3 and 4) are higher in sodium, unless they are specifically labeled as "low sodium." Canned foods are high in sodium.

Test-Taking Strategy: Focus of the issue: a low-sodium food. Eliminate options 3 and 4 first because they are similar and are processed foods. Recalling that canned foods are high in sodium will assist in eliminating option 1. Review the foods that are high and low in sodium and the various test-taking strategies if you had difficulty with this question.

Level of Cognitive Ability: Application
Client Needs: Physiological Integrity
Integrated Process: Teaching/Learning
Content Area: Fundamental Skills

Reference
Williams S: *Basic nutrition & diet therapy,* ed 11, St Louis, 2001, Mosby, p 119.

---

252. A clear liquid diet has been prescribed for a client. The nurse offers which item to the client?
1   Apple juice
2   Ice cream without nuts
3   Orange juice
4   Tomato juice

Answer: 1
Rationale: A clear liquid diet consists of foods that are relatively transparent. The food items in options 2, 3, and 4 would be included in a full liquid diet.

Test-Taking Strategy: Eliminate options 2, 3, and 4 because they are similar and are items allowed on a full liquid diet. Remember that a clear liquid diet consists of foods that are relatively transparent. Option 1 is the only food item that is transparent. Review food items allowed on clear liquid and full liquid diets and the various test-taking strategies if you had difficulty with this question.

Level of Cognitive Ability: Application
Client Needs: Physiological Integrity
Integrated Process: Nursing Process/Implementation
Content Area: Fundamental Skills

Reference
Williams S: *Basic nutrition & diet therapy*, ed 11, St Louis, 2001, Mosby, p 321.

---

253. A nurse is teaching a client about a low-fat diet. The nurse tells the client to avoid which food item?
   1 Tomato soup
   2 Watermelon
   3 Cream of mushroom soup
   4 Low-fat yogurt

Answer: 3
Rationale: One-cup of cream of mushroom soup contains 14 g fat, whereas tomato soup contains 2 g. Low-fat yogurt contains 2 g fat. Fresh fruits and vegetables are low in fat.

Test-Taking Strategy: Note the keyword *avoid*. Eliminate option 2 first because it is a fruit and eliminate option 4 because of the words *low-fat*. From the remaining options, noting the word *cream* in option 3 will direct you to this option. Review the foods high in fat and the various test-taking strategies if you had difficulty with this question.

Level of Cognitive Ability: Application
Client Needs: Physiological Integrity
Integrated Process: Teaching/Learning
Content Area: Fundamental Skills

Reference
Mitchell M: *Nutrition across the life span*, ed 2, Philadelphia, 2003, WB Saunders, p 361.

---

254. A nurse provides dietary instructions to a client with cholecystitis. The nurse determines that the client understands the instructions if the client states that which of the following food items is acceptable in the diet?
   1 Angel food cake
   2 Ice cream
   3 Barbecued chicken
   4 Baked potato with broccoli and cheese

Answer: 1
Rationale: The client with cholecystitis should decrease the overall intake of dietary fat. Angel food cake contains negligible amounts of or no fat. Ice cream, barbecue sauce, and cheese contain fat and should be avoided.

Test-Taking Strategy: Recall that the client with cholecystitis needs to consume a low-fat diet. Eliminate options 2, 3, and 4 because they are similar and all contain fat. Review the appropriate dietary measures for the client with cholecystitis and the various test-taking strategies if you had difficulty with this question.

Level of Cognitive Ability: Analysis
Client Needs: Physiological Integrity
Integrated Process: Teaching/Learning
Content Area: Adult Health/Gastrointestinal

Reference
Mitchell M: *Nutrition across the life span*, ed 2, Philadelphia, 2003, WB Saunders, p 360.

255. A nurse has taught a client with a new colostomy about measures to control stool odor in the ostomy drainage bag. The nurse determines that the client understood the information if the client states to include which of the following foods in the diet?

1 Fish
2 Onions
3 Parsley
4 Asparagus

Answer: 3

Rationale: Deodorizing foods for the ostomy client include spinach, beet greens, parsley, buttermilk, cranberry juice, and yogurt. Fish, onions, and asparagus can cause problems with odor in the stool.

Test-Taking Strategy: Focus on the issue: measures to control stool odor. Recalling the effect of various foods on the gastrointestinal tract of the client with an ostomy will direct you to option 3. Review the foods that cause odor or gas, foods that have a deodorizing effect, and the various test-taking strategies if you had difficulty with this question.

Level of Cognitive Ability: Analysis
Client Needs: Physiological Integrity
Integrated Process: Teaching/Learning
Content Area: Adult Health/Gastrointestinal

Reference
Ignatavicius D, Workman M: *Medical-surgical nursing: critical thinking for collaborative care*, ed 4, Philadelphia, 2002, WB Saunders, p 1253.

---

256. A nurse provides dietary instructions to a client diagnosed with iron deficiency anemia. The nurse tells the client to increase the intake of which of the following foods?

1 Plums
2 Egg whites
3 Red apples
4 Kidney beans

Answer: 4

Rationale: The client with iron deficiency anemia should increase intake of foods that are naturally high in iron. Foods high in iron include kidney beans, soybeans, chickpeas, lima beans, cooked swiss chard, red meat, liver and other organ meats, blackstrap molasses, lentils, egg yolk, spinach, kale, turnip tops, beet greens, carrots, raisins, and apricots.

Test-Taking Strategy: Focus on the issue: a food high in iron. Eliminate options 1 and 3 first because they are similar and are fruit items. From the remaining options, it is necessary to recall either that beans are high in iron or that egg yolk (not egg white) is high in iron. This will direct you to option 4. Review foods high in iron and the various test-taking strategies if you had difficulty with this question.

Level of Cognitive Ability: Application
Client Needs: Physiological Integrity
Integrated Process: Teaching/Learning
Content Area: Fundamental Skills

Reference
Mitchell M: *Nutrition across the life span*, ed 2, Philadelphia, 2003, WB Saunders, p 380.

---

257. A nurse instructs a client taking a potassium-sparing diuretic about the foods high in potassium that should be included in the daily diet.

Answer: 2

Rationale: Meats, some dairy products, dried fruits, bananas, cantaloupe, kiwi, and oranges are high in potassium. Vegetables that are high in potassium include avo-

The nurse determines that the client needs further instruction if the client states that which food is high in potassium?

1 Kiwi
2 Celery
3 Dried fruit
4 Oranges

cados, broccoli, dried beans or peas, lima beans, mushrooms, potatoes, seaweed, soybeans, and spinach. Celery is a vegetable that is low in potassium.

Test-Taking Strategy: Note the keywords *needs further instruction.* These words indicate a false response question, and that you need to select the option that is an incorrect client response. Eliminate options 1, 3, and 4 because they are similar and are fruit items. Review the foods that are high and low in potassium content and the various test-taking strategies if you had difficulty with this question.

Level of Cognitive Ability: Analysis
Client Needs: Physiological Integrity
Integrated Process: Teaching/Learning
Content Area: Fundamental Skills

Reference
Ignatavicius D, Workman M: *Medical-surgical nursing: critical thinking for collaborative care,* ed 4, Philadelphia, 2002, WB Saunders, p 180.

---

258. The registered nurse tells a nursing assistant that a client recovering from a myocardial infarction requires a complete bed bath. During the bath, the registered nurse would intervene if the nurse observed the nursing assistant

1 Washing the client's perineal area
2 Giving the client a back rub
3 Asking the client to wash his legs
4 Washing the client's chest

Answer: 3
Rationale: A complete bed bath is for clients who are totally dependent and require total hygiene care. Total care may be necessary for a client recovering from a myocardial infarction to conserve client energy and reduce oxygen requirements. The nurse would intervene if he or she observed the nursing assistant asking the client to wash his own legs. Options 1, 2, and 4 are components of providing a complete bed bath.

Test-Taking Strategy: Note the words *the registered nurse would intervene.* This indicates that this is a false response question, and that you need to select the option that identifies an incorrect action by the nursing assistant. Focusing on the words *complete bed bath* will direct you to option 3, because in this option the nurse asks the client to participate in the bathing process. Review the procedure for giving a complete bed bath and the various test-taking strategies if you had difficulty with this question.

Level of Cognitive Ability: Application
Client Needs: Safe, Effective Care Environment
Integrated Process: Nursing Process/Implementation
Content Area: Leadership/Management

Reference
Potter P, Perry A: *Fundamentals of nursing,* ed 6, St Louis, 2005, Mosby, p 1022.

---

259. A client requires a partial bed bath. The registered nurse gives instructions to a nursing assistant about

Answer: 4
Rationale: A partial bed bath involves bathing the body parts that would cause discomfort or odor if left unbathed. These body parts may include the axillary areas, perineal

the partial bed bath and tells the nursing assistant to
1. Just wash the client's hands and face
2. Let the client decide what she wants washed
3. Provide mouth care and perineal care only
4. Be sure to bathe the client's body parts that would cause discomfort or odor if left unbathed

areas, and any skinfold areas. Options 1, 2, and 3 do not completely address a partial bed bath.

Test-Taking Strategy: Note the keywords *partial bed bath.* Eliminate option 1 because of the word *just* and eliminate option 3 because of the word *only.* From the remaining options, recalling the definition of a partial bed bath will direct you to option 4. Review the components of a partial bed bath and the various test-taking strategies if you had difficulty with this question.

Level of Cognitive Ability: Application
Client Needs: Physiological Integrity
Integrated Process: Nursing Process/Implementation
Content Area: Leadership/Management

Reference
Potter P, Perry A: *Fundamentals of nursing,* ed 6, St Louis, 2005, Mosby, p 1022.

---

260. A nurse notes documentation in a client's medical record that the client is experiencing anuria. On the basis of this notation, the nurse determines that the client
1. Is unable to produce urine
2. Has a diminished capacity to form urine
3. Has difficulty having a bowel movement
4. Has episodes of alternating constipation and diarrhea

Answer: 1

Rationale: Anuria is the term used to describe an inability to produce urine. Oliguria is a diminished capacity to form urine and is most likely the result of a decrease in renal perfusion. Options 3 and 4 do not relate to urinary tract dysfunction.

Test-Taking Strategy: Note the word *anuria* and use medical terminology skills to answer the question. Recalling that the prefix *a-*refers to absence and the suffix *-uria* refers to urine will direct you to option 1. Review the description of anuria and the various test-taking strategies if you had difficulty with this question.

Level of Cognitive Ability: Analysis
Client Needs: Physiological Integrity
Integrated Process: Nursing Process/Assessment
Content Area: Fundamental Skills

Reference
Potter P, Perry A: *Fundamentals of nursing,* ed 6, St Louis, 2005, Mosby, p 1326.

---

261. A nurse is caring for a client who has a fever and is diaphoretic. The nurse monitors the client's intake and output and expects that
1. The client's output will be decreased
2. The client's urine will be dilute
3. The client's urine production will be increased
4. The majority of the client's fluid will be excreted through the skin

Answer: 1

Rationale: Febrile conditions affect urine production. The client who is diaphoretic loses fluids through insensible water loss, which decreases urine production. However, the increased body temperature associated with fever increases accumulation of body wastes. Although urine volume may be reduced, it is highly concentrated. Options 2, 3, and 4 are incorrect.

Test-Taking Strategy: Noting that the client has a fever and is diaphoretic will direct you to option 1, because this client will be losing some fluid through the skin. Review the conditions that affect fluid balance and the various test-taking strategies if you had difficulty with this question.

Level of Cognitive Ability: Analysis
Client Needs: Physiological Integrity
Integrated Process: Nursing Process/Assessment
Content Area: Fundamental Skills

Reference
Potter P, Perry A: *Fundamentals of nursing*, ed 6, St Louis, 2005, Mosby, p 1327.

---

262. A nurse provides instructions to a female client regarding the procedure for collecting a midstream urine sample. The nurse tells the client to do which of the following?
1 Douche before collecting the specimen.
2 Cleanse the perineum from front to back.
3 Collect the urine in the cup as soon as the urine flow begins.
4 Collect the specimen before bedtime and bring it to the laboratory the next morning.

Answer: 2
Rationale: As part of correct procedure, the client should cleanse the perineum from front to back with the antiseptic swabs that are packaged with the specimen kit. The client should begin the flow of urine, collecting the sample after starting the flow of urine. The specimen should be sent to the laboratory as soon as possible and not be allowed to stand. Improper specimen handling can yield inaccurate test results. It is not normal procedure to douche before collecting the specimen.

Test-Taking Strategy: Noting the name of the type of sample, *midstream*, will assist in eliminating option 3. Recalling that the specimen should be sent or brought to the laboratory immediately after collection will assist in eliminating option 4. From the remaining options, use basic principles related to hygiene to assist in directing you to option 2. Review the procedure for collecting a midstream urine specimen and the various test-taking strategies if you had difficulty with this question.

Level of Cognitive Ability: Application
Client Needs: Safe, Effective Care Environment
Integrated Process: Teaching/Learning
Content Area: Fundamental Skills

Reference
Potter P, Perry A: *Fundamentals of nursing*, ed 6, St Louis, 2005, Mosby, pp 1336–1339.

---

263. A physician has prescribed a cleansing enema for an adult client. The registered nurse provides directions to a nursing assistant who is trained and certified to administer enemas and tells the nursing assistant that the maximum volume of fluid that can be administered is
1 100 mL
2 300 mL
3 500 mL
4 1000 mL

Answer: 4
Rationale: Cleansing enemas promote complete evacuation of feces from the colon. They act by stimulating peristalsis through the infusion of a large volume of solution or through local irritation of the colon's mucosa. For an adult client, 750 to 1000 mL solution is used. Therefore, the maximum volume of solution for an adult is 1000 mL.

Test-Taking Strategy: Note the keywords *maximum volume* and note that the question addresses an adult client. Recalling the anatomy of the colon in an adult client and the procedure for administering a cleansing enema will direct you to option 4. Review this procedure and the various test-taking strategies if you had difficulty with this question.

Level of Cognitive Ability: Application
Client Needs: Physiological Integrity
Integrated Process: Nursing Process/Implementation
Content Area: Leadership/Management

Reference
Potter P, Perry A: *Fundamentals of nursing*, ed 6, St Louis, 2005, Mosby, p 1399.

---

264. A nurse develops a plan of care for a client recently admitted to the hospital who reports difficulty sleeping. The nurse most appropriately includes which intervention in the plan of care?
1   Provides the client with a snack at bedtime
2   Offers the client a sleeping pill at night
3   Asks the client what he or she does to prepare for sleep
4   Leaves the television on in the client's room at a low volume

Answer: 3
Rationale: The nurse would most appropriately ask the client what he or she does to prepare for sleep. The nurse needs to assess habits that are beneficial to the client compared with those that disturb sleep. Options 1, 2, and 4 provide interventions without assessing what measures would be helpful to the client.

Test-Taking Strategy: Use the steps of the nursing process. The only option that addresses assessment is option 3. Review care to the client who has difficulty sleeping if you had difficulty with this question.

Level of Cognitive Ability: Application
Client Needs: Physiological Integrity
Integrated Process: Nursing Process/Assessment
Content Area: Fundamental Skills

Reference
Potter P, Perry A: *Fundamentals of nursing*, ed 6, St Louis, 2005, Mosby, p 1213.

---

265. A client asks a nurse about the use of a complementary or alternative measure that will assist in promoting sleep. The nurse suggests which of the following?
1   Acupuncture sessions
2   Herbal therapy
3   Muscle relaxation techniques
4   Traditional Chinese medicine sessions

Answer: 3
Rationale: A simple relaxation technique such as muscle relaxation can help reduce any existing anxiety and promote sleep. Acupuncture is an invasive procedure that is a method of stimulating certain points on the body by the insertion of special needles to modify the perception of pain, normalize physiological functions, or treat or prevent disease. Traditional Chinese medicine focuses on restoring and maintaining a balanced flow of vital energy, and interventions include acupressure, acupuncture, herbal therapies, diet, meditation, and Tai Chi and Qigong (exercise that focuses on breathing, visualization, and movement). Herbal therapy involves the use of herbs (plant or a plant part). Some herbs have been determined to be safe, yet other herbs, even in small amounts, can be toxic; the nurse would not recommend their use to a client. If the client is taking prescription medications, the client should consult with the health care provider regarding the use of herbs, because serious herb–medication interactions can occur.

Test-Taking Strategy: Note the relation between the words *promoting sleep* and option 3. Also note that options 1, 2, and 4 are similar in that they include invasive measures. Review complementary and alternative therapies that will assist in promoting sleep and the various test-taking strategies if you had difficulty with this question.

Level of Cognitive Ability: Application
Client Needs: Physiological Integrity
Integrated Process: Teaching/Learning
Content Area: Fundamental Skills

Reference

Potter P, Perry A: *Fundamentals of nursing*, ed 6, St Louis, 2005, Mosby, p 1217.

Index

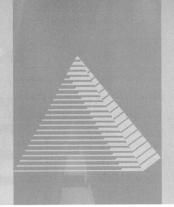

Page numbers followed by f indicate figures; t, tables.